BIODENTAL ENGINEERING II

PROCEEDINGS OF THE 2ND INTERNATIONAL CONFERENCE ON BIODENTAL ENGINEERING, BIODENTAL 2012, PORTO, PORTUGAL, 7–8 DECEMBER 2012

Biodental Engineering II

Editors

R.M. Natal Jorge, J.C. Reis Campos, João Manuel R.S. Tavares, Mário A.P. Vaz & Sónia M. Santos
Universidade do Porto, Porto, Portugal

CRC Press
Taylor & Francis Group
Boca Raton London New York Leiden

CRC Press is an imprint of the
Taylor & Francis Group, an **informa** business
A BALKEMA BOOK

Published by:
CRC Press/Balkema
P.O.Box 447, 2300 AK Leiden, The Netherlands
e-mail: Pub.NL@taylorandfrancis.com
www.crcpress.com – www.taylorandfrancis.com

ISBN: 978-1-138-00131-2 (Hardback)
ISBN: 978-1-315-79826-4 (eBook PDF)

Typeset by MPS Limited, Chennai, India

Biodental Engineering II – Natal Jorge et al (Eds)
© 2014 Taylor & Francis Group, London, ISBN 978-1-138-00131-2

Table of contents

Biodental Engineering II – Natal Jorge et al (Eds)
© 2014 Taylor & Francis Group, London, ISBN 978-1-138-00131-2

Acknowledgements

The editors and the Conference co-chairs acknowledge the support towards the publication of the Book of Proceedings and the organization of the 2nd International Conference on Biodental Engineering BIODENTAL 2012 to the following organizations:

- Universidade do Porto (UP)
- Faculdade de Engenharia da Universidade do Porto (FEUP)
- Faculdade de Medicina Dentária da Universidade do Porto (FMDUP)
- Instituto de Engenharia Mecânica – Pólo FEUP (IDMEC-Polo FEUP)
- Instituto de Engenharia Mecânica e Gestão Industrial (INEGI)
- Laboratório de Biomecânica do Porto (LABIOMEP)
- Fundação para a Ciência e a Tecnologia (FCT)
- Associação Portuguesa de Mecânica Teórica Aplicada e Computacional (APMTAC)

Biodental Engineering II – Natal Jorge et al (Eds)
© 2014 Taylor & Francis Group, London, ISBN 978-1-138-00131-2

Preface

This book contains full papers presented at BIODENTAL 2012 – 2nd International Conference on Biodental Engineering, which was held in Porto, Portugal, during the period 7–8 December 2012. The event had 2 invited lectures, and 46 contributed presentations originated from 8 countries: Brazil, Croatia, France, Germany, Iran, Poland, Portugal and Spain

The dentistry is a branch of medicine with its own peculiarities and very diverse areas of action which means that it can be considered as interdisciplinary field. The use of new techniques and technologies is currently the subject of great interest, and this conference was intended to be a privileged space for discussion among all stakeholders.

The purpose of these BIODENTAL Conferences on Biodental Engineering, initiated in 2009, is to solidify knowledge in the field of bioengineering applied to dentistry promoting a comprehensive forum for discussion on the recent advances in the related fields in order to identify potential collaboration between researchers of different sciences. Henceforth, BIODENTAL 2012 brought together researchers representing fields related to Biomechanical disorders, Orthodontics, Implantology, Aesthetics, Dental, Medical device, Medical imaging.

The conference co-chairs would like to take this opportunity to express gratitude to all sponsors, to all members of the Scientific Committee, to all Invited Lecturers, to all Session-Chairs and to all Authors for submitting and sharing their knowledge.

R.M. Natal Jorge
J.C. Reis Campos
João Manuel R. S. Tavares
Mário A.P. Vaz
Sónia M. Santos
(Conference co-chairs)

Biodental Engineering II – Natal Jorge et al (Eds)
© 2014 Taylor & Francis Group, London, ISBN 978-1-138-00131-2

Invited Lectures

During BIODENTAL 2012, were presented Invited Lectures by 2 Expertises:

- Luís Pires Lopes, Faculdade de Medicina Dentária, Universidade de Lisboa, Portugal
- Christoph Bourauel – University of Bonn, Germany

Biodental Engineering II – Natal Jorge et al (Eds)
© 2014 Taylor & Francis Group, London, ISBN 978-1-138-00131-2

Scientific Committee

All works submitted to BIODENTAL 2012 were evaluated by an International Scientific Committee composed by 44 expert researchers from recognized institutions:

- Afonso Pinhão Ferreira, University of Porto, Portugal
- André Correia, University of Porto, Portugal
- Begoña Calvo Calzada, University of Zaragoza, Spain
- Cláudia Barros Machado, CESPU, Portugal
- Cornelia Kober, Hamburg University of Applied Sciences, Germany
- Daniela Iacoviello, Sapienza University of Rome, Italy
- Edson Capello, UNESP, Brazil
- Eduardo Borges Pires, Technical University of Lisbon, Portugal
- Elza Maria Morais Fonseca, Polytechnical Institute of Bragança, Portugal
- Estefânia Peña Baquedano, University of Zaragoza, Spain
- Estevam Las Casas, Federal University of Minas Gerais, Brazil
- Fernanda Gentil, IDMEC – FEUP, Portugal
- Gerhard A. Holzapfel, Graz University of Technology, Austria
- Helena Figueiral Ioannis Misirlis, University of Patras, Greece
- Iracema Braga, Federal University of Minas Gerais, Brazil
- João Carlos Pinho, University of Porto, Portugal
- João Manuel Tavares, University of Porto, Portugal
- João Paulo Flores Fernandes, University of Minho, Portugal
- Joaquim Gabriel, Universidade do Porto, Portugal
- John Middleton, Cardiff University, UK
- Jorge Marinho, IPO, Portugal
- José Antonio de Oliveira Simões, University of Aveiro, Portugal
- José Mário Rocha, University of Porto, Portugal
- Kazem Alemzadeh, University of Bristol, UK
- Leopoldo Forner Navarro, University of València, Spain
- Lídia Carvalho, University of Aveiro, Portugal
- Luis Geraldo Vaz, UNESP, Brazil
- Luís Pires Lopes, Universidade de Lisboa, Portugal
- Marcos Pinotti Barbosa, Federal University of Minas Gerais, Brazil
- Maria Cristina Manzanares Céspedes, University of Barcelona, Spain
- Mário Vasconcelos, University of Porto, Portugal
- Mário Vaz, University of Porto, Portugal
- Miguel Pinto, University of Porto, Portugal
- Oliver Röhrle,University of Stuttgart, Germany
- Pablo Jesús Rodríguez Cervantes, Universitat Jaume I, Spain
- Paula Vaz, University of Porto, Portugal
- Paulo Alexandre Gonçalves Piloto, Polytechnical Institute of Bragança, Portugal
- Paulo Melo, University of Porto, Portugal
- Paulo Rui Fernandes, Technical University of Lisbon, Portugal
- Pedro Mesquita, University of Porto, Portugal
- Pedro Miguel Gomes Nicolau, University of Coimbra, Portugal
- Reis Campos, University of Porto, Portugal
- Renato Natal Jorge, University of Porto, Portugal
- Sampaio Fernandes, University of Porto, Portugal

Biodental Engineering II – Natal Jorge et al (Eds)
© 2014 Taylor & Francis Group, London, ISBN 978-1-138-00131-2

How do dental students perceive profession demands?

M.E. Pinho & M.A. Vaz
FEUP, Porto, Portugal

J. Reis Campos
FMDUP, Porto, Portugal

P.M. Arezes
U. Minho, Guimarães, Portugal

ABSTRACT: This paper aims to study dental students' perceptions on work demands and risk factors for the adoption of awkward working postures, and their association with socio-demographic variables. A self-administered questionnaire survey was carried out among dental students of 4th and 5th class years at the Faculty of Dental Medicine of the University of Porto. Results showed that participants perceive Oral Surgery, Paediatric Dentistry, Endodontics and Fixed Prosthodontics as the most demanding dental activities. Conversely, the majority of respondents reported visual demands, work precision, accessibility to the site to treat, fatigue, tasks duration, support of an assistant, required manual dexterity, stress and working tools location/position as important work-related risk factors for the adoption of awkward working postures. Although some statistically significant associations have been found between socio-demographic variables and either perceived work demands or perceived risk factors for the adoption of awkward working postures, no consistent pattern could be recognized.

1 INTRODUCTION

Despite the improvements in aspects such as technology, ergonomics and work environment (Leggat et al., 2007, Lindfors et al., 2006), dental practitioners are still at higher risk of musculoskeletal disorders (MSDs) than most of the other occupational groups (Akesson et al., 1999, Finsen et al., 1998, Kerosuo et al., 2000). Increased risk of MSDs was also found among dental students, indicating that musculoskeletal symptoms may appear very soon after a short period of clinical training (Melis et al., 2004, Rising et al., 2005, Tezel et al., 2005). However, even if work-related MSDs are recognized as the most concerning occupational health problem among dentists (Chowanadisai et al., 2000), the clinical practice is still centred on patients and little attention is paid to the practitioners while performing the treatments (Pentikis, 1998).

The complexity and multifactorial nature of MSDs may explain some ineffectiveness of "the current methods for identifying and reducing or eliminating MSDs in today's industries" (Allread, 2006). In this context, Allread (2006) highlights the importance of individuals' personal aspects and perceptions of the work environment for the development of MSDs. On the other hand, individuals' awareness on work demands and the perception on risk factors for MSDs are fundamental steps for the adoption of ergonomic principles and in the changing process of attitudes and behaviours which play a central role in the prevention of disease (Abduljabbar, 2008, Rucker & Sunell, 2002, Sunell & Rucker, 2003). Therefore, the purpose of this preliminary study is twofold: (1) to assess dental students' perception on the level of both physical and mental demands associated to dental medicine practice, as well as on the importance of some work-related risk factors for the adoption of awkward working postures (WRRFFAAWP), and (2) to find out if there are significant differences in dental students' perceptions, based on their socio-demographic characteristics.

2 MATERIAL AND METHODS

A self-administered questionnaire survey was carried out, in April–May 2012, among 92 dental students of 4th and 5th class years at the Faculty of Dental Medicine of the University of Porto. Beyond some socio-demographic characteristics, the questionnaire included three different parts. In the two first parts, students were asked to rank, respectively, the physical demands and the mental demands of nine different dental activities included in their curricular plan (Oral Surgery, Dentistry, Endodontics, Preventive Dental Medicine, Occlusion, Paediatric Dentistry, Periodontology, Fixed Prosthodontics, and Removal Prosthodontics), by using a five level Likert-type scale (1 – not demanding at all; 2 – low demand; 3 – average demand; 4 – high demand; 5 – very high demand). In the third part, students were asked to report the

Table 1. Number (and %) of dental students participating in the survey, by gender and class year.

	Students' class year		
Gender	4th year	5th year	Total
Female	20	50	70 (76.1%)
Male	8	14	22 (23.9%)
Total	28 (30.4%)	64 (69.6%)	92 (100.0%)

perceived importance of twelve WRRFFAAWP, using a five level Likert-type scale (1 – not important at all; 2 – low importance; 3 – average importance; 4 – high importance; 5 – very high importance). The twelve work-related risk factors are (1) visual demands, (2) work precision, (3) accessibility to the site to treat, (4) required manual dexterity, (5) dentist chair, (6) working tools location/position, (7) tasks duration, (8) tasks cognitive demands, (9) stress, (10) fatigue, (11) patient chair, and (12) support of an assistant.

The questionnaires were distributed to students during 4th and 5th year classes. The 92 volunteers to participate in the survey were distributed according to Table 1.

Microsoft Office Excel 2007 and IBM SPSS Statistics 20 were used in data analysis. Contingency Tables and Chi-Square Tests were performed to analyse the association between variables under investigation (perceived work physical demands, perceived work mental demands and perceived risk factors for the adoption of awkward working postures) and the socio-demographic variables (age, gender, height, body mass index (BMI), dominant hand, class year, clinical and/or pre-clinical practice hours per week, regular physical exercise practice). Pearson Chi-Square and, when appropriate, Fisher's Exact Test were used. For analysis purpose, all non-dichotomous variables were dichotomised. Two-tailed tests were used and the significance level was set at $\alpha = 0.05$. For the statistically significant associations found, relative risk (RR), and 95% confidence intervals (95% CI) were computed to estimate the effect size.

The study was submitted to and approved by the Commission of Ethics of the Faculty of Dental Medicine of the University of Porto.

3 RESULTS

Response rates of 32.6% in 4th class year and 70.3% in 5th class year were achieved, representing an overall response rate of 52.0% (92/177).

3.1 *Sample characterisation*

Survey participants (92) were mostly female (76.1%), right-handed (94.6%) and a little less than half (46.7%) of them reported to practice regular physical exercise. Other demographic characteristics of survey participants are presented in Table 2.

Table 2. Demographic characteristics of survey participants.

	Gender		
Variable parameters	Female	Male	Total
Age (in years) (n = 88)			
Mean	23.4	23.3	23.4
SD*	3.1	1.9	2.8
Range	21–45	21–30	21–45
Height (in cm) (n = 92)			
Mean	165.3	177.6	168.2
SD*	6.4	6.4	8.3
Range	150–178	170–191	150–191
BMI (in Kg/m^2) (n = 92)			
Mean	21.0	23.6	21.6
SD*	2.5	2.1	2.7
Range	15.2–29.2	20.3–28.9	15.2–29.2

*SD = standard deviation.

3.2 *Physically demanding dental activities*

Oral Surgery (72.8%), Paediatric Dentistry (70.7%), Endodontics (67.0%), Fixed Prosthodontics (63.1%) and Dentistry (58.7%) were perceived as the most physically demanding dental activities by students who ranked them in the "high" or "very high" demand levels. Conversely, Preventive Dental Medicine (68.2%) and Occlusion (65.9%) were perceived as the less physically demanding activities by students who ranked them in the "not demanding at all" or "low demand" levels.

The perceived physical demands (PPD) of Endodontics ($\chi^2 = 6.113$, $p = 0.019$) and Paediatric Dentistry ($\chi^2 = 8.854$, $p = 0.004$) were found significantly associated to students' gender. Female students seem more likely to perceive Endodontics (RR: 1.626, 95% CI: 1.007–2.625) and Paediatric Dentistry (RR: 1.729, 95% CI: 1.076–2.776) as "high" or "very-high" physically demanding than their male colleagues.

On the other hand, the PPD of Paediatric Dentistry was found significantly associated to students' height ($\chi^2 = 5.904$, $p = 0.021$). Students below 170 cm height seem more likely to perceive Paediatric Dentistry (RR: 1.405, 95% CI: 1.043–1.892) as "high" or "very-high" physically demanding than their taller colleagues.

Furthermore, the PPD of Oral Surgery ($\chi^2 = 5.510$, $p = 0.022$), Dentistry ($\chi^2 = 6.255$, $p = 0.021$) and Paediatric Dentistry ($\chi^2 = 5.663$, $p = 0.025$) were found significantly associated to students' class year. 4th year students seem more likely to perceive Oral Surgery (RR: 1.361, 95% CI: 1.093–1.693) as "high" or "very-high" physically demanding while 5th year students seem more likely to perceive Dentistry (RR: 1.710, 95% CI: 1.046–2.795) and Paediatric Dentistry (RR: 1.458, 95% CI: 1.009–2.108) as "high" or "very-high" physically demanding than their counterpart colleagues.

Finally, the PPD of Removal Prosthodontics was found significantly associated to students' BMI (p = 0.030). Overweight students seem more likely to perceive the activity as "high" or "very-high" physically demanding (RR: 3.500, 95% CI: 1.448–8.463) than their colleagues under BMI 25.

Apart from these, no other statistically significant association was found between the PPD of the investigated dental activities and students' socio-demographic characteristics.

3.3 *Mentally demanding dental activities*

Fixed Prosthodontics (73.3%), Endodontics (71.7%), Pediatric Dentistry (57.6%), Occlusion (54.7%) and Oral Surgery (53.3%) were pointed out as the most mentally demanding dental activities by survey participants who classified them in the "high" or "very high" demand levels. Conversely, Preventive Dental Medicine and Periodontology were perceived as the less mentally demanding activities by, respectively, 70.0% and 41.3% of the respondents, which classified them in the "not demanding at all" and "low demand" levels.

The perceived mental demands (PMD) of Endodontics ($\chi^2 = 6.740$, $p = 0.014$) and Fixed Prosthodontics ($\chi^2 = 6.180$, $p = 0.022$) were found significantly associated to students' gender. Female students seem more likely to perceive Endodontics (RR: 1.571, 95% CI: 1.017–2.429) and Fixed Prosthodontics (RR: 1.527, 95% CI: 0.998–2.337) as "high" or "very-high" mentally demanding than their male colleagues.

The PMD of Endodontics ($\chi^2 = 7.077$, $p = 0.010$) and Fixed Prosthodontics ($\chi^2 = 8.200$, $p = 0.006$) were also found significantly associated to students' height. Unexpectedly, students below 170 cm height seem more likely to perceive Endodontics (RR: 1.438, 95% CI: 1.072–1.930) and Fixed Prosthodontics (RR: 1.475, 95% CI: 1.098–1.982) as "high" or "very-high" mentally demanding than their taller colleagues.

On the other hand, the PMD of Dentistry ($\chi^2 = 4.789$, $p = 0.034$), Endodontics ($\chi^2 = 6.112$, $p = 0.022$) and Preventive Dental Medicine ($p = 0.010$) were found significantly associated to students' class year. 4th year students seem more likely to perceive Dentistry (RR: 1.882, 95% CI: 1.085–3.264), Endodontics (RR: 1.394, 95% CI: 1.114–1.743) and Preventive Dental Medicine (RR: 11.071, 95% CI: 1.356–90.424) as "high" or "very-high" mentally demanding than their 5th year colleagues.

Furthermore, the PMD of Dentistry ($\chi^2 = 5.408$, $p = 0.032$) and Endodontics ($\chi^2 = 4.353$, $p = 0.045$) were found significantly associated to clinical and/or pre-clinical practice hours per week. Students practicing up to 15 hours per week seem more likely to perceive Dentistry (RR: 1.940, 95% CI: 1.122–3.353) and Endodontics (RR: 1.326, 95% CI: 1.048–1.679) as "high" or "very-high" mentally demanding than their colleagues with a heavier load of clinical and/or pre-clinical practice.

Apart from these, no other statistically significant association was found between the PMD of the investigated dental activities and students' socio-demographic characteristics.

3.4 *Most important work-related risk factors for the adoption of awkward working postures*

Visual demands (95.6%), work precision (94.5%), accessibility to the site to treat (93.4%), fatigue (65.9%), tasks duration (62.6%), support of an assistant (62.6%), required manual dexterity (59.3%), stress (52.7%) and working tools location/position (50.5%) were perceived as the most important WRRFFAAWP by survey participants who classified them in the "high" or "very high" importance levels. Conversely, tasks cognitive demands, patient chair and dentist chair were perceived as the less important ones.

The perceived importance of the required manual dexterity was found significantly associated with students' gender ($\chi^2 = 4.085$, $p = 0.050$) while the perceived importance of the support of an assistant was found significantly associated with students' height ($\chi^2 = 4.870$, $p = 0.031$). Female students seem more likely to perceive the required manual dexterity as highly or very-highly important WRRFFAAWP (RR: 1.594, 95% CI: 0.937–2.711) than their male colleagues. On the other hand, Students under 170 cm height seem more likely to perceive the support of an assistant as highly or very-highly important WRRFFAAWP (RR: 1.451, 95% CI: 1.020–2.065) than their taller colleagues.

Based on students' socio-demographic characteristics, no other significant differences were found in the perceived importance of the investigated WRRFFAAWP.

4 DISCUSSION

Perceived workload is often used in the assessment of occupational risk factors for MSDs (Vieira & Kumar, 2007), since high perceived workload has been found associated with musculoskeletal symptoms (Bongers et al., 2002). A recent study carried out among Iranian operating room nurses found significant association between PPD and musculoskeletal symptoms (Choobineh et al., 2010). Also dentists participating in a Swedish study reported high levels of perceived workload and work demands (Jonker et al., 2009).

The first aim of this preliminary study was to investigate how dental students perceive the work demands of dental practice. In line with the conclusions of former studies that have showed dental practice as a physically demanding work (Puriene et al., 2008, Rolander, 2010), most of the survey participants perceived Oral Surgery, Paediatric Dentistry, Endodontics, Fixed Prosthodontics and Dentistry as highly or very highly physically demanding. On the other hand, dental practice has also been indicated as requiring high levels of mental demands and a New Zealand's study found them "as the highest general work-related stressor" (Palliser et al., 2005). In the present investigation, most of survey respondents perceived Fixed Prosthodontics, Endodontics, Pediatric Dentistry, Occlusion and Oral Surgery as highly or very highly mentally demanding. Conversely, Preventive Dental Medicine was perceived as either the less physically or the less mentally demanding dental activity what, partially, seems to contradict the findings of a Danish study where the physical load on the musculoskeletal system for the three most common tasks (dental examination, cleaning and filling) performed by the dentists participating in the study, regardless of their technical differences, was similar (Finsen et al., 1998).

Individual factors such as age (Augustson & Morken, 1996) and gender (Lin et al., 2012, Marshall et al., 1997, Puriene et al., 2008) are often indicated as influencing perceived musculoskeletal symptoms. Since these are associated with perceived work demands, it was expected that females and males perceived differently the work demands of the investigated dental activities. However, in the present study, females only perceived Endodontics and Paediatric Dentistry as more demanding (either physically or mentally) than their male colleagues, what seems to indicate an inconclusive relationship between gender and perceived work demands. Conversely, neither perceived work demands of the investigated dental activities nor the perceived importance of the investigated WRRFFAAWP were found significantly associated to students' age, although this may be explained by the small range of students' ages.

On the other hand, a greater body height (e.g. >178 cm) has been indicated as risk factor for musculoskeletal symptoms (Lin et al., 2012). Despite it could be easily understood that "taller individuals probably have to work with more neck flexion to compensate for their body height" (Rolander et al., 2005) and, therefore, survey participants should have perceived the investigated activities as more physically demanding than their shorter colleagues, our findings doesn't support that statement since only a few significant associations were found between students' height category and the perceived work demands of the investigated dental activities. Even so, unexpectedly, it was the students under 170 cm height, and not the tallest, who perceived the activity as more demanding.

Conversely, BMI is often recognized as a risk factor for MSDs (Gilleard & Smith, 2007, Wearing et al., 2006), particularly in some occupations (see e.g. Pensri et al., 2009). A Swedish study seems to indicate that in individuals exposed to higher physical workloads, such as nurses, MSDs in neck-shoulder region are associated to BMI, while in individuals exposed to lower physical workloads (teachers), such an association was not found (Arvidsson et al., 2012). However, in the present study, only the PPD of Removal Prosthodontics was found significantly associated to students BMI, indicating that the higher the students BMI the more demanding they perceive the activity. Neither the PPD of the remaining activities and the PMD of all the investigated dental activities nor the perceived importance of WRRFFAAWP, were found associated to BMI.

On the other hand, despite Tezel et al. (2005) have found that left-handed dental students reported more musculoskeletal symptoms than their right-handed colleagues, other authors did not find significant differences in the reported musculoskeletal symptoms when considering dentists dominant hand (Chamani et al., 2012). Since perceived work demands have been found associated to the musculoskeletal symptoms, the present study seems to support Chamani et al. (2012) findings because none significant difference was found in the investigated variables based on students' dominant hand.

Although significant differences have been found in musculoskeletal symptoms reported by students of different class years (Abou-Atme et al., 2007, Rising et al., 2005, Thornton et al., 2008), in the present study, no consistent pattern could be identified in the relationship between students' class year and the variables under investigation, regardless of some significant associations between the perceived work demands of some of the investigated dental activities and students' class year.

Among dental practitioners, the high perceived physical load is often attributed to the high precision demands and uncomfortable work postures (Rolander, 2010). Since awkward working postures have been indicated as one of the most important risk factors for MSDs (Aarabi et al., 2009, Morse et al., 2010), particularly among professional groups such as dental practitioners (Finsen et al., 1998), it is important to identify the main work-related factors leading to the adoption of such working postures. However, no studies were found on this particular issue. Therefore, this study also aimed to find out how students perceive the importance of some work-related risk factors for the adoption of such postures while performing dental work. The results obtained show that more than 50% of the students perceive visual demands (95.6%), work precision (94.5%), accessibility to the site to treat (93.4%) fatigue (65.9%), tasks duration (62.6%), support of an assistant (62.6%), required manual dexterity (59.3%), stress (52.7%) and working tools location/position (50.5%) as highly or very highly important for the adoption of awkward postures during dental practice. However, only two statistically significant associations were found between the perceived importance of the WRRFFAAWP and students socio-demographic characteristics, indicating an inconsistent pattern.

Due to the difficult access to and visibility inside oral cavity, dental practitioners are often forced to adopt awkward working postures (Al Wassan et al., 2001). High visual demands, work precision, manual dexterity and working with unsupported and elevated arms have been indicated as the main causes for the high frequency of MSDs among dental professionals (Abduljabbar, 2008, Akesson et al., 2000). Despite the multifactorial origin of awkward working postures adopted by dental practitioners, they have often been recognized as a consequence of high work visual demands (Abduljabbar, 2008, Akesson et al., 1999, Marshall et al., 1997, Morse et al., 2010). In the present study, over 93% of the respondents reported visual demands, work precision and accessibility to the site to treat as highly or very highly important risk factor for the adoption of awkward working postures.

On the other hand, a cross-sectional study carried out among female dentists, dental hygienists and dental nurses showed the highest levels of fatigue in dentists (Lindfors et al., 2006) whereas a study carried out among Lithuanian dentists found fatigue (94.7%) as the most prevalent physical complaint reported (Puriene et al., 2008). Although fatigue is often indicated as a common outcome of awkward and/or static working postures, fatigue itself may be a contributing factor for the adoption of non-neutral postures (Anghel et al., 2007). Furthermore, a significant increase of stress amongst dental students has been shown in studies published in the last decades (Alzahem et al., 2011). In the present study, fatigue and stress are among the most important perceived risk factors for the adoption of awkward working postures, what seems to be in line with the findings of those studies.

5 CONCLUSIONS

Dental students of the 4th and 5th years at the Faculty of Dental Medicine of the University of Porto seem to be aware of both physical and mental demands associated to the dental practice and, simultaneously, show an accurate perception concerning WRRFFAAWP. This may indicate that education and training on prevention strategies during undergraduate years could contribute for a better musculoskeletal health and quality of life of future dentists. The results of the present study do not show consistent patterns in the association between socio-demographic variables and either the perceived work demands of the nine dental activities or the perceived importance of WRRFFAAWP. Therefore, further research is needed to understand the mechanisms leading to the adoption of critical working postures. Besides, more comprehensive studies are required to investigate risk factors and identify effective strategies to be implemented in order to avoid awkward and prolonged static working postures and, thus, prevent the development of work-related MSDs.

ACKNOWLEDGEMENTS

The authors express their sincere gratitude to all those who contributed for the questionnaire improvement, in particular to Professor André Correia (FMDUP), and to Professor Helena Figueiral (FMDUP) for her valuable participation in data collection process. Utmost recognition is also due to the dental students participating in the survey for their fundamental and voluntary contribution.

REFERENCES

Aarabi, A.M., Zamiri, B., Mohammadinezhad, C., Rahmanian, F., & Mahmoudi, H. 2009. Musculoskeletal Disorders in Dentists in Shiraz, Southern Iran. *Iranian Red Crescent Medical Journal 11*(4): 464–465.

Abduljabbar, T.A. 2008. Musculoskeletal disorders among dentists in Saudi Arabia. *Pakistan Oral & Dental Journal 28*(1): 135–144.

Abou-Atme, Y.S., Melis, M., Zawawi, K.H., & Cottogno, L. 2007. Five-year follow-up of temporomandibular disorders and other musculoskeletal symptoms in dental students. *Minerva stomatologica 56*(11–12): 603–609.

Akesson, I., Johnsson, B., Rylander, L., Moritz, U., & Skerfving, S. 1999. Musculoskeletal disorders among female dental personnel-clinical examination and a 5-year follow-up study of symptoms. *Int Arch Occup Environ Health 72*(6): 395–403.

Akesson, I., Schutz, A., Horstmann, V., Skerfving, S., & Moritz, U. 2000. Musculoskeletal symptoms among dental personnel; lack of association with mercury and selenium status, overweight and smoking. *Swedish Dental Journal 24*(1–2): 23–38.

Al Wassan, K., Almas, K., Al Shethri, S., & Al Qahtani, M. 2001. Back and neck problems among dentists and dental auxiliaries. *The journal of contemporary dental practice 2*(3): 17–30.

Allread, W.G. 2006. The Role Personality in Ergonomics. In W. S. Marras & W. Karwowski (eds), *Fundamentals and Assessment Tools for Occupational Ergonomics:* 25-01-25-14. Boca Raton: CRC Press.

Alzahem, A., Van Der Molen, H., Alaujan, A., Schmidt, H., & Zamakhshary, M. 2011. Stress amongst dental students: a systematic review. *European Journal of Dental Education 15*(1): 8–18.

Anghel, M., Argesanu, V., Talpos-Niculescu, C., & Lungeanu, D. 2007. Musculoskeletal disorders (MSDs)-Consequences of prolonged static postures. *Journal of Experimental Medical & Surgical Research Year XIV*(4): 167–172.

Arvidsson, I., Simonsen, J.G., Balogh, I., Hansson, G.-å., Dahlqvist, C., Granqvist, L., et al. 2012. Discrepancies in pain presentation caused by adverse psychosocial conditions as compared to pain due to high physical workload? *Work: A Journal of Prevention, Assessment and Rehabilitation 41*(0): 2472–2475.

Augustson, T.E., & Morken, T. 1996. Musculoskeletal discomfort among dental health personnel: A survey in the Public Dentist Services of Hordaland. *Tidsskrift for den Norske Laegeforening 116*(23): 2776–2780.

Bongers, P.M., Kremer, A.M., & ter Laak, J. 2002. Are psychosocial factors, risk factors for symptoms and signs of the shoulder, elbow, or hand/wrist? A review of the epidemiological literature. *American Journal of Industrial Medicine 41*(1): 315–342.

Chamani, G., Zarei, M.R., Momenzadeh, A., Safizadeh, H., Rad, M., & Alahyari, A. 2012. Prevalence of Musculoskeletal Disorders among Dentists in Kerman, Iran. *Journal of Musculoskeletal Pain 20*(3): 202–207.

Choobineh, A., Movahed, M., Tabatabaie, S., & Kumashiro, M. 2010. Perceived demands and musculoskeletal disorders in operating room nurses of Shiraz city hospitals. *Ind Health 48*(1): 74–84.

Chowanadisai, S., Kukiattrakoon, B., Yapong, B., Kedjarune, U., & Leggat, P.A. 2000. Occupational health problems of dentists in southern Thailand. *International Dental Journal 50*(1): 36–40.

Finsen, L., Christensen, H., & Bakke, M. 1998. Musculoskeletal disorders among dentists and variation in dental work. *Applied Ergonomics 29*(2): 119–125.

Gilleard, W., & Smith, T. 2007. Effect of obesity on posture and hip joint moments during a standing task, and trunk forward flexion motion. *International Journal of Obesity 31*(2): 267–271.

Jonker, D., Rolander, B., & Balogh, I. 2009. Relation between perceived and measured workload obtained by long-term inclinometry among dentists. *Applied Ergonomics 40*(3): 309–315.

Kerosuo, E., Kerosuo, H., & Kanerva, L. 2000. Self-reported health complaints among general dental practitioners, orthodontists, and office employees. *Acta Odontologica Scandinavica 58*(5): 207–212.

Leggat, P.A., Kedjarune, U., & Smith, D.R. 2007. Occupational health problems in modern dentistry: A review. *Industrial Health 45*(5): 611–621.

Lin, T.-H., Liu, Y.C., Hsieh, T.-Y., Hsiao, F.-Y., Lai, Y.-C., & Chang, C.-S. 2012. Prevalence of and risk factors for musculoskeletal complaints among Taiwanese dentists. *Journal of Dental Sciences 7*(1): 65–71.

Lindfors, P., von Thiele, U., & Lundberg, U. 2006. Work characteristics and upper extremity disorders in female dental health workers. *Journal of Occupational Health 48*(3): 192–197.

Marshall, E.D., Duncombe, L.M., Robinson, R.Q., & Kilbreath, S.L. 1997. Musculoskeletal symptoms in New South Wales dentists. *Australian Dental Journal 42*(4): 240–246.

Melis, M., Abou-Atme, Y.S., Cottogno, L., & Pittau, R. 2004. Upper body musculoskeletal symptoms in Sardinian dental students. *Journal of the Canadian Dental Association 70*(5): 306–310.

Morse, T., Bruneau, H., & Dussetschleger, J. 2010. Musculoskeletal disorders of the neck and shoulder in the dental professions. *Work: A Journal of Prevention, Assessment & Rehabilitation 35*(4): 419–429.

Palliser, C.R., Firth, H.M., Feyer, A.M., & Paulin, S.M. 2005. Musculoskeletal discomfort and work-related stress in New Zealand dentists. *Work and Stress 19*(4): 351–359.

Pensri, P., Janwantanakul, P., & Chaikumarn, M. 2009. Prevalence of self-reported musculoskeletal symptoms in salespersons. *Occup. Med. 59*(7): 499–501.

Pentikis, J. 1998. Ergonomic issues in dentistry, the US Army perspective. *Advances in Occupational Ergonomics and Safety 2*: 727–730.

Puriene, A., Aleksejuniene, J., Petrauskiene, J., Balciuniene, I., & Janulyte, V. 2008. Self-Reported Occupational Health Issues among Lithuanian Dentists. *Industrial Health 46*(4): 369–374.

Rising, D.W., Bennett, B.C., Hursh, K., & Plesh, O. 2005. Reports of body pain in a dental student population. *Journal of American Dental Association 136*(1): 81–86.

Rolander, B. 2010. *Work conditions, musculoskeletal disorders and productivity of dentists in public dental care in Sweden.* Linköping University. Linköping, Sweden.

Rolander, B., Karsznia, A., Jonker, D., Oberg, T., & Bellner, A.-L. 2005. Perceived contra observed physical work load in Swedish dentists. *Work: A Journal of Prevention, Assessment & Rehabilitation 25*(3): 253–262.

Rucker, L.M., & Sunell, S. 2002. Ergonomic risk factors associated with clinical dentistry. *J Calif Dent Assoc 30*(2): 139–148.

Sunell, S., & Rucker, L. 2003. Ergonomic Risk Factors, Associated with Clinical Dental Hygiene Practice. *Probe 37*(4): 159–166.

Tezel, A., Kavrut, F., Tezel, A., Kara, C., Demir, T., & Kavrut, R. 2005. Musculoskeletal Disorders in Left- and Right–Handed Turkish Dental Students. *International Journal of Neuroscience 115*(2): 255–266.

Thornton, L.J., Barr, A.E., Stuart-Buttle, C., Gaughan, J.P., Wilson, E.R., Jackson, A.D., et al. 2008. Perceived musculoskeletal symptoms among dental students in the clinic work environment. *Ergonomics 51*(4): 573–586.

Vieira, E.R., & Kumar, S. 2007. Occupational risks factors identified and interventions suggested by welders and computer numeric control workers to control low back disorders in two steel companies. *International Journal of Industrial Ergonomics 37*(6): 553–561.

Wearing, S.C., Hennig, E.M., Byrne, N.M., Steele, J.R., & Hills, A.P. 2006. Musculoskeletal disorders associated with obesity: a biomechanical perspective. *Obesity Reviews 7*(3): 239–250.

Biodental Engineering II – Natal Jorge et al (Eds)
© 2014 Taylor & Francis Group, London, ISBN 978-1-138-00131-2

Designing dental implant surfaces by Laser microtexturing

M. Oliveira
Instituto de Engenharia Mecânica e Gestão Industrial, Porto, Portugal

J. Machado & A. Reis
Faculdade de Engenharia, Universidade do Porto, Porto, Portugal

ABSTRACT: This work focus the potential of the ns pulsed Nd:YAG (1064 nm) fiber Laser for the microtexturing of Ti and its alloys, targeting its application for dental implants surfaces. The influence of Laser process parameters, such as pulse width and pulse overlap, on the surface morphology characteristics of TiCP GII and Ti-6Al-4V is analyzed, and its impact to the surface wettability is discussed. The results show that combining different levels of pulse width (10–200 ns), peak power (<10 kW) and pulse overlap (0–90%), three types of surfaces can be created, namely, patterned, isotropic and/or oxidized surfaces, with distinct functional properties. Slight morphological differences observed between TiCP and Ti-6Al-4V and the stronger oxidation in TiCP were seen to have a significant impact on the wetting behavior of these surfaces. Ti-6Al-4V textured with 200 ns pulses presented the lowest contact angles, independently of the pulse overlap rate.

1 INTRODUCTION

1.1 *Surface characteristics*

Current dental implant concepts target osseointegration, understood as the structural, direct and functional bonding between the local bone and the implant surface. Titanium and its alloys are disseminated as the base-material in dental implants manufacturing, as these are bio-inert materials. However, despite all dedicated research, not all implants show effective osseointegration, resulting in high direct and indirect costs (Lavenus et al. 2010).

Surface characteristics determine tissue/implant interaction, affecting implant stability and lifetime, since all reactions take place at the interface. Main surface-related factors affecting osseointegration are the surface morphology, chemical composition and wettability (Guéhennec et al. 2007).

Surface morphology has been considered as the most determinant factor, as the increase on the contact area influences the tissue response at molecular and cellular level. Surface morphology characterization mainly involves the assessment of surface roughness and irregularities' orientation. Most of the commercially available dental implants present isotropic surfaces obtained by plasma spray or sand blasting and acid etching (SLA), while non-isotropic surfaces are usually observed in machined implants (Bonewald et al. 1999; Wennerberg et al. 2004). These are moderately rough surfaces 1.0–2.0 μm, as this is assumed to be the preferable roughness range regarding osseointegration, and excessively high or low roughness levels are usually associated to weaker tissue responses, although this is still unclear. However, surface roughness would be expected to vary along the implant body, with increasing roughness levels from body top to tip, in order to inhibit bacteria adhesion close to the soft tissues on top, and to enhance osseointegration by surface area increase on bottom.

Although surface treatment influences the surface chemical composition, in most cases the natural oxidation of Ti prevails. Ti presents high affinity to O_2, forming a 3–6 nm thick protective oxide layer (mainly TiO_2 with minor amounts of Ti_2O_3 & TiO) of significant adherence and stability. During osseointegration, the TiO_2 layer behaves as the receptor of a series of reactions promoting cell adhesion to pure Ti. On the other hand, for small body diameters, Ti implants present reduced mechanical resistance. In alternative, Ti alloys, such as Ti-6Al-4V, provide for higher mechanical properties, but osseointegration seems to be significantly compromised (Ballo & Omar 2011).

Surface wettability is affected by both, morphology and chemical composition. This is quantified by observing the contact angle between a fluid drop placed over the surface. Contact angles below 90° indicate partial surface wetting, characteristic of a hydrophilic surface, which enhances adhesion of biological particles and favors osseointegration. Theoretical models are used to describe the influence of roughness in the contact angle. The Cassie-Baxter model (1944) assumes that the presence of air in the rough surface' cavities restricts its wettability by the liquid. Considering such surface as a composite substrate, where $\O_S$ is the fraction of solid in contact with the liquid, the contact angle would be determined by (1):

$$\cos\theta_{CB} = -1 + \O_S\,(1 + \cos\theta) \qquad (1)$$

As $\O_S$ is always lower than 1, this model foresees a higher effective θ_{CB}, independently of θ.

1.2 *Surface Laser microtexturing*

Laser micro-processing offers high accuracy and fine selectivity of the surface treatment conditions per unit area, enabling the creation of a wide range of roughness profiles, microstructures and irregularities resolution, which can be adjusted according to the required surface-tissue interaction level (Esposito & Thomsson 2008).

In-between the available Laser systems, pulsed fiber Laser systems had a remarkable grown in the last years, being seen as an industrial tool with a great potential for new microapplications. Pulsed Nd:YAG fiber Lasers are particularly interesting for metals processing, overcoming their high reflectivity with the short wave length (1064 nm), leading to stronger energy absorption in reduced material volume, and minimizing the impact of thermal conduction to the neighboring areas. Surface microtexturing is one of the most interesting application fields for these pulsed Lasers, as they enable a tight control of Laser/material interaction. Different types of surfaces with controlled material removal can be created according to the application specific requirements.

During process, Laser energy is focused and concentrated at the metal surface, being partly absorbed on a fine surface layer. The absorbed energy diffuses by conduction and a part of it is converted in thermal energy. As surface temperature rises above the evaporation temperature threshold, Laser ablation occurs, understood as a complex process involving melting, vaporization and material expel phenomena. The result is an ionized ablation plume, leaving behind a well-defined ablation crater. The morphological characteristics of this crater are determined by the Laser parameterization. The quantification of the material damage induced typically includes the estimation of irradiance and fluence, respectively the power and energy density reaching the surface. When defining the Laser power density required for ablation, and considering that a Gaussian profile is the most common distribution of the transversal beam intensity I. Such a profile induces a temperature gradient at the Laser/material interaction spot, and the consequent melt flow in the radial direction.

Besides the beam diameter (D), defined by the optical setup and focus position, the critical parameters in the operation of a pulsed Laser beam are: the pulse width (ns), beam intensity (kW), pulse repetition frequency (PRF; kHz), scanning speed (SS; mm/s) and hatch step (h; μm) between consecutive scans. These later 2 parameters are particularly critical in surface micro-texturing, as they determine the total pulse overlap ratio, as follows (2):

$$\%\ \text{Pulse overlap} = (1 - L/D) * 100 \qquad (2)$$

where L = SS/PRF. For a constant beam diameter, reduction in pulse width is associated to higher peak power and, consequently, irradiance values, at the expenses of the average Laser power. The main benefit is the reduction of the Laser-material interaction, minimizing the thermal load over the material, and the risk of overheating.

1.3 *Ti Laser microtexturing*

Several studies have been dedicated to the surface microtexturing of Ti and its alloys using pulsed Lasers operating in the nanosecond range (ns), and to the applicability of these surfaces for biomedical uses, considering their tight requirements regarding cell adhesion.

The creation of patterns of individualized craters with different diameters and inter-distances, on Ti surfaces, has been explored (Pecora et al. 2009), demonstrating their positive influence to cell adhesion. Others, exploring the microtexturing of Ti-6Al-4V with short Laser pulses (Trtica et al. 2006; Palmquist et al. 2009), highlighted the impact of irradiance and fluence level on the surface texture, roughness level and cell adhesion. Irradiance and fluence threshold values to be considered for Laser ablation of Ti have also been provided by others (Lavisse et al. 2009), who studied its dependency on the Laser wavelength, i.e., on the beam absorption of the material, and the morphology of the interaction spots created. For TiCP and a 1064 nm pulsed laser, 0.32 GW/cm^2 is indicated as the irradiance threshold required to achieve melting and vaporization of Ti. The increase on power or energy density was seen to result on stronger hydrodynamic effects, such as smoother surfaces of the craters and higher amount and size of melt drops solidified at the spot edges.

In what concerns wettability, Ti-based surfaces were shown to be hydrophilic, but the range of the contact angle values presented in the literature is quite broad. These studies have mainly tested TiCP and Ti-6Al-4V with H_2O, glycerol, blood or other fluids simulating plasma or blood, comparing polished and textured surfaces with different roughness levels. In general, strong reductions on the contact angle with the textured surfaces were observed and this effect has been attributed to the impact of higher surface roughness and/or O_2 content (Narendra et al. 2010).

2 METHODS & EXPERIMENTS

2.1 *Laser test conditions*

The ns Laser is a MOPA-M-HP-20 model by Multiwave Photonics. The laser operates at 1064 nm, and

Table 1. Input power and pulse energy values related to Laser conditions tested. Estimated irradiance, fluence and surface temperature values are also included.

PRR [kHz]	Pulse Width [ns]	
36.5	10	200
	Power Level [%]	
Settings	80	27.5
Peak Power [kW]	9.60	2.50
Pulse Energy [mJ]	0.088	0.138
Irradiance [GW/cm^2]	0.76	0.20
Fluence [J/cm^2]	7.00	10.94
Temperature [10^4 °C]		
TiCP (Grade II)	1.4	3.6
Ti-6Al-4V	1.1	2.7

has a range of 10 to 200 ns in pulse width, with PRF ranging from single shot up to 500 kHz. Average power is up to 20 W, peak power up to 12 kW, and pulse energy is up to 0.6 mJ. Detailed calibration of the Laser, together with the flexibility in the choice of pulse width, PRF and average power allows for the generation of any desired pulse peak power and pulse energy combination.

Two ns pulse widths were used for these tests, namely 10 ns and 200 ns pulses, operating at the same PRR of 36.5 kHz. These two values are at opposite ends of the ns spectrum of the Laser, enabling a comparison of the effect of a relatively low energy pulse with that of a longer and higher energy pulse. Peak power was adjusted by adjusting the average power setting of the fiber laser while keeping track of pulse energy. Scanning speed and hatch step were defined to maintain similar values of pulse-to-pulse overlap ratios, as well as, line-to-line overlap ratios in the range 0–90%.

Commercially pure titanium Grade II (TiCP) and Ti-6Al-4V thin sheets have been used. Test areas of 5*5 mm^2 have been produced. Power rate was adjusted as 80%, for 10 ns pulses, and 27.5% for the 200 ns pulses, corresponding to the pre-defined spot size (33 μm), as this is understood to accommodate the size of osteoblasts. The irradiance and fluence values corresponding to these conditions are presented in Table 1; these values are significantly above the threshold values collected from the literature, insuring the required processability. The maximum surface temperature achieved is also shown.

As depicted, in the conditions used, the surface irradiance achieved with a 10 ns pulse is about 4–5 times higher than that coming from a 200 ns pulse. On the other hand, the 200 ns pulse energy is about 50% higher and, consequently, the resulting surface temperature is about 2.5 times higher, independently on the material. The influence of the thermal and optical properties of the materials to the surface temperature increase is also made evident. The temperature reached in TiCP is about 30% higher than that in Ti-6Al-4V. Despite the higher thermal conductivity and diffusivity of TiCP, its higher absorption of the 1064 nm Laser beam justifies this difference.

2.2 *Surface morphology characterization*

The Laser-textured surfaces were examined by optical microscopy. Surface morphology was acquired using a stylus profilometer (Hommelwerke, Germany), stylus model TKL300/17, mounted on a T8000 Tester.

Depending on the pulse overlap and the hatch step, the textured surface created formed either a periodic pattern of evenly spaced craters, or a more irregular surface structure. In the first, parallel measurements clearly yield different results, thus requiring 3D surface measurements. Although 3D roughness parameters are not standardized, these are calculated using conditions inherited from the 2D standards. Most common 3D roughness parameter is the surface arithmetic average roughness, S_a, which indicates the average distance from the profile to the center line over the total measurement length in each direction. Average peak (S_p), average valley (S_v) and average peak-to-valley (S_z) height values were also calculated. The roughness measurement values shown were averaged over a scan area of 480 μm × 480 μm, with incremental measurement steps of 2.5 μm, and applying a filter of 80 μm to limit waviness effects.

2.3 *Surface wettability characterization*

Laser-textured surfaces were tested with a neutral fluid, deionized H_2O, in order to assess their hydrophilic character. All samples have been previously cleaned with ethanol under ultrasonic bath, and properly dried.

Wettability tests have been executed using the sessile drop method, in a contact angle measuring system integrating proper image acquisition and calculation *software* (OCA 20 & SCA20, Dataphysics). The Laplace method was used to calculate the contact angle, as a function of the fluid drop volume (2 μL, for each fluid). The H_2O drop deposition rate was 1.0 μL/s, and the total measuring time was 300 s. The test was reproduced in 3 surface areas for each Laser condition.

3 RESULTS & DISCUSSION

3.1 *Surface morphology characterization*

Figure 1 presents the type of crater created in TiCP by the interaction with the pulsed Laser.

The strong influence of pulsed Laser transmission conditions is here evident. The interaction of TiCP with the short and high peak power 10 ns pulse resulted in a low depth crater with an inner wave-like surface, typical from the rapid solidification of the melt. Solidified drops, expelled during the complex ablation process, are spread along the crater edge. The diameter and inner surface of the crater created in Ti-6Al-4V were

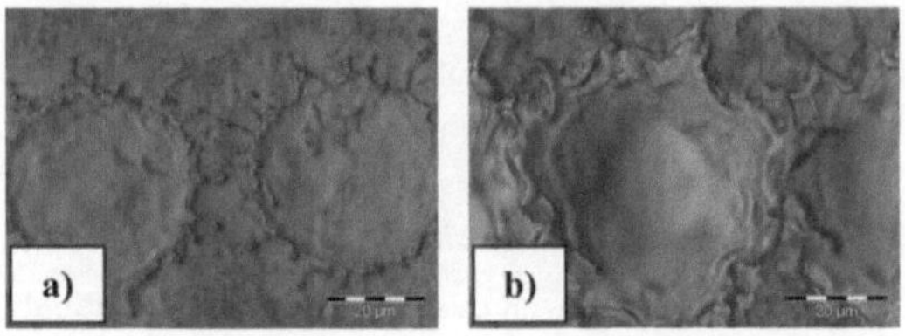

Figure 1. Influence of the Laser pulse width on the characteristics of a crater formed on the TiCP surface: a) 10 ns, b) 200 ns.

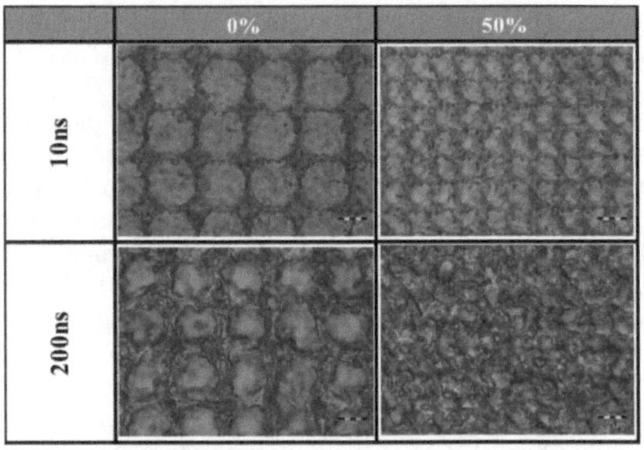

Figure 2. Optical images of the microstructures of the Laser-textured surfaces obtained in TiCP, with 10 ns and 200 ns pulses, and 0% and 50% pulse overlap.

similar to that observed in TiCP. However, the level of melt spreading and scattered drops surrounding the crater is lower, as expected from the lower surface temperature estimated. In contrast, the crater formed in TiCP with the 200 ns pulse showed a quite smooth inner surface, but the spreading is much higher than that observed with the 10 ns pulses. This is justified by the high pulse energy inherent to the longer pulses and, consequently, by the higher temperature induced (Table 1).

As advanced, the morphology of the Laser-processed surfaces is mostly determined by the pulse overlap ratio applied and type of surface, as further discussed. Figure 2 presents the patterns observed in TiCP, obtained with a 0% pulse overlap, i.e., creating adjacent craters, and 50% pulse overlap. Pulse overlap ratios till 50% resulted in the appearing of well-defined patterns, outlined by the accumulated solidified melt at the craters edge, as observed by others [10,11,14,16]. The values of the main 3D roughness parameters measured on these surfaces are presented in Figure 3.

The average arithmetic roughness (S_a) found on the surface textured with 0% overlap of 200 ns pulses (1.8 μm) is about 3x higher than that obtained with 10 ns pulses. These surfaces presented peak he ight values (S_p) much higher than the depth of the valleys (S_v); higher values were found on the TiCP when compared to the Ti-6Al-4V, particularly regarding S_p (>20%), reflecting the higher melt volume solidified at the edges.

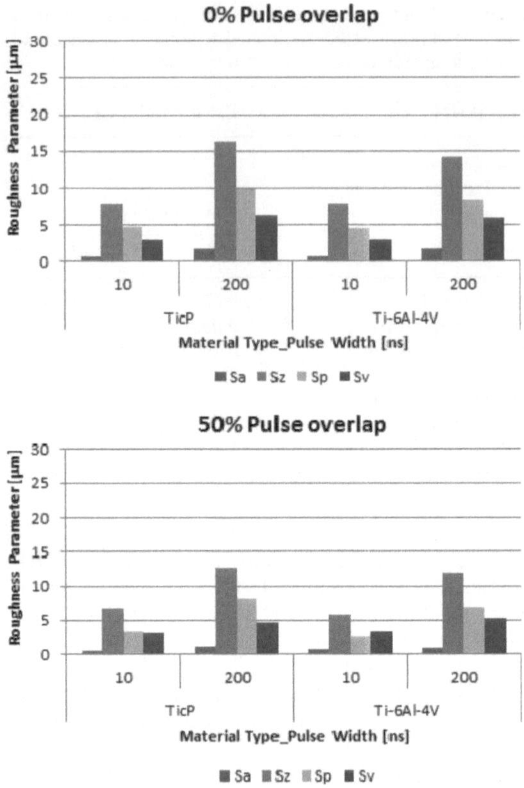

Figure 3. Roughness parameters (3D) values obtained with 0% and 50% pulse overlap, as a function of material type and Laser pulse width.

The 50% pulse overlap resulted in finer patterns and the pulse width was also here determinant to the roughness values of the textured surfaces. With 10 ns pulses, these surfaces presented similar S_a, S_z and S_v values to those observed a 0% overlap. However, the peak height values are about 20% lower with 50% pulse overlap, when compared to that observed with non-overlapping craters, revealing the more uniform distribution of the melt at the overlapping crater' edges. In the 200 ns surfaces, the increase on pulse overlap effectively results in finer and less rough structures, as S_a was seen to reduce in about 50% in both materials. The peaks' height (S_p) also reduced significantly, as observed with the short pulses, followed by a slight decrease in the valley's depth (S_v).

Figure 4 presents the microstructures observed with 80% and 90% pulse overlap for TiCP. The 3D roughness parameters values associated to these surfaces and those of Ti-6Al-4V in similar conditions are shown in Figure 5. At 80% pulse overlap, the S_a values are close to those obtained with 0% pulse overlap. In particular, the surfaces textured with 10 ns pulses present the finest roughness observed, either in terms of S_a (0.4 μm) or S_z (5.9 μm) and S_p (2.7 μm), though slightly oriented in the direction of the Laser scan. However, the application of longer and energetic 200 ns pulses resulted in the increase of all parameters

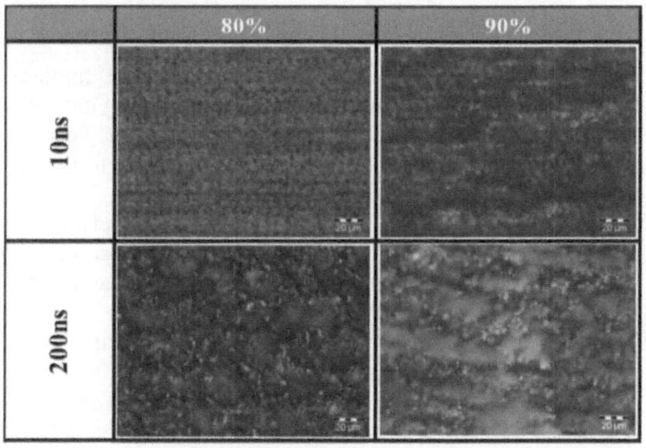

Figure 4. Optical images of the microstructures of the Laser-textured surfaces obtained in TiCP, with 10 ns and 200 ns pulses, and 80% and 90% pulse overlap.

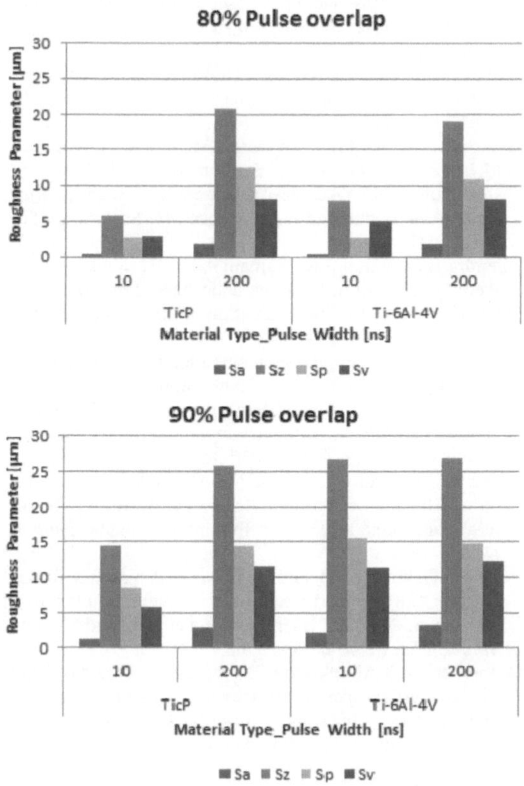

Figure 5. Roughness parameters (3D) values obtained with 80% and 90% pulse overlap, as a function of material type and Laser pulse width.

assessing the deviations of the irregularities, namely S_p, S_v and S_z, particularly in the later, which accumulates the slighter increments of S_p and S_v. TiCP tends to present higher values of S_p, when compared to Ti-6Al-4V, independently on the pulse width used. The 90% pulse overlap resulted in significantly irregular textures, as validated by the high roughness values, in terms of any of the parameters analyzed, as a result

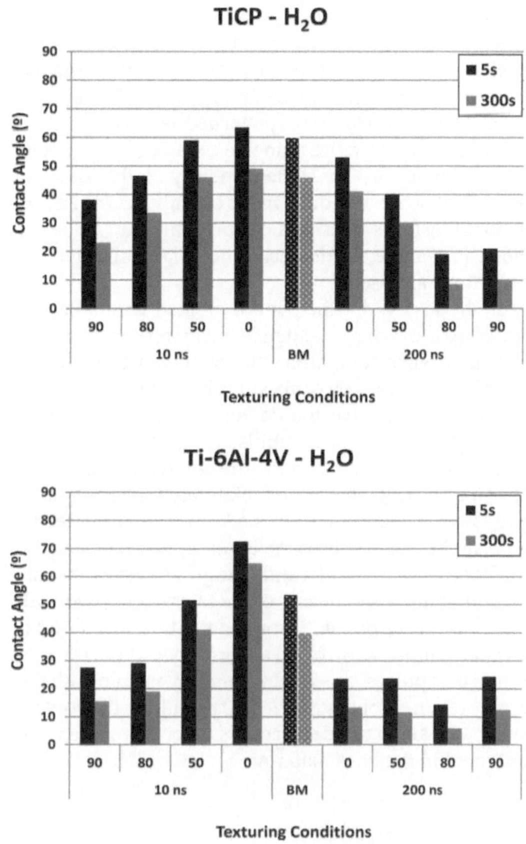

Figure 6. Influence of texture on surface wettability, as a function of material type and Laser process conditions (pulse width and pulse overlap; BM: base-metal.

from the energy accumulation related with the high pulse overlapping.

The differences observed between both materials when worked with 10 ns are to be highlighted. In this condition, the presence of an oxide layer at the surface of TiCP is revealed by the intense color observed, while in the Ti-6Al-4V alloy, the type of texture and the roughness level is similar to that obtained with 200 ns pulses. This can be explained by the higher affinity of TiCP to oxygen, when compared to the Ti-6Al-4V alloy, and the related hue should be associated to the oxide layer thickness. The resultant irregularities level is similar to that observed in conditions of shorter pulse overlap.

3.2 *Surface wettability*

The influence of texture on the surface wettability can be analyzed from Figure 6 presenting the contact angles measured on the Laser-textured surfaces with H_2O, as a function of base materials and Laser texturing conditions (pulse width and pulse overlap). Non-textured surfaces were also assessed and values obtained are here used as reference. It can be observed that the general evolution of the contact angle with the

Laser texture conditions is similar for both materials. Independently of the material type or Laser parameters, $\theta < 90°$ was observed in all cases, confirming the hydrophilic character of these materials. In general, lower pulse overlap rates (patterned texture) resulted in higher contact angles than that obtained in the irregular isotropic surfaces, independently on the material type, fluid or pulse width. On the other hand, the 200 ns textured surfaces clearly tend to present lower values of the contact angle, particularly when high pulse overlap conditions are used.

In the Ti-6Al-4V, the pattern created with adjacent craters (0% overlap) resulted in the increase of the contact angle when compared with the base metal, though on TiCP this effect was only slightly visible. Moreover, it must be noted that the decreasing rate of the contact angle with time was similar for all samples tested with H_2O. Particularly with the longer 200 ns pulse conditions, which presented relatively high roughness and lower oxidation levels, the Wenzel models seems here applicable, as the contact angle decreases as the surfaces become significantly rough. However, the formation of thick and denser oxide layers observed with the 10 ns pulses on TiCP would deter this. The Ti-6Al-4V seems more sensitive to the presence of the texture. With 10 ns pulses, this effect is mostly visible with the grainy textures, but, with the 200 ns pulses, the contact angle with all textured surfaces is much lower than that observed in the base material.

4 CONCLUSIONS

The potential of pulsed Laser to obtain Ti-based surfaces microtextures with distinct morphologies and wetting behaviors has been demonstrated. The pulse width and pulse overlap were the main factors evaluated, determining the type of texture obtained. Isotropic structures of fine roughness, as low as 0.4 μm, can be obtained with 80% pulse overlap. Higher overlap values increase the irregularities deviations on these surfaces, and the roughness level obtained is mostly influenced by the accumulated fluence induced on the surface. However, on TiCP, high pulse overlap conditions, particularly when combined with shorter pulses, enhances surface oxidation, and this effect should not be neglected as it prevails over the topography of the base metal. Such surfaces tend to be poorly wetted when compared to those chemically more close to the base material. High Ti-6Al-4V surface wetting was observed, particularly when processed with long pulses and high pulse overlap.

REFERENCES

Ballo A. & Omar O. 2011, Palmquist A. Dental Implant Surfaces – Physicochemical Properties, Biological Performance, and Trends. *Implant Dentistry – A Rapidly Evolving Practice*, Ilser Turkyilmaz (Ed.) InTech; ISBN: 978-953-307-658-4.

Bonewald L., Boyan B., Dean D., Lohmann C., Oefinger J. & Schwartz Z. 1999. Implant surface characteristics modulate differentiation behavior of cells in the osteoblastic lineage. *Adv Dent Res.*; 13:38–48.

Esposito M & Thomsson M. 2008. A retrospective case series evaluating Branemark BioHelix implants placed in a specialist private practice following 'conventional' procedures. One-year results after placement. *Eur J Oral Implantol*; 1: 229–234.

Guéhennec L., Soueidan A., Layrolle P. & Amouriq Y. 2007. Surface treatments of titanium dental implants for rapid osseointegration. *Dent Materials*; 23:844–854.

Gyorgy E., Mihailescu I.N., Serra P., Pino A.P. & Morenza J.L. 2002. Single pulse Nd:YAG Laser irradiation of titanium: influence of laser intensity on surface morphology. *Surf Coat Tech*; 154: 63–67.

Lavenus S., Louarn G. & Layrolle P. 2010. Nanotechnology and Dental implants. *Int J Biomaterials*, doi:10.1155/201/915327.

Lavisse L., Sahour M.C., Jouvard J.M., Pillon G. & Lucas M.C.M. 2009. Growth of titanium oxinitride layers by short pulsed Nd:YAG laser treatment of Ti plates: Influence of the cumulated laser fluence. *Ap. Surf. Sci.*; 255: 5515–5518.

Narendra B.D., Paital S.R., Samant A.N. & Daniel C. 2010. Wetting behavior of laser synthetic surface microtextures on Ti-6Al-4V for bioapplication. *Phil R Soc A*; 368: 1863–1889.

Palmquist A., Lindberg F., Emmanuelsson L., Brånemark R., Engqvist A. & Thomsen P. 2009. Biomechanical, histological, and ultra-structural analyses of laser micro- and nano-structured titanium alloy implants: A study in rabbit. *J Bio Mat Res A*; doi: 10.1002/jbm.a.32439.

Pecora G., Ceccarelli R., Bonelli M., Alexander H. & Ricci J. 2009. Clinical evaluation of Laser microtexturing for soft tissue and bone attachment to dental implants. *Implant Dent*; 18/1.

Trtica M., Gakovic B., Batani D., Desai T., Panjan P. & Radak B. 2006. Surface modifications of a titanium implant by a picosecond Nd:YAG laser operating at 1064 and 532 nm. *Ap. Surf. Sci.*; 253: 2551–2556.

Wennerberg A., Albrektsson T, Andersson B. 2004. Oral implant surface: Part 1 – Review focusing on telegraphic and chemical properties of different surfaces an in vivo response of them. *Int J Prosthondont*; 17:356–543.

Biodental Engineering II – Natal Jorge et al (Eds)
© 2014 Taylor & Francis Group, London, ISBN 978-1-138-00131-2

Three-dimensional visualization of teeth by magnetic resonance imaging during speech

Sandra R. Ventura
Área Técnico-Científica da Radiologia, Escola Superior de Tecnologia da Saúde – Instituto Politécnico do Porto, Portugal

Diamantino R. Freitas
Departamento de Engenharia Electrotécnica e de Computadores, Faculdade de Engenharia, Universidade do Porto, Portugal

Isabel M. Ramos
Departamento de Radiologia do Centro Hospitalar de S. João EPE, Faculdade de Medicina, Universidade do Porto, Portugal

João Manuel R.S. Tavares
Instituto de Engenharia Mecânica e Gestão Industrial, Departamento de Engenharia Mecânica, Faculdade de Engenharia, Universidade do Porto, Portugal

1 INTRODUCTION

Teeth morphology and oral cavity visualization through imaging techniques enables an accurate vocal tract assessment in speech research, especially when by Magnetic Resonance Imaging (MRI) [1].

Magnetic Resonance Imaging has been successfully applied on real-time analysis of the articulators during speech production, along the whole vocal tract, with good signal-to-noise ratio and without ionizing effects. As such, several MRI techniques provided the calculation of cross-sectional areas and volumes directly from static postures during sustained articulations [2] or using multiple repetitions [3, 4].

Currently, the application of MRI in speech research provides useful and accurate qualitative and quantitative analysis of speech articulation [5]. The role of teeth during speech is important not only to the evaluation of dental and lingual sounds, but also for measuring the vocal tract shape in three dimensions (3D) and the mouth acoustic opening [6].

The vocal tract is similar to an inverted L-shaped tube, with a significant length, which extends from the vocal folds to the lips and with a side branch leading to the nasal cavity [7] and nostrils. The articulators include the lips, the tongue, the teeth, the palate and the pharynx, and establish a set of cavities for air stream modification during speech. Because of the wide range of movements and flexibility of some articulators, in particularly of the tongue, it is difficult to observe and assess their movements and deformations.

Some methods for teeth observation have been attempted intending the qualitative and quantitative analysis of speech articulation using different techniques [1, 8], mainly using MRI; however, with some drawbacks, especially for speech production assessment purposes, as summarized in Tables 1 and 2.

As found during the literature review, teeth visualization by MRI is growing and in different directions, being the results promising, not only for dentistry and orthodontics, but also for speech research purpose.

The aim of this study was to describe and present an effective and useful method to extract the teeth morphology in MRI images that facilitates the MRI based qualitative and quantitative analysis concerning speech articulation.

2 MATERIAL AND METHODS

In this section, the procedures adopted to visualize teeth using MR images are described. Thus, the MRI equipment and protocol adopted in the acquisition process is specified; afterwards, the image data processing and analysis accomplished is described.

2.1 *Teeth visualization*

During this study, some experiments, including one similar to the one described in [1], were attained to improve teeth visualization using MRI; however, due to the discomfort implied to the subjects and the indirect visualization of the dental crows, these experiments were discarded.

Due to the lack of signal from teeth produced by MRI and considering only the methods that could be

Table 1. Current methods concerning the teeth visualization using MRI.

Study	Purpose and drawbacks
Wakumoto et al., 1997 [*cited in 9, 10*]	1st trial performed using MRI. Paired plates containing contrast medium to visualize dental crown. Image-by-image manual segmentation of teeth boundaries. Indirect visualization of teeth crowns. Cannot be used during speech articulation, especially of some fricative consonants.
Tutton & Goddard, 2002 [11]	MRI appearances of the anatomy of pathology of the dento-alveolar region. Reveals that the best technique for demonstrating the crowns of the teeth is with the subject with his mouth close and refrain swallowing during the scan. Cannot be used during speech articulation.
Olt & Jakob, 2004 [8]	Contrast-enhanced dental MRI for 3D visualization of the oral cavity, jaw and teeth. Pure water was used as contrast medium inside the oral cavity. Isosurface reconstructions (3D) of the teeth and jaw were performed. Indirect visualization of teeth crowns. Subject effort and discomfort; artifacts can occur. Cannot be used during speech articulation.
Takemoto et al., 2004 [1]	Three steps: 1st dental scans for extracting digital jaw casts with the subject holding blueberry juice inside the mouth; 2nd the superimposition of teeth in the images collected during speech based on the position matching of the reference landmarks; 3rd extraction of 3D vocal tract shape. Some errors in landmark sampling, due to the different body positions of the subject (prone position during the 1st scan and then supine position for speech production scans) and motion. Indirect visualization of teeth crowns. Subject effort and discomfort due to long acquisition times.
Ventura et al., 2009 [5]	Two steps: 1st an acquisition of a midsagittal high resolution image with the tongue in full contact with the tooth for manual extraction of teeth shape; 2nd superimposition of tooth in further sagittal images collected during speech production using manual editing and pasting. Misalignments errors and time consuming method. Indirect visualization of incisors crowns. Not possible to obtain 3D models of teeth due to reduced volume image data.
Idiyatullin et al., 2011 [12]	*In vitro* and *in vivo* teeth MRI to assess a recent technique – Sweep Imaging with Fourier Transform (SWIFT). Images acquired using a 9.4T and 4.0T systems and further compared with other techniques. Offers simultaneous 3D hard and soft tissues imaging of the teeth. High cost of SWIFT-based MRI systems. Low affordability of MRI systems and ultra-high fields not approved for patient clinical management. Cannot be used during speech articulation due to long acquisition times.
Kitamura et al., 2011 [10]	Measurement of the tooth shape separately from MRI data acquisition during speech production. Thermoplastic elastomer dental mouthpiece used to measure the 3D tooth shape. The proposed method requires two MRI acquisitions and the correction of the chemical shift artifact to reconstruct the volume data. Imposes less physical strains on subjects. Cannot be used during speech articulation.
Ng et al., 2011 [6]	A custom-made retainer filled with the jelly form of ferric ammonium citrate was used for superimposition of the incisor boundary into sequential images of MRI movie. Landmarks on the forehead, nasal root, nasal tip and points along the cranium were used for superimposition of the upper incisor. Direct visualization of incisors crowns. Detailed geometry relationships between tongue and tooth were observed during the production of some consonants. Not possible to obtain 3D models of teeth.

possible to use during speech, we pursued the use of materials with the following requirements:

- Biocompatibility in oral cavity, easy and effective to use;
- Biosafety in MRI environment;
- High intensity on conventional brain MR images, especially T1-weighted images using either spin echo or gradient-echo sequences;
- Possible to use during phonation without affect the speech articulation;
- Availability and affordability of the material.

For this purpose, with the collaboration of a medical dentist, four solutions were tested although without the expected results: 1) fluorine coating, (2) orthodontic adhesive, (3) plastic mouthpiece coating with whitening gel and (4) thin-layer (of 2 mm) molded silicone mouthpiece for the upper jaw.

Considering the good adhesion of the silicone mold to the teeth and because it is subject custom-made, we decided to improve this solution. Therefore, after some experiments, the new solution was to coat the molded silicone mouthpiece of the upper jaw with a thin-layer of petroleum jelly. This substance was chosen because it is a hydrophobic hydrocarbon, is insoluble in water, provides high intensity on T1-weighted images and is an effective oral contrast. The silicone mouthpiece developed can be seen in Figure 1.

Cod liver oil capsules were used as head surface landmarks in order to facilitate the localization of the molded silicone mouthpiece along the acquired volumetric MRI data for the subsequent image processing and analysis.

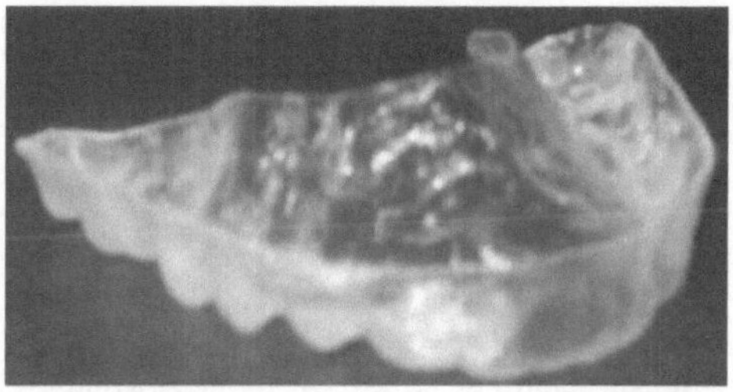

Figure 1. The molded silicone mouthpiece of the upper jaw coated with a thin-layer of petroleum jelly.

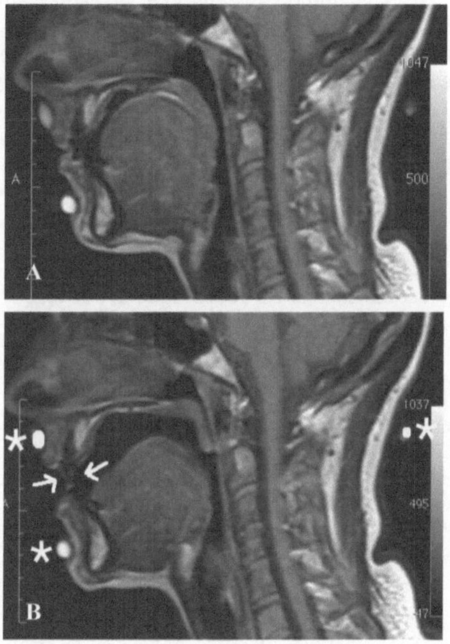

Figure 2. MR T1-weighted images depicting the teeth boundaries (indicated by *arrows*) and cod liver oil capsules used as head surface landmarks (indicated by *asterisks*), with mouth according to the rest position (A) and during the speech production (B).

2.2 *MR system and protocol imaging*

The MRI data was acquired using a clinical 3.0 Tesla MRI system at the Radiology Department of the Hospital S. João, Porto, Portugal. Experiments were performed with one female subject during some speech production tasks and according to the specific safety procedures.

The first images were acquired using a turbo spin echo 2D sequence, and consisted of one T1-weighted 4 mm thick midsagittal slice. Two tasks were performed during the image acquisition with the subject in a supine position: 1) with the mouth in rest position and then 2) demand to sustain the sound /a/. The remainder imaging acquisition parameters adopted were the following: a repetition time of 400 ms, an echo time of 10 ms, an echo train length of 5, a square field of view of 240 mm, a matrix size of 512 × 512 pixels, a

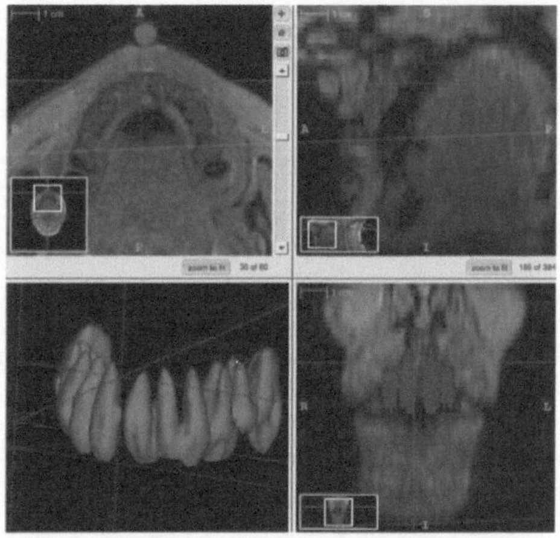

Figure 3. Image processing and 3D reconstruction of teeth from volumetric MRI data accomplished using the ITK-SNAP software.

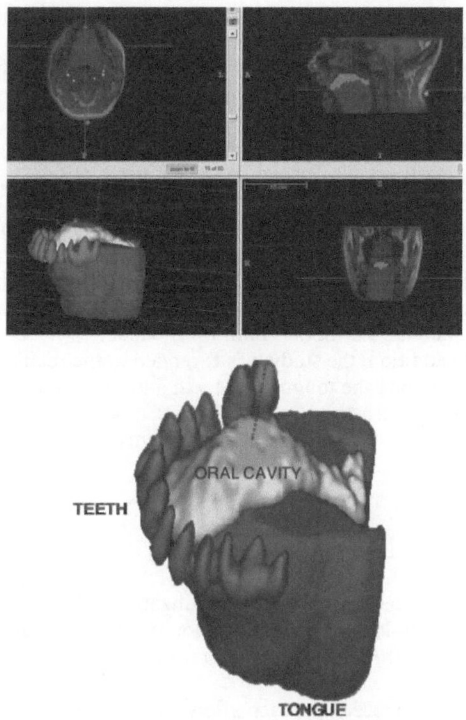

Figure 4. Image processing and 3D reconstruction of the teeth, tongue and oral cavity from volumetric MRI data accomplished using the ITK-SNAP software.

resolution of 2.133 pixels per mm and a pixel size of 0.469 × 0.469 mm. The acquisition time lasted around 8.07 seconds for each task.

Afterwards, a 3D volumetric MRI of the vocal tract resonance cavities was carried out using a flash gradient echo sequence during the speech task. A single 120 mm thick midsagittal slab was acquired according to the following parameters: repetition time of 5.8 ms, echo time of 2.17 ms, flip angle equal to 10°, a square field of view of 270 mm, a matrix size of 256 × 256 pixels, a resolution of 0.948 pixels per mm and a pixel size of 1.05 × 1.05 mm. The acquisition time lasted around 16.12 seconds.

2.3 *Image processing and analysis*

The image-based reconstruction of the 3D dental shapes was carried out using the ITK-SNAP software (version 2.1.4-rc1) developed by the Penn Image Computing and Science Laboratory (PICSL). The 3D models of the teeth were automatically built using *snakes* to segment each slice and posterior interpolation of the resultant contours.

3 RESULTS AND DISCUSSION

By means of this MRI-based, method the entire vocal tract was imaged resulting in two sagittal slices that permit to visualize the teeth boundaries. Figure 2 depicts the images acquired from the subject with the mouth in rest position, i.e. mouth and lips closed, and during the production of the sound /a/.

As can be observed in Figure 2, the teeth boundaries are clearly visible during the speech production.

From the 3D volumetric MRI data acquired, a total of 60 transversal images corresponding to slices with 2 mm of thickness was analysed. The image processing and reconstruction results are depicted in Figure 3. The display windows included show the segmented dental area and the 3D models built for the teeth.

In addition, the study was extended to the relationships among the tongue, the teeth and the oral cavity during speech production. The 3D models built for the tongue, the teeth and the oral cavity are shown in Figure 4.

4 CONCLUSIONS

Our approach allows the visualization of the dental morphology and the extraction of 3D information related with speech articulators, for speech research purposes.

The proposed approach allows the visualization of the teeth in both static and dynamic MRI acquisitions during speech production; in addition, it is feasible and affordable.

Through the present development, volumetric MRI can be successfully applied to obtain 3D models, and measurable data concerning the vocal tract resonance cavities and all the articulators involved, including for the first time the teeth. This knowledge is especially important for speech studies based on MRI.

As future work, more experiments in different subjects must be addressed in order to evaluate spatial and temporal relationships among articulators during speech.

The proposed approach may also be effective and easy to apply in other medical fields such as dentistry and orthodontics.

ACKNOWLEDGMENTS

The authors would like to express their gratitude to Dr Augusta Marques, from Arrábida Hospital, Vila Nova de Gaia, in Portugal, for her kind collaboration.

The images used in this work were acquired at the Radiology Department of Hospital S. João EPE, in Portugal. The authors would like to express their gratitude to the Hospital technical staff.

The first author would like to thank the support and contribution of the PhD grant from Escola Superior de Tecnologia da Saúde (ESTSP) and Instituto Politécnico do Porto (IPP), in Portugal.

This work was partially done in the scope of the project "Methodologies to Analyze Organs from Complex Medical Images – Applications to Female Pelvic Cavity", with reference PTDC/EEA-CRO/103320/2008, financially supported by Fundação para a Ciência e a Tecnologia, in Portugal.

REFERENCES

[1] Takemoto, T., Kitamura, T., Nishimoto, H., Honda, K., A method of tooth superimposition on MRI data for accurate measurement of vocal tract shape and dimensions, *Acoustical Sciences & Technology*, **25(6)**: 468–474, 2004.

[2] Kim, Y-C., Narayanan, S.S., Nayak, K.S., Accelerated Three-Dimensional Upper Airway MRI Using Compressed Sensing, *Magnetic Resonance in Medicine*, 61: 1434–1440, 2009.

[3] Stone, M., Davis, E.P. Douglas, A.S., NessAiver, M., Gullapalli, R., Levine, W.S., Lundberg, A., Modeling the motion of the internal tongue from tagged cine-MRI images, *Journal of the Acoustical Society of America* 109(6): 2974–2982, 2001.

[4] Shadle, C.H., Mohammad, M., Carter, J.N., Jackson, P.J.B., Multi-planar Dynamic Magnetic Resonance Imaging: New Tools for Speech Research. In *International Congress of Phonetics Sciences* (ICPhS99), San Francisco, 623–626, 1999.

[5] Ventura, S.R., Freitas, D.R., Tavares, J.M., Application of MRI and biomedical engineering in speech production study, *Computer Methods in Biomechanics and Biomedical Engineering*, 12(6): 671–681, 2009.

[6] Ng, I.W., Ono, T., Inoue-Arai, M.S., Honda, E., Kurabayashi, T., Moriyama, K., Application of MRI movie for observation of articulatory movement during fricative /s/ and a plosive /t/, *Angle Orthodontist*, 81(2): 237–244, 2011.

[7] Ventura, S.R., Freitas, D.R., Tavares, J.M., Toward Dynamic Magnetic Resonance Imaging of the Vocal Tract During Speech Production, *Journal of Voice*, 25(4): 511–518, 2011.

[8] Olt, S. & Jakob, P.M., Contrast-Enhanced Dental MRI for visualization of the Teeth and Jaw, *Magnetic Resonance in Medicine*, 52:174–176, 2004.

[9] Masaki, S., Nota, Y., Takano, S. Takemoto, H., Kitamura, T., Honda, K., Integrated magnetic resonance imaging methods for speech science and technology, *The Journal of the Acoustical Society of America,* 123(5): 5083–5088, 2008.

[10] Kitamura, T., Nishimoto, H., Fujimoto, I., Shimada, Y., Dental imaging using magnetic resonance visible mouthpiece for measurement of vocal tract shape and dimensions, *Acoustical Sciences & Technology*, 32(5): 224–227, 2011.

[11] Tutton, L.M. & Goddard, P.R., MRI of the teeth, *The British Journal of Radiology*, 75: 552–562, 2002.

[12] Idiyatullin, D., Corum, C., Moeller, S., Prasad, H.S., Garwood, M., Nixdorf, D.R., Dental magnetic resonance imaging: making the invisible visible, *Journal of Endodontics*, 37(6): 745–752, 2011.

Biodental Engineering II – Natal Jorge et al (Eds)
© 2014 Taylor & Francis Group, London, ISBN 978-1-138-00131-2

Backscattered electron imaging for the interface analysis of dental biomaterials

Sebastiana Arroyo Bote & Javier Martínez Osorio
Department of Odontostomatology, HUBc, University of Barcelona

Javier Martínez Arroyo
Nuclear Engineer

Patricia Carvalho Lobato & Mª Cristina Manzanares Céspedes
Human Anatomy and Embryology Unit, HUBc, University of Barcelona

ABSTRACT: Observation of samples using a Scanning Electron Microscope (SEM) is one of the most common investigation methods for the morphological study of the interphases created between dental materials and tooth structure. This technique allows us to obtain images with the Secondary Electron Image detector (SEI) and/or the backscattered electron image detector (BSE). Interpretation of these observations is often hard, leading to misinterpretations and false results. A methodology to obtain reliable observations is presented in this paper, clarifying the potential concerns raised when using SEI or BSE detectors, varying the polarities of the BSE detector.

1 INTRODUCTION

The best available method to study surfaces is the scanning electron microscope (SEM).

The main components of a scanning electron microscope are:

1. A fast-electron source (high-energy electrons)
2. A series of electromagnetic lenses responsible for reducing the diameter of the electron beam
3. A scanning system that allows the electron beam to traverse the surface of the sample
4. A series of detectors responsible for gathering information from the electromagnetic signals produced by the sample-electron interaction (secondary, backscattered and x-ray)
5. A vacuum pump system, which prevents interaction between the emitted electrons and gas molecules in order to facilitate beam directionality.

Images obtained by the SEM and observed through a monitor (cathode ray tube or digital) are obtained due to the interaction between the electron beam that traverses the sample surface.

When the electron beam interacts with the sample atoms a series of electromagnetic radiations are emitted. In order to obtain a greater conductivity of the sample, it has to be coated with a thin layer of a conductor material, generally gold or carbon (Mahajan A. et al. 2012).

Scanning electron microscopy techniques are fundamentally based in two different types of signals (J. I. Goldstein):

1. The electron beam emitted by the SEM (primary electrons emitted by the source. Due to the low energy of these secondary electrons and the intrinsic irregularities of the sample surface, the total amount of electrons detected is different depending on the orientation: for areas oriented towards the detector, the detected amount of electrons is high, while it is almost inexistent for holes or areas oriented in the opposite direction. Images produced using this method provides a similar output to that perceived by the human eye: three-dimensional.
2. The electron beam emitted by the source is backscattered after suffering an elastic interaction with the sample's atoms, without producing any ionization. Primary electrons are backscattered with the same energy as the source electrons (millions of Volts). These fast electrons are detected using a specific electron detector, BSE. The backscattering cross section (probability of an electron to suffer an elastic interaction with a given atom) increases proportionally to the average atomic number in the sample. If a sample has different chemical components, and therefore atoms with different atomic number and electronic density, the fraction of backscattered electrons will be inhomogeneous. Areas with greater atomic density, higher atomic number, will show a greater density of backscattered electrons. Thus a backscattered electron image provides information on chemical composition of the different phases present in the studied surface.

Accordingly, two different images are obtained when observing the same sample (one provides topographic contrast and the other chemical contrast) helping us to interpret and clarify potential doubts

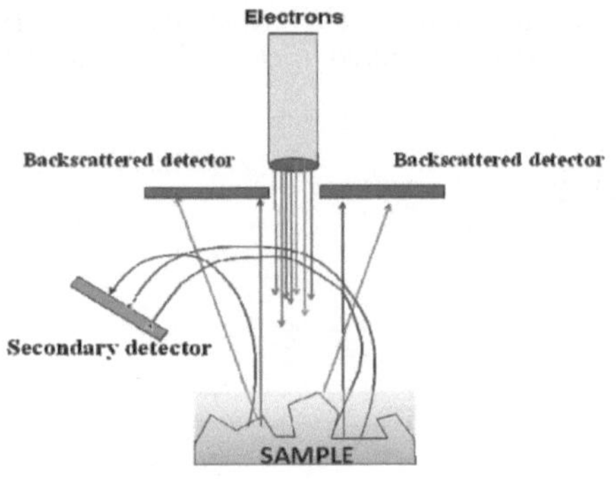

Figure 1. Schema of a scanning electron microscope.

or concerns regarding the dental materials and its interaction with the tooth structure.

If the SEM features an adequate microanalysis sensor an analysis of the sample's atomic composition can be performed (Kotula P.G. et al. 2012).

2 MATERIALS AND METHODS

A Cambridge S-360 scanning electron microscope SEM has been used for this study, observing samples included in resin, polished and coated with a sub-nanometric gold layer to improve the electrical conductivity of the surfaces.

Samples have been prepared using extracted human molars, on which we have conducted Black I type cavities, which have been sealed with different sealing materials:

SAMPLE 1: Xeno V, SDR™, Ceram X Duo™ (Dentsply)

SAMPLE 2: Clearfil S Bond plus, Majesty F y P (Clearfil)

SAMPLE 3: Futurabond M, X-trabase, Grandioso (VOCO)

Once the cavities have been sealed according to the manufacturer's instructions for each product, polishing of the restorations was performed using diamond burs and fine grain silicone cups. Then we performed a longitudinal occlusal-to-apical slitting and a longitudinal medial-to-distal slitting in the center of the seals, in all samples, obtaining two halves of each sample, which were then included in epoxy resin by exposing to the outside of the interface zone. Finally samples were polished using mirror polishing.

Samples were attached to the microscope sample holder, and after coating them with gold, were observed using the SEM under the following conditions.

Images of the samples were both obtained with the secondary electron detector and, without moving the sample, with the backscattered electron detector. Once the first images are obtained, the conditions of the backscattered electron detector are modified: the detector is divided into four sectors, each one being activable or polarizable.

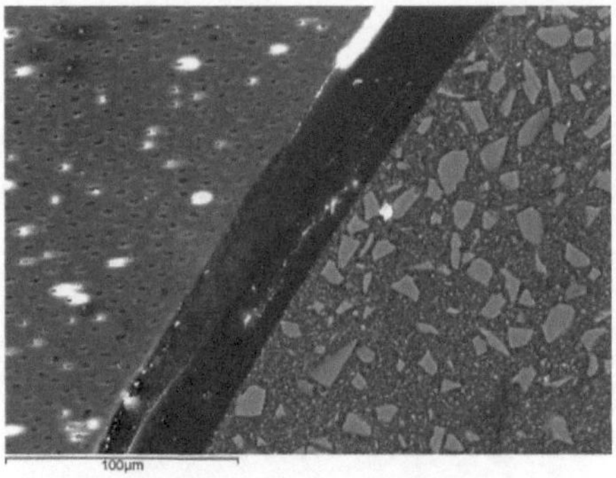

Figure 2. INTERFASE X500 secondary electrons.

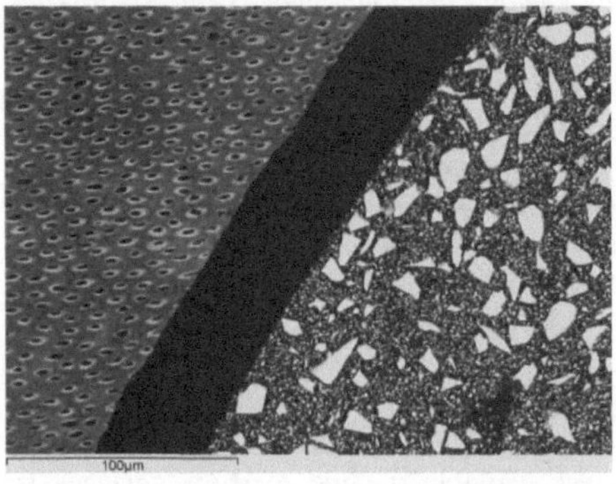

Figure 3. INTERFASE X500 backscattered electrons, 4 sectores.

When the four sectors of the backscattered electron detector are polarized a pure chemical image is obtained. On some occasions, when two consecutive sectors are inversely polarized, a chemical-topographic contrast image is obtained.

3 RESULTS

SAMPLE 1: Cavity type I performed in inferior molars sealed with Xeno V, SDR™ y Ceram X Duo™ (Dentsply).

In Figure 2 a microphotography of the interphase created between the dentin, Xeno V and SDR can be appreciated. On the top side of the image a white line can be observed, probably due to the electrostatic charge of the sample or a fracture between the adhesive material and the dentin. Another non-interpreted line is also present in the adhesive material. On the dentin, some small white particles can be observed, what could probably be interpreted as artifacts ejected during the sample polishing. Nevertheless, the fact that these particles are only present in the dentin suggests that these might be residual particles of the sealing material inside the dentinal tubules.

When the sample is observed under the backscattered electron detector (Figure 3), which provides us with a grey-scale image that provides the chemical composition of the materials, we appreciate that the

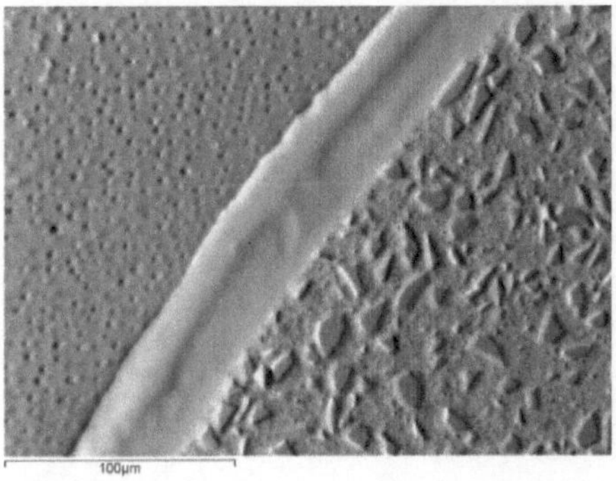

Figure 4. INTERFASE X500 backscattered electrons, 2 sectores.

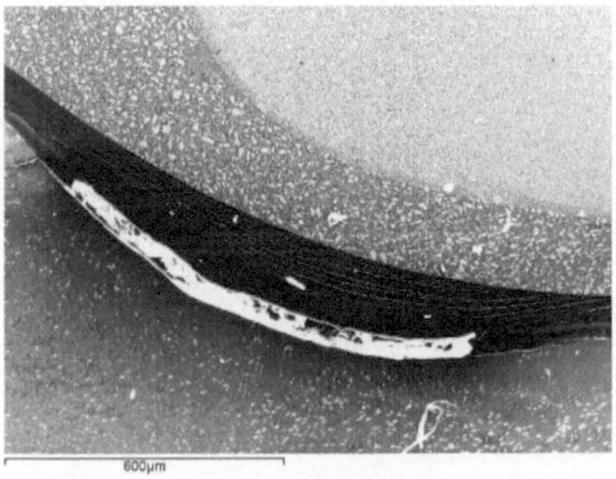

Figure 5. INTERFASE X100 secondary electrons.

white line previously observed on the top of the image has disappeared, as well as the white line observed in the adhesive, which suggests that the interphase fracture previously envisioned does not exist, concluding that these lines to the superelevation of the interphase electrostatically charged.

The white particles that were dispersed throughout the dentin have also disappeared, indicating that there was no contamination or leftovers of other materials on the dentin, so the hypothesis of polishing artifacts is discarded.

When the backscattered electron detector sectors are manipulated in such a way that the upper right and bottom right sectors are turned off a three-dimension image is obtained (Figure 4), helping us to confirm the assumptions made. This new two-right-sector image allows us to guarantee that there is no fracture between the dentin-adhesive interphase, or inside the adhesive. In addition, Figure 4 provides a detailed image of the dentin and its dentinal tubules filled with adhesive, with a thickness of 120 microns from the interphase, making clear the presence of residual inorganic particles of the cavity-lining material SDR protruding from the inorganic resin mass.

Figure 5 allows the observation of an area that corresponds to the cavity angle formed between the cavity floor and one of the lateral walls. The image is obtained using the secondary electron detector, observing, again, a white line between the interphase

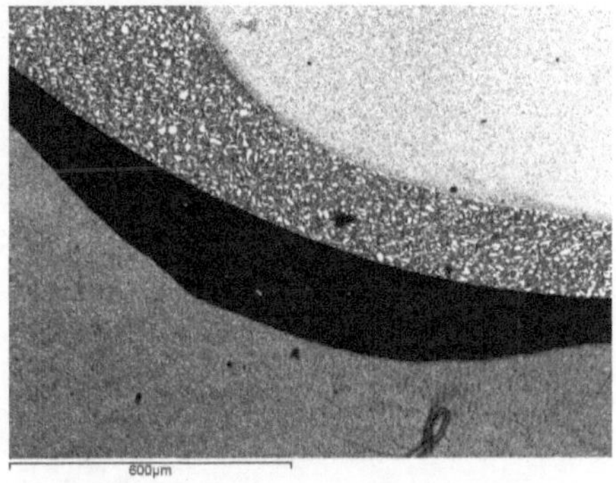

Figure 6. INTERFASE X100 backscattered electrons, 4 sectors.

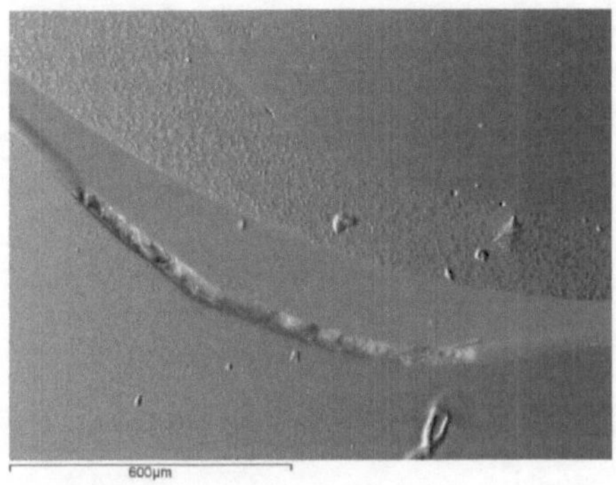

Figure 7. INTERFASE X100 backscattered electrons, 2 sectors.

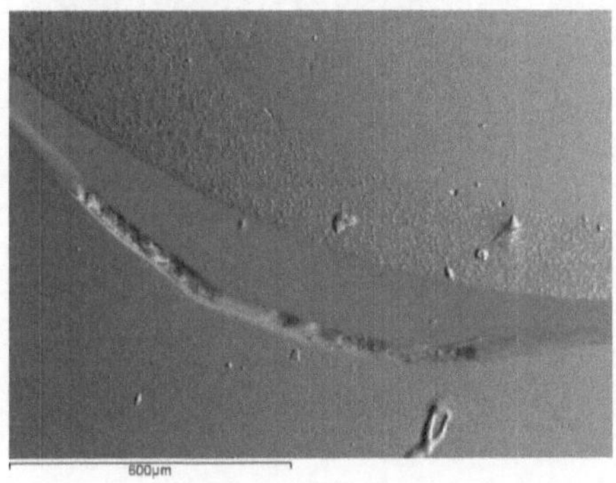

Figure 8. INTERFASE X100 backscattered electrons, 2 sectors.

created between adhesive and dentin, and the presence of small white particles in the bottom-right side of the image and inside the cavity-lining material. When the same sample image is taken with the backscattered electron detector (Figure 6) these characteristics are maintained, observing a change of color tone in the adhesive layer of the cavity angle region, which leads us towards the hypothesis of a real fracture between the adhesive material and the dentin. This hypothesis is confirmed while switching the sectors' configuration of the backscattered electron detector (Figures 7

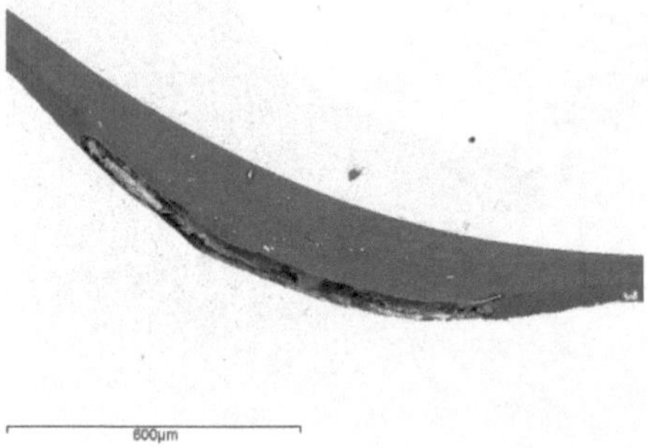

Figure 9. INTERFASE X100 backscattered electrons (4 sectors inverted).

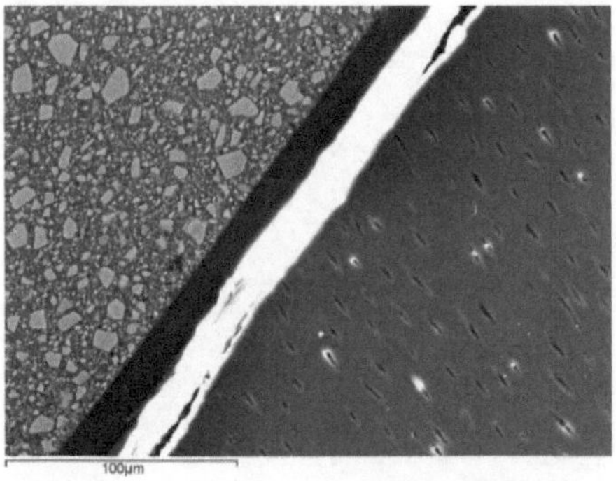

Figure 10. INTERFASE X500 secondary electrons.

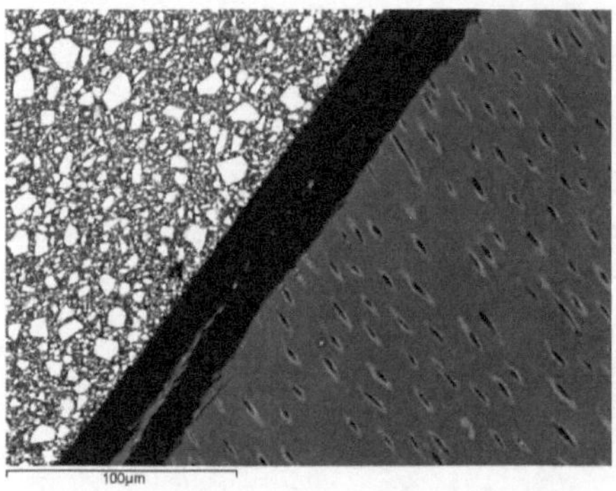

Figure 11. INTERFASE X500 backscattered electrons (4 sectors).

and 8) both in terms of activation and polarization, obtaining a grey-scale image that perfectly shows the fracture in the adhesive interphase.

SAMPLE 2. Cavity type I performed in inferior molars sealed with Clearfil S Bond plus, Majestic flow and Majestic posterior (Clearfil).

The interphase created between the dentin and the adhesive material is also studied in sample 2. In the secondary electron image (Figure 10) a 15-micron black fringe corresponding to the adhesive material is observed and a similar white fringe is also present,

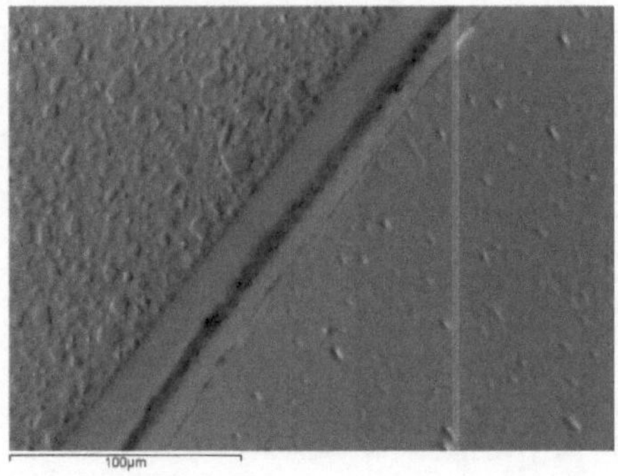

Figure 12. INTERFASE X500 backscattered electrons (2 sectors).

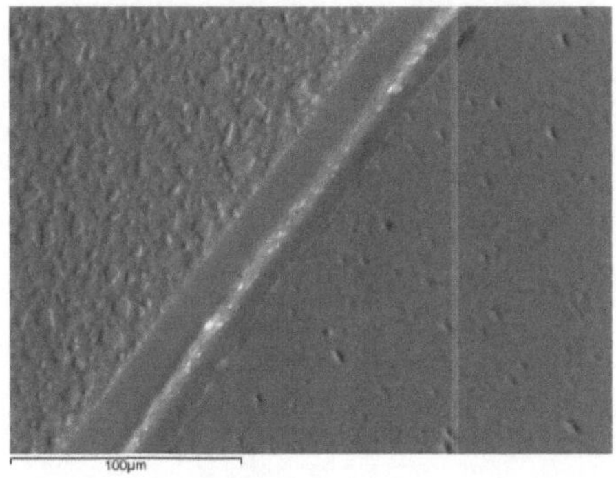

Figure 13. INTERFASE X500 backscattered electrons (2 sectors).

which may correspond to a fracture in the dentin-adhesive interphase, which would imply the failure of the adhesive technique due to the interpretation of an adhesive fracture between the adhesive system and the dental tissue. Nevertheless, when observing the backscattered electron image of the sample (Figure 11) it is clear that there is no such fracture because the line of junction between the adhesive and dentin is created by a high density material, observing only a small fracture in the thickness of the adhesive layer, which is totally clear when new images are obtained with the backscattered electron detector varying the sectors' configuration (Figure 12 and 13), allowing us to sustain that the sample presents a cohesive fracture in the adhesive layer, but that it clearly remains attached to the dentin obtaining a perfect seal.

SAMPLE 3. Cavity type I performed on inferior molars sealed with Futurabond M, X-tra base y Grandioso (VOCO).

The interphase created between the enamel and the dental materials is studied in sample 3. The secondary electron image (Figure 14) allows us to appreciate a white line, of approximately one third of the adhesive layer's thickness, that could be interpreted as a fracture in the junction, two brightness areas can also be observed on the upper-right side of the image. When observing the same sample under the backscattered electron detector (Figure 15) the hypothesis of

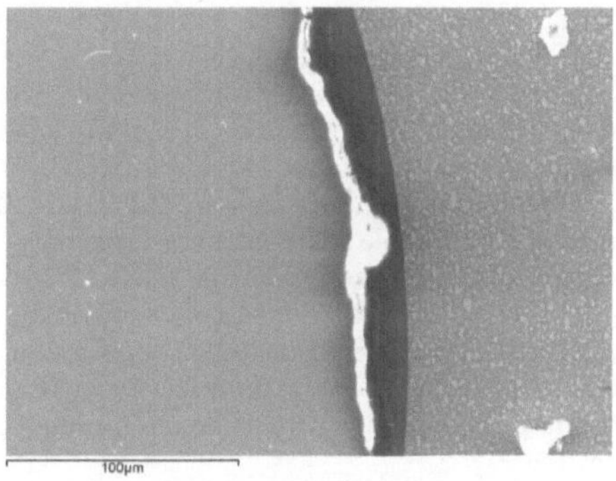

Figure 14. INTERFASE X500 secondary electrons.

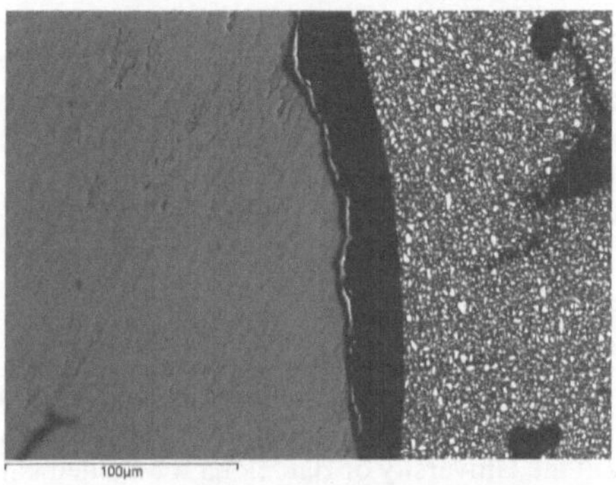

Figure 15. INTERFASE X500 backscattered electrons (4 sectores).

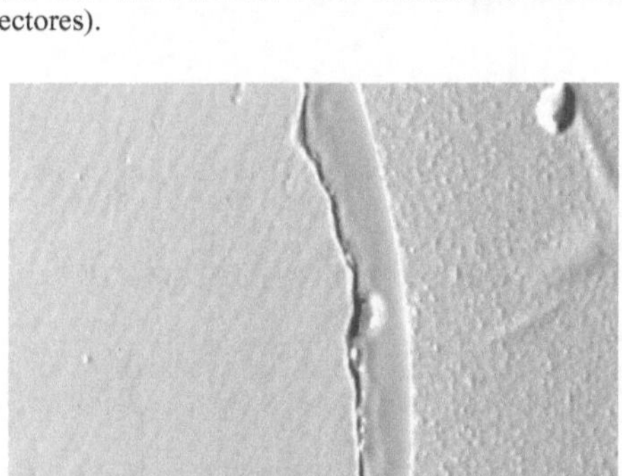

Figure 16. INTERFASE X500 backscattered electrons (2 sectors).

a detachment between the adhesive material and the enamel is confirmed, but with a much lesser thickness than the secondary electron image could suggest. If the secondary electron image is studied in detail (Figure 14), a brighter zone can be appreciated within the white line observed in the enamel-adhesive interphase, corresponding to the pore in the adhesive, a pore that can be clearly identified in Figure 16. Additionally, it is also possible to confirm that the brighter areas observed in the upper-right side of the image correspond to artifacts or contamination of the sample (Figures 16 and 17).

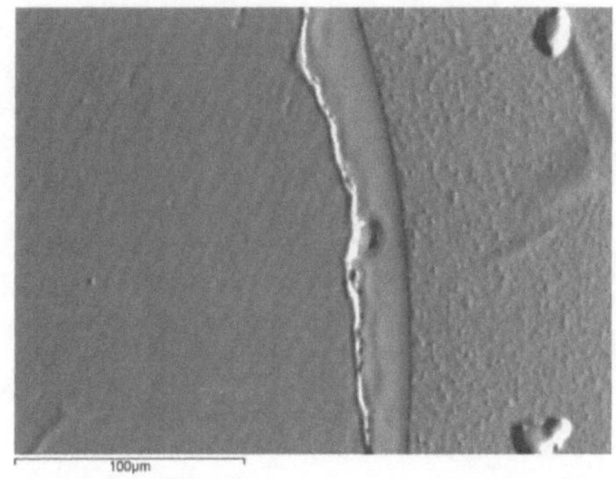

Figure 17. INTERFASE X500 backscattered electrons (2 sectors).

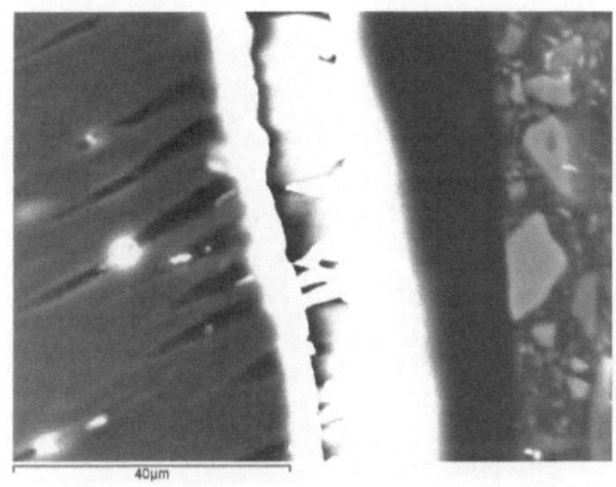

Figure 18. INTERFASE X1500 secondary electrons.

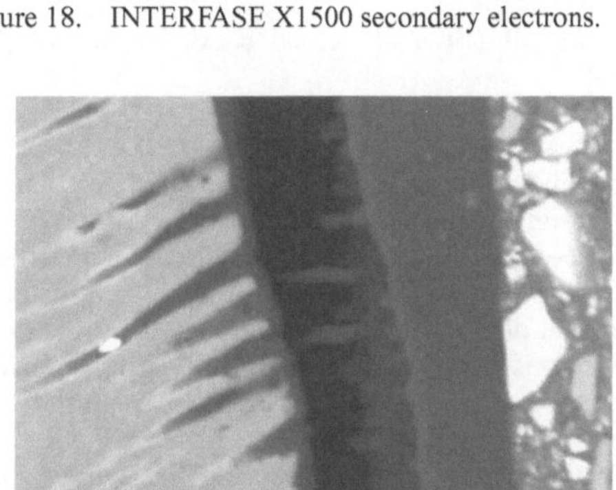

Figure 19. INTERFASE X1500 backscattered electrons (4 sectors).

Figures 18, 19, 20 and 21 provide a detail of the interphase created between the dentin, adhesive and composite at x1500 increases. Figure 18, obtained using the secondary electrons detector, provides an image of the junction between the composite and the adhesive, attached without solution of continuity, allowing the observation of a brighter white are between the adhesive and dentin with an irregular dark line in the middle of the brighter zone suggesting the lack of attachment between both materials, of approximately 38 microns. The observation of the

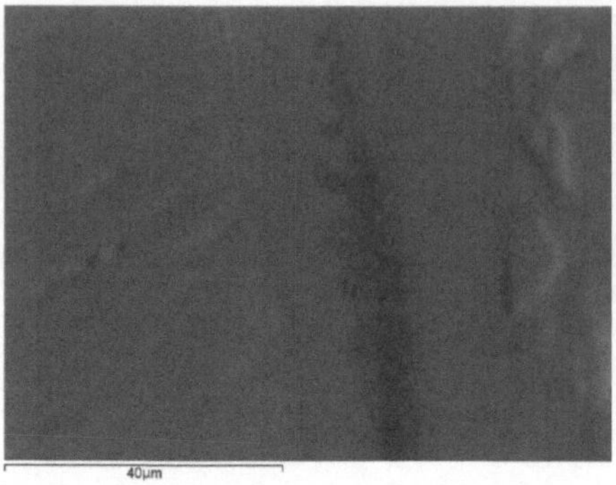

Figure 20. INTERFASE X1500 backscattered electrons (2 sectors).

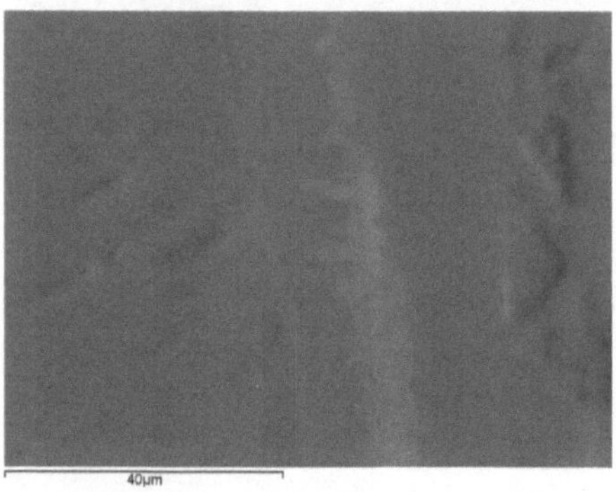

Figure 21. INTERFASE X1500 backscattered electrons (2 sectors).

sample under the backscattered electron detector clarifies the image and allows a better observation of the adhesive-dentin fracture, of about 18 microns, and the observation of the presence of adhesive material within the dentinal tubules creating a layer of about 3–4 microns that coats the dentin. In addition, inside the crevice some artifacts of adhesive material that have left the dental tubules can be observed. All these observations allow us to assess that the cause of the fracture has been the lack of adhesive and cohesive junction between materials.

4 DISCUSSION

The use of SEM is a useful and reliable technique to study material surfaces (Silva Soares, 2012), as well as for interphases created between dental materials (Son Y-H., et al. 2012, Yousry, M.M. et al. 2011) and coating dental materials (Beyeret M. et al. 2012).

Images obtained with the SEI have some electrostatic charges areas (white areas) that could lead us to misinterpretations, an effect specially observed in Figures 10 and 18 where a significant gap could be interpreted on the adhesive layer. The observation of samples under the BSE provides greater details of the interphase areas, helping us to objectivize the quantity and quality of the interphase.

Polishing of the samples helps its cleaning, even if new techniques that allow the study of samples without polishing are being developed (McKenzie M.B., et al. 2012), nevertheless some artifacts are still present as a consequence of sample manipulation, especially relevant in Figure 14, where 3 artifacts are observed, and, after observation of the sample with BSE, we can conclude that these are material deposits on the composite layer and a pore on the adhesive layer (Figure 16), impossible to identify using a traditional SEI (Figure 14).

5 CONCLUSION

Morphological study of interphases created between dental materials and tooth structure requires the observation of samples using a SEI and a BSE, obtaining a substantial added-value to the observations when the polarity of the BSE sectors is modified.

ACKNOWLEDGMENTS

The authors thank posthumously Dr. Ramón Fontarnau i Griera, director of the scanning electron microscopy unity at the University of Barcelona for his dedication and teaching in the use and application of SEM as a research method.

REFERENCES

Beyeret M, et al. "Morphology and structure of polymer layers protecting dental enamel against erosion" dental materials, 28: 1089–1097, 2012

Goldstein JI. Scaning Electron Microscopy and X-Ray Microanalysis

Kotula PG, Klenov DO & Von Harrach HS 2012. Challenges to Quantitative Multivariate Statistical Analysis of Atomic-Resolution X-Ray Spectral. Microscopy and Microanalysis, 18, pp. 691–698

Mahajan A, Iftekharul Haque R, Vilarinho PM & Kingon A. 2012. Microscopy Studies of Carbon Nanotubes/ Ferroelectric Composites for Microelectronics. Microscopy and Microanalysis, 18 (Suppl. 5) , pp. 107–108

McKenzie MB, et al. "Application of Electron Backscatter Diffraction for Crystallographic Characterization of Tin Whiskers". Microscopy and Microanalysis, 18: 876–884, 2012

Silva Soares LE, Ribeiro Cortez L, de Oliveira Zarur R & Abrahão Martin A. 2012 "Scanning Electron Microscopy and Roughness Study of Dental Composite Degradation." Microscopy and Microanalysis, 18: 289–294

Yong-Ha Son, et al. "Influence of internal-gapwidth and cement type on the retentive force of zirconia copings in pullout testing" Journal of dentistry 40: 866–872, 2012

Yousry, MM, et al. "Microshear bond strength and interfacial morphology of etch-and-rinse and self-etch adhesive systems to superficial and deep dentin". Quintessence International 42: 96–106, 2011.

Biodental Engineering II – Natal Jorge et al (Eds)
© 2014 Taylor & Francis Group, London, ISBN 978-1-138-00131-2

Finite element analysis applied to a dental implant-supported structure

U. Garitaonaindia
Department of Mechanical Engineering, Escuela Politécnica de San Sebastián, University of the Basque Country, Spain

J.L. Alcaraz
Department of Mechanical Engineering, E.T.S. de Ingeniería de Bilbao, University of the Basque Country, Spain

ABSTRACT: In this paper a dental implant-supported structure has been analyzed by means of a finite element method. A 3-D geometry with tetrahedral finite elements has been used. The structure material is titanium and is assumed as homogeneous and isotropic. Different acting forces are considered as mastication forces. Boundary conditions are imposed on the implant regions in order to prevent their displacement. According to the obtained results higher stresses and displacements are found in the longest cantilever part of the structure. The reaction forces produced in the implant zones as a function of the application point of the mastication force are also illustrated. As a main conclusion the performed analysis of the selected implant-supported structure shows a satisfactory behaviour under the applied mastication forces. Besides, the most sensitive part of the structure is found at the junction between the longest cantilever part and the corresponding insert location.

1 INTRODUCTION

At present manufacturing fixed dental prostheses especially designed for every patient has become possible through CAD/CAM technology. The aim of this research is to analyse a given implant structure subjected to a mastication load and to evaluate whether the resulting stresses and strains are within admissible limits.

The reaction forces acting at the implant insert location will also be analyzed as a function of the application point of the mastication force. Besides, the most relevant structure features are considered to gain insight of the mechanical behaviour applicable to other designs.

2 MATERIAL AND METHODS

The implant structure shown in Figure 1 and designed by CREATECH MEDICAL, S.L. Company has been analyzed by a 3D finite element model. The structure is supported on 4 implants and Tet-10 elements are used in the modelling, similarly to the models employed in other works (Kimura et al. 2006), (Nagasao et al. 2002), (Correa et al. 2012). The material structure under homogeneous, isotropic conditions is titanium (Young's modulus, E = 110 GPa; Poisson's ratio, $\nu = 0.35$; 0.2% yield point, $\sigma_Y = 830$ MPa; ultimate limit, $\sigma_U = 950$ MPa; maximum elongation, $\varepsilon_{max}(\%) = 15\%$) (Bonnet et al. 2009).

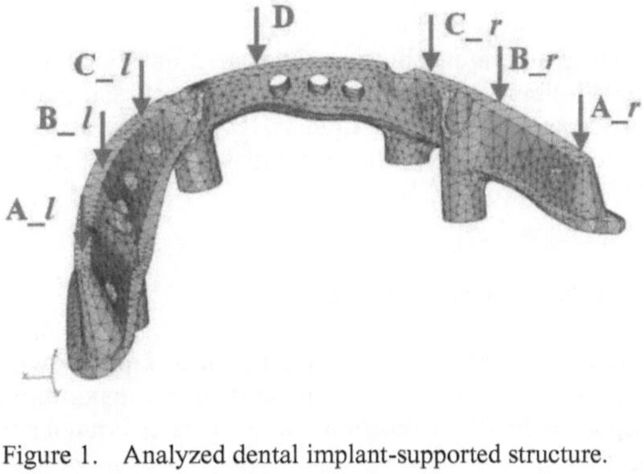

Figure 1. Analyzed dental implant-supported structure.

The mastication forces used in the literature are between 50 and 150 N. In this work the applied loads will be 75 N in the cantilever parts as loading cases A_*l* and A_*r*, for left and right application, respectively (Kayabaşı et al. 2006). Besides, load values of 100 N, 55 N and 40 N will be applied in molar, canine and incisor zones, plotted as loading cases B_*l* and B_*r*, C_*l* and C_*r*, and D, respectively (Daas et al. 2008). Finally, a case with a total force of 400 N is simulated, corresponding to the 80% of the sum of the previously described loads (Manda et al. 2010), (Uysal et al. 2005).

As for the boundary conditions, fixed displacements are imposed to nodes in contact with implants. Boundary conditions are labeled as BC_1 to BC_4, as shown in Figure 2.

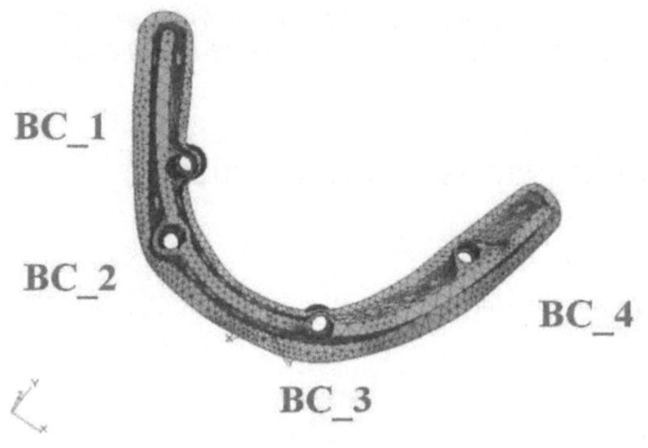

Figure 2. Boundary Conditions defined in the model.

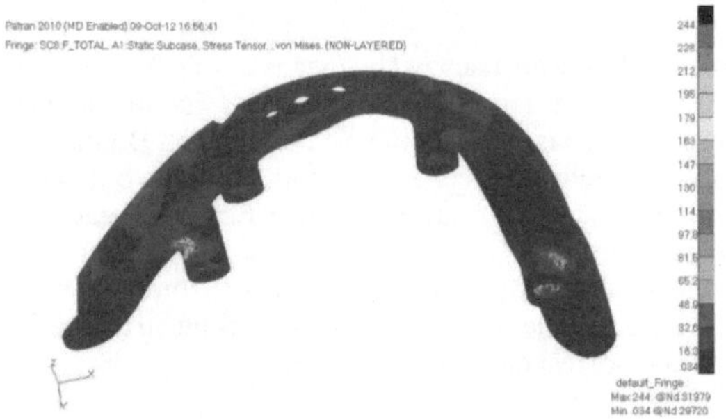

Figure 3. Von Mises stresses for the total loading case of 400 N.

The resultant meshing provides a 32,680-node and 19,047-element model. Pre- and post-processing are carried out with MSC.Patran 2010 for MD Nastran, while the analysis is performed with MSC.MD Nastran 2008 software.

3 RESULTS AND DISCUSSION

The obtained results from the simulations are shown as maximum von Mises equivalent stress, maximum displacements and reaction force in each boundary condition.

Figure 3 shows the von Mises stress contours for the total loading case of 400 N. The highest values are obtained in the junction area between the implant insertion posts and the cantilever part of the structure. The maximum stress attained is 244 MPa for the joint between the most distal implant and the right cantilever.

The displacements for the case of applying a force of 75 N on the right cantilever are plotted in Figure 4. As can be noticed the highest value obtained is 0.023 mm and there are almost no displacements in the left zone of the structure.

Table 1 shows the maximum von Mises equivalent stresses (MPa) and maximum displacements (mm) in all of the eight loading cases.

The highest von Mises stress attained is 244 MPa for the case of a total loading of 400 N. This value lies

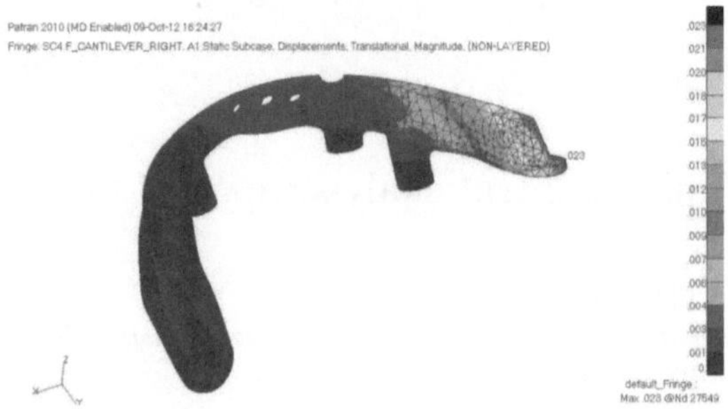

Figure 4. Displacements for the load of 75 N acting on the right cantilever.

Table 1. Maximum von Mises equivalent stress (MPa) and maximum displacement (mm).

	Force	σ_{VM} (MPa)	Displ. (mm)
A_*l*	75 N	102	0.011
B_*l*	100 N	143	0.011
C_*l*	55 N	73.4	0.005
D	40 N	41.2	0.003
C_*r*	55 N	63.9	0.002
B_*r*	100 N	125	0.011
A_*r*	75 N	166	0.023
Total	400 N	244	0.026

below the titanium yield point. On the other hand, the maximum displacement of 0.026 mm is also achieved for this loading case.

The stresses and displacements nearer the maximum are attained in the cantilever longest part, which is the right cantilever, with values of 166 MPa and 0.023 mm, respectively. This proves that the cantilever parts are the most sensitive ones in this kind of structures, as also concluded in other works (Holst et al. 2008).

This cantilever effect could be lessened if the implant insertion at more distal zones were performed with some inclination angle to the mesial direction so that the cantilever part length could be reduced (Takahashi et al. 2010).

As to the reaction forces produced at the inserts, the different force components have been considered: axial (X), buccal-lingual (Y) and mesial-distal (Z) directions. For this purpose, a local coordinate system (Bonnet et al. 2009) is applied for each boundary condition, as shown in Figure 5.

In general the values obtained for the three components in the eight analyzed loading cases are in the same range as those reported in other works (Kayabaşı et al. 2006).

For the A_*r* and A_*l* cases with forces applied on the cantilever parts, a higher reaction force is obtained in the nearest insertion post. Moreover the most relevant force component is the axial one. On the other hand, for both A_*r* and A_*l* cases a tension force results in the insertion post following the nearest one, as noticed in the values included in Table 2.

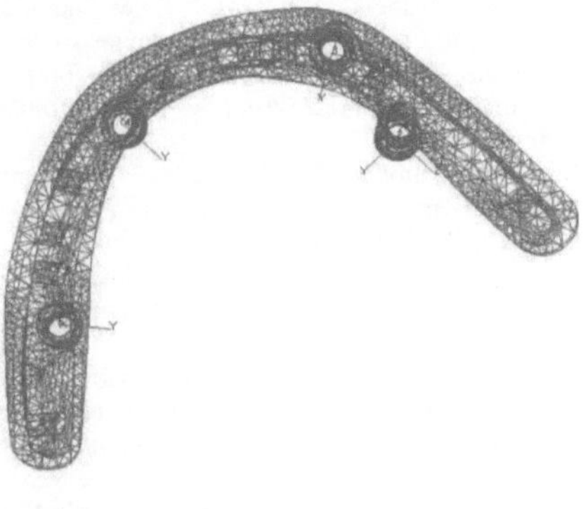

Figure 5. Local coordinate systems for each BC.

Table 2. Reaction force components in each implant insert for loads applied on cantilever parts.

Force	Dir	BC_1	BC_2	BC_3	BC_4
A_*l*	X	0.15	−0.07	−18.90	95.37
75 N	Y	0.27	−0.53	−13.50	2.36
	Z	0.05	0.66	17.51	−27.26
A_*r*	X	125.76	−47.98	−6.98	1.33
75 N	Y	8.83	−11.26	−12.98	1.29
	Z	51.08	−16.80	−4.76	−1.01

Table 3. Reaction force components in each implant insert for loads applied on molars.

Force	Dir	BC_1	BC_2	BC_3	BC_4
B_*l*	X	1.73	−5.32	27.01	75.59
100 N	Y	1.06	−7.61	13.89	1.72
	Z	−0.22	5.19	−11.80	1.03
B_*r*	X	90.56	9.36	−5.44	0.61
100 N	Y	4.61	16.58	−12.44	1.03
	Z	20.69	10.12	−5.94	−1.72

According to Table 2, the resultant force increases with the cantilever length. Values for the three reaction force components in BC_1 on applying 75 N on the right cantilever are higher than those in BC_4 on applying the same force on the left cantilever.

Implant location can vary according to the physiological features of each patient and consequently the application point of the mastication force in relation to the implant inserts. In the case analyzed in this paper, the mastication force of 100 N produced in the left molar zone is applied between two implant inserts while in the right zone is acting directly on the cantilever. Table 3 shows the results for the reaction force components with B_*l* and B_*r* loads applied on molars (left and right, respectively).

From Table 3 it can be seen that when the molar force of 100 N is applied between implants (B_*l* case), this load is absorbed by BC_4 at about 75% and by BC_3 at 27%. On the contrary, when the molar force is applied on the cantilever zone (B_*r* case) about 90% of the mastication force is supported by BC_1 implant while BC_2 implant only absorbs around 9% of the total force.

In relation to the loading cases on canine zones, the reaction forces are located between the implants BC_1 and BC_2, and between BC_3 and BC_4, for right and left application of the loads, respectively. Table 4 shows such reaction forces.

The axial component is distributed on the nearer implants in proportion to the distance from the application point of the load. On the other hand, the bucco-lingual and mesial-distal components assume more significant values than in previous cases. This can be assigned to the inclination angle of the implants.

Finally Table 5 shows the results for the reaction force components in the case of applying a load of 40 N on the incisor zone. It is also included in Table 5

Table 4. Reaction force components in each implant insert for loads applied on canines.

Force	Dir	BC_1	BC_2	BC_3	BC_4
C_*l*	X	0.27	−3.45	44.08	13.55
55 N	Y	0.47	−6.66	13.25	0.85
	Z	0.25	6.36	−13.98	5.62
C_*r*	X	20.21	32.84	−1.08	−0.13
55 N	Y	1.37	17.11	−3.85	0.22
	Z	−1.12	12.78	−2.49	−0.90

Table 5. Reaction force components in each implant insert for loads applied on incisor zones and on the whole structure.

Force	Dir	BC_1	BC_2	BC_3	BC_4
D	X	−6.81	17.66	28.34	−3.76
40 N	Y	−2.67	12.82	12.56	−1.29
	Z	1.09	−9.19	10.91	−2.20
Total	X	185.49	2.44	53.63	146.05
400 N	Y	11.16	16.35	−2.46	4.94
	Z	57.44	7.29	−8.44	−21.14

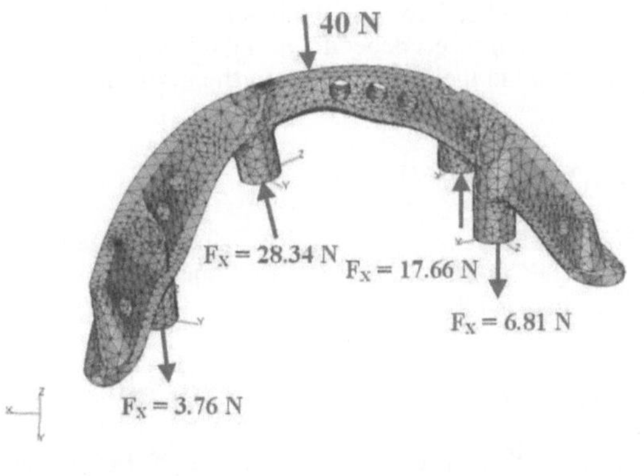

Figure 6. Axial components of the reaction force for the incisor load.

the case of a total force of 400 N applied on the whole structure.

For the incisor load it is noticed that axial components are positive at the implant inserts nearer the application point of the load (BC_2 and BC_3) and negative at the farther ones (BC_1 and BC_4), as illustrated in Figure 6.

For the case of a total load of 400 N, the axial component of the reaction force is positive at all of the implants, as shown in Table 5. The maximum values of the reaction force components are likewise higher than those obtained for the case of a load of 75 N on the cantilever parts.

4 CONCLUSIONS

The analysis performed for the given dental implant-supported structure allows us to conclude that the geometry as well as the employed material are adequate under the assumed mastication loads.

The most relevant conditions are obtained for the case of applying a load to the whole structure and for the case of a load applied on the longest cantilever zone. In all cases higher stresses as well as displacements result in this longest cantilever zone.

It is also verified how the reaction force varies at each implant insert depending on the load application point and the inclination angle of the insert post.

ACKNOWLEDGMENTS

The authors are gratefully acknowledged to CREATECH MEDICAL, S.L. for their valuable assistance in providing the geometry.

REFERENCES

Bonnet, A. S., Postaire, M., & Lipinski, P. 2009. Biomechanical study of mandible bone supporting a four-implant retained bridge: Finite element analysis of the influence of bone anisotropy and foodstuff position. *Medical Engineering & Physics*, *31*(7), 806–815.

Correa, S., Ivancik, J., Isaza, J. F., & Naranjo, M. 2012. Evaluation of the structural behavior of three and four implant-supported fixed prosthetic restorations by finite element analysis. *Journal of Prosthodontic Research*, *56*(2), 110–119.

Daas, M., Dubois, G., Bonnet, A. S., Lipinski, P., & Rignon-Bret, C. 2008. A complete finite element model of a mandibular implant-retained overdenture with two implants: Comparison between rigid and resilient attachment configurations. *Medical Engineering & Physics*, *30*(2), 218–225.

Holst, S., Geiselhoeringer, H., Wichmann, M., & Holst, A. I. 2008. The effect of provisional restoration type on micromovement of implants. *The Journal of Prosthetic Dentistry*, *100*(3), 173–182.

Kayabaşı, O., Yüzbasıoğlu, E., & Erzincanlı, F. 2006. Static, dynamic and fatigue behaviors of dental implant using finite element method. *Advances in Engineering Software*, *37*(10), 649–658.

Kimura, A., Nagasao, T., Kaneko, T., Tamaki, T., Miyamoto, J., & Nakajima, T. 2006. Adaquate fixation of plates for stability during mandibular reconstruction. *Journal of Cranio-Maxillofacial Surgery*, *34*(4), 193–200.

Manda, M., Galanis, C., Georgiopoulos, V., Provatidis, C., & Koidis, P. 2010. Effect of varying the vertical dimension of connectors of cantilever cross-arch fixed dental prostheses in patients with severely reduced osseous support: A three-dimensional finite element analysis. *The Journal of Prosthetic Dentistry*, *103*(2), 91–100.

Nagasao, T., Kobayashi, M., Tsuchiya, Y., Kaneko, T., & Nakajima, T. 2002. Finite element analysis of the stresses around endosseous implants in various reconstructed mandibular models. *Journal of Cranio-Maxillofacial Surgery*, *30*(3), 170–177.

Sertgoz, A. & Guvener, S. 1996. Finite element analysis of the effect of cantilever and implant length on stress distribution in an implant-supported fixed prosthesis. *The Journal of Prosthetic Dentistry*, *76*(2), 165–169.

Takahashi, T., Shimamura, I. & Sakurai, K. 2010. Influence of number and inclination angle of implants on stress distribution in mandibular cortical bone with All-on-4 Concept, *Journal of Prosthodontic Research*, *54*, 179–184.

Uysal, H., Kurtoglu, C., Gurbuz, R., & Tutuncu, N. 2005. Structure and mechanical properties of cresco-ti laser-welded joints and stress analyses using finite element models of fixed distal extension and fixed partial prosthetic designs. *The Journal of Prosthetic Dentistry*, *93*(3), 235–244.

Biodental Engineering II – Natal Jorge et al (Eds)
© 2014 Taylor & Francis Group, London, ISBN 978-1-138-00131-2

Design of orthodontic mini-implants contributing to implantation torque

V. Katić
Private Dental Practice, Zagreb, Croatia

S. Špalj
Dental Study at Medicine Faculty, Rijeka, Croatia

M. Opalić & Z. Domitran
Faculty of Mechanical Engineering and Naval Architecture, Zagreb, Croatia

ABSTRACT: Aim was to determine contribution of design characteristics of orthodontic mini-implants on Maximum Insertion Torque (MIT), vertical force at MIT and maximum vertical force during implantation, with cortical bone thickness as covariate. Ten specimens of six types of cylindrical self-drilling orthodontic mini-implants (Dual Top) with diameters from 1.4 to 2.0 mm and length of 6 and 8 mm were measured using optical stereomicroscope, and then manually inserted into the swine ribs. Cortical bone thickness was measured with a digital sliding caliper. The MIT and vertical forces were recorded, and interpreted with ANOVA and F Value. Cortical bone thickness ($p < 0.0001$), length of implant ($p = 0.0065$) and lead angle of thread ($p = 0.0003$) have significant influence on the MIT, R-Squared = 0.5520, F Value = 1.41. Maximum vertical force during implantation depends on length of screw ($p = 0.0493$), and lead angle of thread ($p < 0.0001$), with R-Squared = 0.5962 and F Value = 1.13.

1 INTRODUCTION

1.1 *Temporary anchorage devices and stability*

The success of orthodontic treatment greatly depends on appropriate, stable anchorage, and a number of temporary anchorage device (TAD) systems are invented to assist with stability. The need for supplemental anchorage is particularly visible in low-compliant patients, periodontal problems and hypodontia (Kanomi 1997). There are many advantages for use of mini-screw type implants in various areas of oral cavity, since their insertion and removal are easy, and surgery is atraumatic.

The initial stability is crucial for the maintenance of the anchorage, if it is to be loaded immediately (Aparicio et al. 2006). If mini-screw has poor primary stability at insertion, it cannot be engaged in therapy for next 6–8 weeks, and result is prolonged orthodontic treatment (Su et al. 2009). Mini-screws have a lower success rate (80%–85%) than osseointegrated implants (Cheng et al. 2004). The cause of displacement of a screw can be inflammation of surrounding tissue, or poor bone-screw interface. Meredith (1998) suggested that excessive insertion torque, heat at the border between the screw and bone, and mechanical injury can cause degeneration of the bone at the implant-tissue interface.

1.2 *Investigation objectives*

Manufacturers mainly offer their TADs with handheld screwdrivers, which make them widely applicable by oral surgeons, orthodontists, and general practitioners, and inexpensive (Motoyoshi 2011). Machine insertion is preferred by researchers (Pithon et al. 2011, Wilmes & Drescher 2011) because it lessens possibility of human error, but it doesn't imitate everyday in-office insertion, its results reflect ideal conditions.

Objective of this study was to identify factors of mini-implant design in conditions similar to those of everyday in-office procedures. Control of mini-implant design characteristics could be used to avoid failure of TADs in manual insertion procedure.

Multiple linear regression model was used to determine contribution of individual geometrical design characteristics of orthodontic mini-screws (length and diameter of screw, depth, pitch and lead angle of thread, and thread shape factor (TSF)) on maximum insertion torque (MIT), vertical force at MIT and maximum vertical force during implantation, with cortical bone thickness as covariate. Our hypothesis is that length, TSF and lead angle of the thread are significant predictors of MIT.

2 MATERIAL AND METHODS

2.1 *Material*

The following six cylindrical self-drilling orthodontic mini-implant types, bracket like head (all made of titanium alloy grade 5, Ti-6Al-4V) were investigated in this study: Dual Top (Jeil Medical Corp., Seoul, S. Korea): 1.4 mm × 6 mm, 1.6 mm × 6 mm,

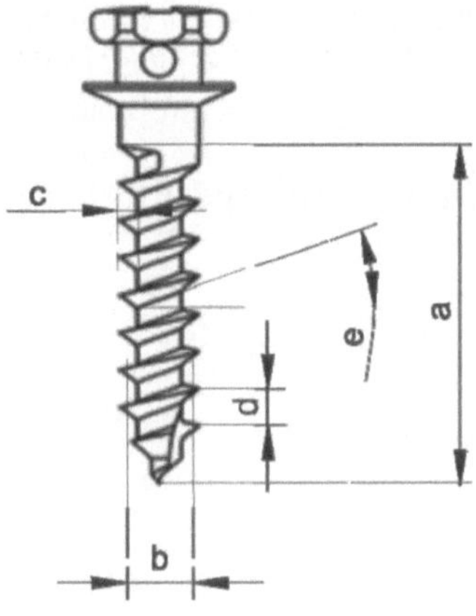

Figure 1. Geometrical design characteristics.

2.0 mm × 6 mm, 1.4 mm × 8 mm, 1.6 mm × 8 mm, 2.0 mm × 8 mm. Ten specimens of each mini-implant type were tested.

Bone samples, each 20 × 15 mm in size, were prepared from spinal part of swine ribs. Fresh swine ribs were deperiosted, cut into bone samples with water-cooling surgical engine and stored in physiological solution at 4°C until further conduct.

2.2 *Methods*

Precise measurement of all orthodontic mini-screws was conducted using the optical stereomicroscope Olympus SZX16 (Olympus, Tokyo, Japan) with 8× and 20× magnifications. Each microscoped sample was photographed alongside calibrated chart, and the measurement was read on photographs. Length (a) and outer diameter (b) of the screw thread; depth (c), pitch (d) and lead angle (e) of the thread (Fig. 1) are geometrical design characteristics measured in this study. All implants were found to have asymmetric overall thread shape type. Thread shape factor (TSF) was calculated as depth – pitch ratio for each mini-screw.

Sixty orthodontic miniscrews were manually inserted perpendicular to the bone surface using a handheld screwdriver of the respective mini-implant system, without pre-drilling of a pilot hole. Each mini-implant was screwed into one bone sample. Manual insertion was completed when miniscrew's thread was no longer visible and the implant neck was in slight contact with the bone surface.

Cortical bone thickness measurements were performed at both ends of cross-section of each bone sample using a digital sliding caliper (Levior S. R. O., Prerov, Czech Republic). The accuracy of the sliding caliper was ±0.03 mm. Mean value of the measurements of cortical bone thickness of each sample was used for further statistical analysis.

Torque measuring device (IGH, Zagreb, Croatia) consists of fixed body with four sensors connected to high resolution PicoScope oscilloscope (Pico Technology Ltd, St Neots, UK) and a custom made docking unit for the bone samples (Fig. 2). The MIT, vertical force at MIT and maximum vertical force were measured and recorded during complete insertion and obtained measurement values of MIT (Nmm) and vertical forces are digitalized and saved in a software PicoLog 5.14.6 (Pico Technology Ltd, St. Neots, UK) in a personal computer.

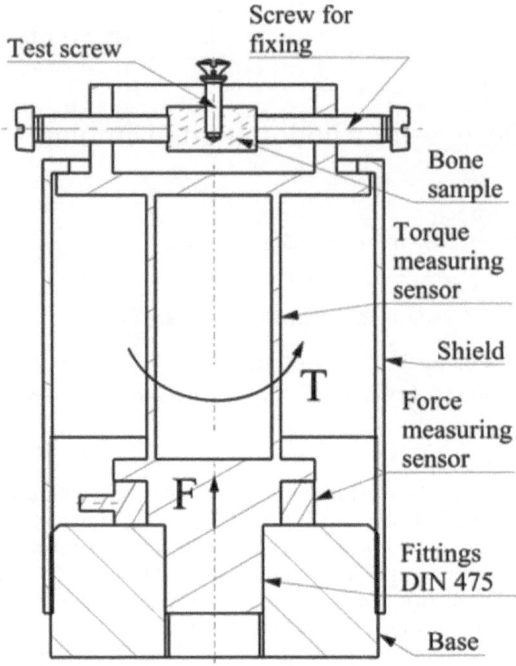

Figure 2. Scheme of torque measuring device.

2.3 *Statistical analysis*

Analysis of variance (ANOVA), lack of fit F value and regression analysis were used to assess how well the factors of miniscrew geometrical design and cortical thickness predict the outcome variables i.e. the MIT and vertical forces.

Statistical analysis were carried out using statistics software Design Expert 7.1.6 (Stat-Ease Inc., Minneapolis, USA), statistical significance was preset to $p < 0.05$.

3 RESULTS AND DISCUSSION

3.1 *Geometrical design characteristics*

Values for length and outer diameter of the screw thread provide every manufacturer, but rarely, there are manufacturer's data regarding depth, pitch, and lead angle of the thread. Mean values and standard deviations of measurement data for design characteristics of every mini-implant type tested are shown in Table 1. Results of all measured geometrical design characteristics show very small variations within same screw type.

Table 1. Results of measured geometrical design characteristics.

Mini-screw type		Thread diameter [mm]	Thread depth [mm]	Thread pitch [mm]	Lead angle [°]	Thread length [mm]
6 × 1.4	mean	1.370	0.198	0.660	8.718	6.025
	Std.dev.	0.000	0.004	0.014	0.184	0.007
8 × 1.4	mean	1.370	0.180	0.660	8.722	8.010
	Std.dev.	0.028	0.007	0.014	0.361	0.071
6 × 1.6	mean	1.572	0.255	0.721	8.307	6.028
	Std.dev.	0.0015	0.008	0.011	0.133	0.039
8 × 1.6	mean	1.558	0.255	0.733	8.512	8.014
	Std.dev.	0.019	0.011	0.007	0.139	0.076
6 × 2	mean	1.990	0.330	0.835	7.608	6.045
	Std.dev.	0.014	0.007	0.007	0.117	0.007
8 × 2	mean	1.950	0.318	0.835	7.762	7.975
	Std.dev.	0.000	0.011	0.007	0.065	0.021

Table 2. Pearson bivariate correlations between MIT, vertical forces, geometrical design characteristics and cortical thickness.

Variable	MIT [Nmm]	Vert. force at MIT [N]	Max vert. force [N]
MIT	1	−0.313*	−0.302*
Cortical thickness	0.672*	−0.122 NS	−0.064 NS
Thread length	0.302*	−0.049 NS	−0.049 NS
Lead angle	−0.320*	0.262*	0.753*
Thread diameter	0.376*	−0.271*	−0.776*
Thread depth	0.376*	−0.271*	−0.776*
Thread pitch	0.318*	−0.203 NS	−0.711*
TSF	0.389*	−0.294*	−0.778*
Vert. force at MIT	−0.313*	1	0.519*
Max vert. force	−0.302*	0.519*	1

*$p < 0.05$. NS-not significant.

3.2 *The MIT and vertical forces*

In-office decision making regarding specific implant type is related to host characteristics, namely bone density and cortical thickness (Ikumi & Tsutsumi 2005), and choosing the right geometrical screw design combination enhances primary stability of TAD, thus success of orthodontic therapy.

Our results (Table 2) show that in bivariate correlations all geometrical design characteristics and cortical thickness are significantly correlated with MIT ($p < 0.05$), and cortical thickness has the highest correlation ($r = 0.627$).

In multiple linear regression model, cortical bone thickness ($p < 0.0001$), length of implant ($p = 0.0065$) and lead angle of thread ($p = 0.0003$) are best predictors of the MIT (R-Squared = 0.5520; lack of fit F Value = 1.41; regression equation: MIT = 262.9 + 81.3 × corticalis + 13.5 × screw length − 42.4 × lead angle). Cortical thickness accounts for 32% of variability of MIT, lead angle for 11.8 and screw length for 6.4%. Screw diameter, lead angle, pitch, depth and TSF demonstrated high intercorrelations ($r > 0.882$) so to resolve problem of multicolinearity in regression model lead angle was included since it resulted in best fitting of the model.

Maximum vertical force during implantation is best predicted by length of screw ($p = 0.0493$), and lead angle of thread ($p < 0.0001$) (R-Squared = 0.5962; lack of fit F Value = 1.13; regression equation: MVF = −20.0 + 0.4× lead angle − 0.4 × screw length).

Vertical force at MIT is best predicted by lead angle of thread ($p = 0.0436$) (R-Squared = 0.0684; lack of fit F Value = 1.35; regression equation: VF at MIT = −4.6 + 1.6 × lead angle).

It is widely accepted that MIT is important and measurable factor of primary stability of orthodontic miniscrews (Meredith 1998, Miyawaki et al. 2003, Aparicio et al. 2006). The other measurements described in literature are radiological examination, Periotest® (Medizintechnik Gulden, Modautal, Germany), removal torque (Okazaki et al. 2008, Pithon et al. 2011), and the resonance frequency analysis (RFA) by Osstell. The RFA is currently not applicable for orthodontic mini-implants, while other test methods deliver only insufficiently precise measurements (Aparicio et al. 2006). Previous studies have demonstrated that larger thread surface (represented through TSF) resists better to pullout forces (Okazaki et al. 2008, Pithon et al. 2011).

3.3 *Manual insertion and MIT*

All of the implantations were done manually, with no pilot hole, because all of the manufacturers recommend direct implantation for self-drilling miniscrews in most bone areas in oral cavity. According to manufacturers' recommendation, a pilot drill, or cortical bone punch is supplied for mandibular and palatal areas with dense cortical bone. Motoyoshi et al. (2006) recommend insertion without a guiding hole for self-drilling implants diameters up to 1.6 mm. Others, like Meredith (1998), state that diameter smaller than 1.5 mm significantly increases risk for implant fracture. Several studies showed that self-drilling mini-implants have better primary stability when inserted without a pilot hole (Miyawaki et al. 2003, Motoyoshi 2011). Majority of everyday in-office routine placement of orthodontic mini-implants is being done manually. It is also the fact that the measurement of MIT is not possible in every situation, and that often orthodontic implantation proceeds until no thread is visible and transmucose neck is seated in surrounding soft tissue. Therefore, practitioners have available just one "measure" for primary stability, and that is the feeling of resistance of the bone during insertion, especially final resistance, which is in fact MIT. Results for MIT in this study are far bellow fracture torque values of respective mini-implant types shown in study of Wilmes et al. (2011), but somewhat higher from recommended insertion torques (Motoyoshi et al.

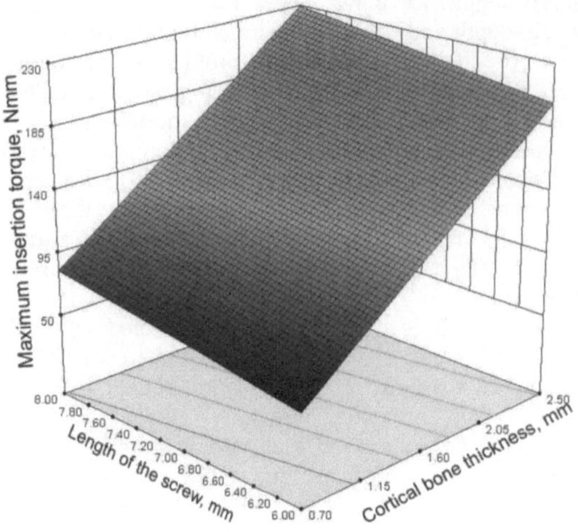

Figure 3. Graph of multiple linear regression model for prediction of MIT.

2006). Primary stability of mini-screw is important for immediate loading, and its purpose is temporary, so it is preferable to achieve better primary stability (Pithon et al. 2011, Motoyoshi et al. 2006).

3.4 *The cortical bone*

Ratio between cortical bone and spongious part of swine ribs is similar to those in alveolar processes of maxilla and mandible (Kim et al. 2010, Friberg et al. 1995). The cortical bone thickness was on average 1.5 mm ± 0.4 mm. Variations in tested biological material are similar to the range in human jaw bones, thus enabling analysis of the influence of variability of cortical bone thickness on overall MIT values (Ikumi & Tsutsumi 2005). Wilmes & Drescher (2011) concluded that excessive insertion forces cause latter bone necrosis. Representative curve for manual insertion of orthodontic mini-implants shows oscillations in insertion torque, as result of repositioning of screwdriver in surgeon's hand. Intermittent force and torque reduces chance for heat at the border between the screw and bone, which is one of the factors for failure of implantation. On the other hand, excessive insertion torque and mechanical injury can only be controlled by operator's subjective judgment. Future research might compare results in equal conditions with different operators, for further analysis of factors influencing successful implantation.

Findings from this study indicate possible choices regarding implant design and host characteristics, in order to achieve proper primary stability without compromising long-term stability, as all measurements were conducted trying to imitate in-office conditions (Fig. 3).

The MIT values can be controlled by choosing implant length and lead angle of the thread according to limitations of assessed thickness of cortical bone and available space (for example, in between tooth roots).

4 CONCLUSIONS

Geometrical design characteristics are highly intercorrelated. Thicker cortical bone, lower lead angle of thread and higher length of screw are significant predictors of higher MIT in linear regression model.

Higher lead angle is significant predictor of vertical force at MIT and higher lead angle and shorter screw length are significant predictors of maximum vertical force during implantation.

REFERENCES

Aparicio C, Lang N P, Rangert B. 2006. Validity and clinical significance of biomechanical testing of implant/bone interface. *Clinical Oral Implants Research* 17(2): 2–7.

Cheng SJ, Tseng IY, Lee JJ, Kok SH. 2004. A prospective study of the risk factors associated with failure of mini-implants used for orthodontic anchorage. *International Journal of Oral & Maxillofacial Implants* 19: 100–106.

Friberg B, Sennerby L, Roos J, Johansson P, Strid CG, Lekholm U. 1995. Evaluation of bone density using cutting resistance measurements and microradiography: an in vitro study in pig ribs. *Clinical Oral Implants Research* 6: 164–171.

Ikumi N, Tsutsumi S. 2005. Assessment of correlation between computerized tomography values of the bone and cutting torque values at implant placement: a clinical study. *International Journal of Oral & Maxillofacial Implants* 20: 253–260.

Kanomi R. 1997. Mini-implant for orthodontic anchorage. *Journal of Clinical Orthodontics* 31: 763–767.

Kim SJ, Yoo J, Kim YS, Shin SW. 2010. Temperature change in pig bone during implant site preparation by low-speed drilling. *Journal of Applied Oral Science* 18: 522–527.

Meredith N. 1998. Assessment of implant stability as a prognostic determinant. 1998. *International Journal of Prosthodontics* 11: 491–501.

Meredith N. 1998. A review of nondestructive test methods and their application to measure the stability and osseointegration of bone anchored endosseous implants. *Critical Reviews in Biomedical Engineering* 26: 275–91.

Miyawaki S, Koyama I, Inoue M, Mishima K, Sugahara T, Takano-Yamamoto T. 2003. Factors associated with the stability of titanium screws placed in the posterior region for orthodontic anchorage. *American Journal of Orthodontics and Dentofacial Orthopedics* 124: 373–378.

Motoyoshi M, Hirabayashi M, Uemura M, Shimizu N. 2006. Recommended placement torque when tightening an orthodontic mini-implant. *Clinical Oral Implants Research* 17: 109–114.

Motoyoshi M. 2011. Clinical indices for orthodontic mini-implants. Review. *Journal of Oral Science* 53(4): 407–412.

Okazaki J, Komasa Y, Sakai D, Kamada A, Ikeo T, Toda I, Suwa F, Inoue M, Etoh T. 2008. A torque removal study on the primary stability of orthodontic titanium screw mini-implants in the cortical bone of dog femurs. *International Journal of Oral and Maxillofacial Surgery* 37: 647–650.

Pithon MM, Nojima MG, Nojima LI. 2011. In vitro evaluation of insertion and removal torques of orthodontic mini-implants. *International Journal of Oral and Maxillofacial Surgery* 40: 80–85.

Su YY, Wilmes B, Honscheid R, Drescher D. 2009. Comparison of self-tapping and self-drilling orthodontic mini-implants: An animal study of insertion torque and displacement under lateral loading. *International Journal of Oral & Maxillofacial Implants* 24: 1–8.

Wilmes B, Drescher D. 2011. Impact of bone quality, implant type, and implatation site preparation on insertion torques of mini-implants used for orthodontic anchorage. *International Journal of Oral and Maxillofacial Surgery* 40: 697–703.

Wilmes B, Panayotidis A, Drescher D. 2011. Fracture resistance of orthodontic mini-implants: a biomechanical *in vitro* study. *European Journal of Orthodontics* 33(4): 396–401.

Biodental Engineering II – Natal Jorge et al (Eds)
© 2014 Taylor & Francis Group, London, ISBN 978-1-138-00131-2

Effectiveness of passive ultrasonic irrigation time in the smear layer removal

F. Tadeu, R. Madureira & O. Oliveira
Instituo Superior de Ciências da Saúde – Norte, Gandra – Paredes – Porto, Portugal

L. Forner
University of València, València, Spain

ABSTRACT: The purpose of the present study was to evaluate the remaining amounts of debris and smear layer on canal walls in the apical third after preparation with ProTaper instruments in combination with 20% of citric acid associated to the Passive Ultrasonic Irrigation (PUI) by different periods time. After the instrumentation with ProTaper instruments the 60 teeth were randomly divided in three distinct groups in accordance to the established final protocol rinse. Data were recorded and analyzed statistically with Kruskal Wallis test and LSD Fisher methods by SPSS software. Citric acid is an irrigant solution widely used in root canal treatment because of its chelating properties and ability to dissolve inorganic tissue. Therefore, a combination of citric acid and PUI reported to be suitable for removing smear layer.

1 INTRODUCTION

Currently the cleaning and disinfection of the root canal are achieved with the assistance of instruments and irrigating solutions. However, obtaining a root canal completely free of smear layer and debris it is an utopia and is recognized by several authors. To get a successful root canal therapy it is important to regarding the combination of proper instrumentation, irrigation, and obturation of the root canal. During the mechanical preparation, the instruments cut the dentin and produce a mass composed of inorganic and organic material that was called smear layer, having a thickness which ranges from 1 to 5 μm. In case if there are blocking the entrance of dentinal tubules, it is called smear plug, possessing constitution identical to smear layer. Furthermore, studies have shown that removal of this layer promotes the permeability of the dentine by improving the diffusion and action of drugs into the conduct, allowing greater penetration and producing one of sealers in lateral root canals and dentinal tubules.

The mechanical preparation of the root canal requires the simultaneous use of an irrigating solution, in order to facilitate and assist the act itself. For this reason, the use of a liquid during root canal instrumentation has always been present since the beginning of Endodontics. The auxiliary solutions, along with mechanical instruments, ie the action of the instruments form a single process, simultaneous, continuous and indivisible, which is the chemomechanical preparation of the root canal.

The use of irrigating solutions is necessary to promote the dissolution of pulpal remnants, hydraulic drive of smear layer, cleaning, lubrication, disinfection and neutralization of bacterial toxins. Furthermore, should effectively remove both the smear layer and the smear plug, allowing penetration of the sealer in the dentinal tubules and hermetically sealing the root canal. The ideal irrigant should possess, in addition to all these properties, low toxicity and be easy to purchase.

Regarding irrigating solutions, it can be said that they are essential in endodontics, because the canals have many ramifications that can only be achieved by them, so it should be used in abundance.

Around the world, sodium hypochlorite (NaOCl) in several concentrations is used to irrigate root canals because it meets all specifications mentioned above. This solution operates in tissue promoting protein denaturation and their replacement of hydrogen and oxygen molecules by chlorine, forming water soluble chloramines. This action is restricted to the organic portion of the tooth.

Several kinds of acids have been investigated to evaluate the dentin demineralization and removal of the smear layer. Citric acid in different concentrations has been suggested as chelating substance for root canal final irrigation.

Citric acid in different concentrations has been suggested as chelating substance for final root canal irrigation. The chelating solutions, associated with sodium hypochlorite, effectively remove the smear layer and smear plug formed during instrumentation of the root canal system.

Numerous investigations have demonstrated the limitation of root canal irrigation regarding the overall quality of cleaning[1].

With endodontic procedures at our disposal it is impossible to fully clean the root canal. This is mainly due to the complex anatomy of the root canal system. The irregularities of the root canal wall, in particular, are a major concern, including oval extensions, isthmus and apical delta.

In fact, into the oval conducts, only 40% of the apical area of the root canal walls may be contacted by instruments, when a rotary technique is used. Therefore, irrigation is an essential part of the root canal treatment because it allows more effective cleaning that the instruments.

PUI is based on the transmission of acoustic energy or oscillatory through a file or thin metal wire, for irrigating the root canal. The energy is transmitted through ultrasonic waves and can induce a streaming through the irrigant causing acoustic cavitation.

These problems have resulted in a wide search for innovative solutions and techniques to obtain a clean, disinfected, debris-free canal for obturation[2,3,4].

The purpose of the present study was to evaluate the remaining amounts of debris and smear layer on canal walls in the apical third after preparation with ProTaper instruments in combination with 20% of citric acid associated to the passive ultrasonic irrigation (PUI) by different periods time.

2 MATERIAL AND METHODS

Sixty distal and palatin roots of mandibular and maxillary molars extracted human teeth with closed apices were used. None of the teeth had received restorative or endodontic therapy. Following extraction, the teeth were stored at 9°C in 0.1% thymol solution to avoid the dissolution of organic tissue. The existence of a single root canal, a necessary condition for the application of the methodology proposed in this work, was evaluated using radiographs taken in mesio-distal of the tooth. Twenty-four hours prior to use they were washed in flowing water until its manipulation to eliminate any residual trace of thymol.

The biomechanical preparation of the conduct was performed using the endodontic motor VDW.SILVER® RECIPROC® (VWD GmbH, Munich, Germany), 250 rpm and 2.0 Ncm of torque for files ProTaper.

During instrumentation with ProTaper system root canals were irrigated with 3 mL of 3% NaOCl between each instrument and kept flooded with irrigant during the instrumentation phase. Then the teeth were randomly divided in three distinct groups in accordance to the established final protocol rinse. There were used ESI points from EMS in Piezon Master400 during 30 seconds for Group 1, 60 seconds for Group 2 and 90 seconds for Group 3.

Then the teeth were prepared for SEM examination. Photomicrographs at x400 (for debris score) and x3000 (for the smear layer) were taken in the apical thirds of the canals. The rating system used was proposed by Hülsmann et al. (1997) graded from 1 to 5[5]. Data were recorded and analyzed statistically with Kruskal Wallis test and LSD Fisher methods by SPSS software.

3 RESULTS AND DISCUSSION

Although the ideal is the removal of debris from the root canal, in most cases, what is achieved is only a significantly reduced. Various studies and researches have shown that no technical instrumentation and irrigation existing nowadays is able to promote a complete cleaning of the root canal system is in agreement with the result obtained in this research study.

Another reason the authors give for the occurrence of these failures are the variations of internal anatomy of the root canal, interfering with the final result, because the remaining tissue can persist in isthmuses, ramifications and reentrances making it difficult to execution of instrumentation and irrigation techniques.

The new methods of root canal irrigation, using energy generated by ultrasonic irrigation allow a continuous high volume of irrigating solution. The technique of ultrasonic irrigation reduces the amount of necrotic debris from the interior of the canal and is helped, significantly, for a continuous high volume flow of irrigating solution, supporting the results obtained.

The irrigating solutions are potencialized both physically and chemically, when used with ultrasound. The action of cavitation displaces debris and creates a vacuum effect, sucking them from the ramifications of the conduct. Moreover, the intense movement of irrigant flow drags such debris out of the canal. The energy given by ultrasound increases the solvency of citric acid, due to heating produced.

The use of the rotary instrumentation resulted in a substantial amount of smear layer. This smear layer consists of dentine particles and pulp tissue closely compacted against the root canal wall and extending into the dentinal tubules. The smear layer produced by instrumentation should be removed, because it could contain bacteria and increase leakage of the canal filling[6,7,8].

Previous investigations generally conclude that chemi-mechanical preparation leaves smear layer within the root canal. Several studies have shown that any existing irrigation protocol is not able to promote a total cleaning of the root canal system. Irrigation solutions when used with ultrasonic devices have a better effect. With the increased of ultrasonic activation time, we obtain a canal without smear layer in both thirds, for values of $p < 0.0002$.

Irrigation plays a key role in successful debridement and disinfection. Citric acid is an irrigant solution widely used in root canal treatment because of its chelating properties and ability to dissolve inorganic tissue. Therefore, a combination of citric acid and PUI reported to be suitable for removing smear layer[9].

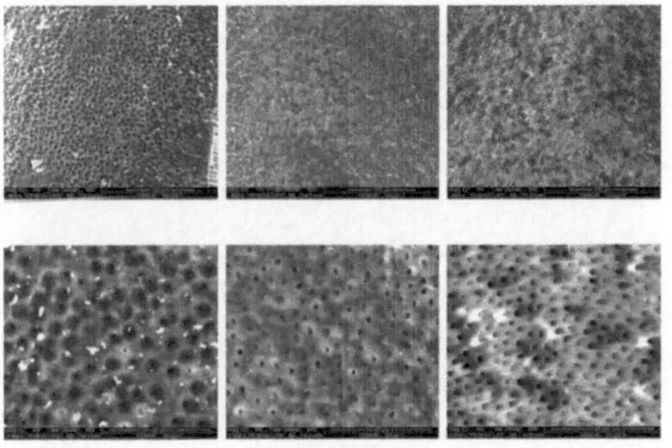

Figure 1. SEM Photomicrographs of apical third with magnification of x400 and x3000 of groups 1, 2 and 3.

At the end of instrumentation, root canal diameters have been adequately enlarged to a funnel-form shape that provides easier and superior penetration of the irrigants in the apical portions. At this stage, no further instrumentation is required and, consequently no more smear layer is produced. This allows the irrigating solutions, which are activated and agited for period of time, to efficiently remove the remaining debris[10].

4 CONCLUSIONS

In the middle third, passive ultrasonic irrigation for 60 seconds removed smear layer better than with 30 seconds.

Statistical analysis showed that the ultrasonic irrigation in the apical area during 90 seconds is the most effective in the smear layer removal.

Passive ultrasonic irrigation for 30 to 60 seconds do not remove the smear layer in the apical third, without statistically significant differences between them.

The results of the present study showed that rotary instrumentation followed by a specific final irrigation by PUI for 90 seconds could produce good canal cleanliness. In most cases, canal surfaces were smooth and free of pulpal remnants (Fig. 1). However it would be important to study if this affected the surface of root dentine walls.

REFERENCES

[1] Garberoglio R, *et al, Oral Surg Oral Med Oral Pathol*, **78**:359–67, 1994.
[2] Khedmat S, *et al, J Endod*, **34**:599–602, 2008.
[3] Scelza MF, *et al, Oral Surg Oral Med Oral Pathol Oral Radiol Endod*, **98**:499–503, 2004.
[4] Lui JN, *et al, J Endod*, **33**:472–5, 2007.
[5] Hulsmann M, *et al, J Endod*, **23**:301–6, 1997.
[6] Dadresanfar B, *et al. J Oral Sci*, **53**:31–6, 2011.
[7] Qian W, *et al, J Endod*, **37**:1437–41, 2011.
[8] Blank-Goncalves LM, *et al, J Endod*, **37**:1268–71, 2012.
[9] Caron G, *et al, J Endod*, **36**:1361–6, 2010.
[10] van der Sluis L, *et al, Quintessence Int*, **40**:875–9, 2009.

Biodental Engineering II – Natal Jorge et al (Eds)
© 2014 Taylor & Francis Group, London, ISBN 978-1-138-00131-2

Impact of fluoride agents on mechanical properties of orthodontic wires

V. Katić
Private Dental Practice, Zagreb, Croatia

S. Špalj
Dental Study at Medicine Faculty, Rijeka, Croatia

J. Leder Horina
Faculty of Mechanical Engineering and Naval Architecture, Zagreb, Croatia

D. Vikić-Topić
Rudjer Bošković Institute, Zagreb, Croatia

ABSTRACT: Effects of fluoride prophylactic agents on mechanical properties of regular and nitrified nickel-titanium (Ni-Ti) Bioforce Sentalloy wires were investigated. Specimens (25 × 0.508 × 0.508 mm) were immersed in Elmex gelée, MI Paste Plus and dH2O (control) for 1 hour at 37°C. After immersion, the loading and unloading elastic modulus (E) and yield strength (YS) of ten samples from each group were measured with a 3-point bending test in a thermal chamber at 37°C. ANOVA and Games-Howell post-hoc test were used in statistical analysis. The unloading YS of Ni-Ti for Elmex gelée is significantly higher in respect to dH2O ($p = 0.007$). In dH2O, Ni-Ti showed significantly lower results in unloading YS, when compared to nitrified Ni-Ti ($p = 0.029$). Dark discolorations are visible in all tested groups. Elmex gelée affects significantly unloading mechanical properties of regular Ni-Ti wire. MI Paste Plus has no significant effect on mechanical properties of tested wires.

1 INTRODUCTION

1.1 *Superelastic properties of Ni-Ti alloys*

Ni-Ti archwires are shape memory alloys, and that is the main reason they are used in orthodontics. The property of superelasticity allows applying low constant forces to the dentition over a long period of activation and the final result is tooth movement to desired position by combining rotation and translatation. Superelasticity results from a stress-induced phase transformation. The formation of martensitic phase in the alloy is initiated by cooling material below M_s which can be defined as the temperature at which the martensitic transformation begins. M_f is temperature at which the martensitic transformation ends. This transformation is reversible, being the A_s the temperature at which the reverse austenitic transformation starts upon heating, and A_f the temperature at the end of the reverse austenitic transformation. When a stress is applied to the parent phase material above its A_f temperature, a mechanically elastic martensite is stress-induced in alloy. That means that the deformed material reverts to its original shape when the stress is released. This effect is called pseudoelasticity or superelasticity. The critical stress increases with increasing temperature while the yield stress of the parent phase decreases with increasing temperature. Due to their superelastic properties Ni-Ti archwires are able to produce teeth movement with greater efficiency and in a shorter time in comparison to other orthodontic alloys. They are especially indicated in situations that require large deflections of an orthodontic archwire such as the leveling and alignment stage of orthodontic therapy (Gil et al. 2012).

1.2 *Properties of fluoride prophylactic agents*

Orthodontic treatment lasts 2–3 years on average and imposes need for better caries prophylaxis (Lucchese & Gherlone 2012). Application of high concentrations of fluoride leads to the formation of a CaF2 layer on the enamel surface (ten Cate 1997). The different fluoride formulations have different dissolution properties: NaF is instantly dissociating in saliva; amine fluoride may bind to organic constituents in saliva and plaque and releases fluoride slower than the stannous fluoride; and casein phosphopeptides (CPP) binds to amorphous calcium phosphate fluoride (ACPF) in metastable solution, thus facilitating remineralization of both surface and subsurface enamel (Robertson et al. 2011).

1.3 *Alloy corrosion*

While fluoride helps prevent development of caries and protects dental enamel, it also can cause corrosion and discoloration of titanium-based orthodontic wires. Titanium-based alloys have high corrosion resistance because they form a thin, stable oxide layer. This investigation studied effects of two different commercially available fluoride prophylactic agents with different chemical formulations of fluoride and pH, on mechanical properties of nickel-titanium (Ni-Ti) orthodontic archwires with different surface coatings (regular Ni-Ti and nitrified Ni-Ti). Mechanical properties and qualitative surface changes were observed. Analysis of all data contributes to better understanding how these changes affect orthodontic therapy.

The hypotheses tested were: 1. the loading and unloading modulus of elasticity (E) will be changed as a result of exposure to prophylactic fluoride agents, 2. the loading and unloading yield strength (YS) will be changed as a result of fluoride exposure, and 3. there will be a qualitative difference in the topography of the wire surface as a result of fluoride exposure.

2 MATERIAL AND METHODS

2.1 *Material preparation and immersion*

Two types of preformed rectangular (0.508 × 0.508 mm) BioForce Sentalloy (Dentsply GAC Int., NY, USA) orthodontic wires were investigated in study:

- regular Ni-Ti – with untreated surface
- nitrified Ni-Ti (IonGuard) with surface treated by nitrogen ion implantation.

Specimens, each 25 mm long, were cut from the straight ends of preformed archwires for every wire type. Ten specimens of every wire type were immersed in Elmex gelée (Gaba, Lörrach, Germany), MI Paste Plus (GC, Tokyo, Japan), and distilled, deionized water (dH2O) as negative control, for 1 hour at 37°C. The immersion time was calculated on average exposure of single orthodontic wire to this type of prophylactic agents (5 minutes per week × 12 weeks between changes of wires). Elmex gelée has 12,500 ppm fluoride content in form of amine fluorides/sodium fluoride in 3/2 ratio. MI Paste Plus is made of casein phosphopeptide-amorphous calcium phosphate (CPP-ACP) with added 900 ppm of fluoride in form of NaF. The pH values of tested solutions were measured at 37°C with pH meter MP 220 (Mettler Toledo Int., Greifensee, Switzerland) measuring device. The fluoride agents were high fluoride-ion concentration gels, and were chosen because of their commercial availability, identical methods of application, various fluoride ion concentrations, various chemical formulations, and differences in pH.

After immersion, the specimens were removed from their respective solutions, rinsed with dH2O, and placed in new, clean, individually coded protective shields.

2.2 *Three-point bending test*

The loading and unloading elastic modulus (E) and yield strength (YS) of ten wires from each group were measured with a 3-point bending test in a thermal chamber at 37°C. Mechanical testing was based on research of Miura et al. (1986), and according to current standards of American Society for Testing and Materials (2010) and ANSI/ADA Specification No. 32 (2000). The three-point bending test demonstrates the spring back (superelastic) properties and simulates the application of a wire force on the teeth in the oral cavity. Support span of Texture Analyser TA.HD.plus (Stable Micro Systems, Godalming, UK) was set to 12 mm, loaded with low force cell (factory calibrated), and set in custom made thermal chamber. Temperature during measurements was set to 37°, regulated automatically and controlled with calibrated infrared measurment instrument Mini Temp FS (Raytek Co., Santa Cruz, USA). Each specimen was loaded to a deflection of 3.1 mm and then unloaded to zero deflection at a cross-head speed of 0,0167 mm/s. Load, in newtons (N), and deflection, in millimeters (mm), were collected every 5 ms for both loading and unloading of each specimen by using the Texture Exponent software program (Stable Micro Systems, Godalming, UK) and stored in a personal computer. Load-deflection curves were generated from these data and used for further analysis.

To calculate elastic modulus (E) and yield strength (YS) it has been used engineering beam theory. The software of the machine gives load-deflection curves where it can be seen loading segment to the value of 3.1 mm for the deflection, and afterwards unloading to the zero of deflection. The maximum of value for force and m (slope of the straight-line portion of deflection curve) was read off at each part of the curve, both loading and unloading.

2.3 *Microscopic observation*

Microscopic observation was used to characterize the effects of the fluoride treatment on the wire topography. After the mechanical testing, 3 representative specimens were selected from each wire/experimental condition group for digital microscope analysis to qualitatively characterize the topography of the wire surface. The specimens were observed by using a Dino-Lite digital microscope (AnMo Electronics, Taipei, Taiwan), photomicrographs were made at 725.4 × magnification by use of DinoCapture 2.0 software program, and stored in a personal computer. This qualitative analysis was applied to provide a potential link between the effect of fluoride on the wire surface topography and any associated degradation of mechanical properties.

Table 1. Results of loading and unloading E (mean ± standard deviation) of tested Ni-Ti wires.

Wire	Treatment	Loading E (GPa)	Unloading E (GPa)
Ni-Ti	dH2O	61.9 ± 6.3	61.0 ± 5.9
	MI Paste Plus	60.2 ± 4.7	59.4 ± 4.5
	Elmex geleé	61.2 ± 4.7	60.9 ± 4.6
Nitrified Ni-Ti	dH2O	60.2 ± 5.0	60.1 ± 4.7
	MI Paste Plus	59.3 ± 6.3	58.7 ± 5.4
	Elmex geleé	60.6 ± 5.2	60.4 ± 5.1

Table 2. Results of loading and unloading YS (mean ± standard deviation) of tested Ni-Ti wires

Wire	Treatment	Loading YS (MPa)	Unloading YS (MPa)
Ni-Ti	dH2O	506.8 ± 28.9	193.5 ± 18.7^{a}
	MI Paste Plus	516.4 ± 32.0	211.3 ± 23.7^{ab}
	Elmex geleé	528.1 ± 12.6	219.2 ± 13.0^{b}
Nitrified Ni-Ti	dH2O	518.9 ± 22.5	209.6 ± 10.6
	MI Paste Plus	513.3 ± 35.5	198.8 ± 34.9
	Elmex geleé	525.7 ± 24.0	218.5 ± 17.9

Values that do not share the same superscript letters differ at $p < 0.05$.

2.4 *Statistical analysis*

ANOVA and Games-Howell post-hoc test were used in statistical analysis. Statistical analysis were carried out using statistics software SPSS 10.0 (SPSS Inc., Chicago, USA), statistical significance was preset to $p < 0.05$.

3 RESULTS AND DISCUSSION

3.1 *The pH values*

The pH values of tested solutions at the temperature of experiment (37°C) were as follows: Elmex gelée 5.5; MI Paste Plus 6.6; dH2O 6.1.

3.2 *Mechanical properties*

Present experiment shows that there are no significant differences in elastic modulus between wires in loading and unloading for both archwires type or between wires exposed to different agents (Table 1). It demonstrates that surface treatment by nitrogen ion implantation and exposure to fluoride agents does not alter elasticity of the wire. An elastic modulus is the mathematical description of an object or substance's tendency to be deformed elastically when a force is applied to it. The elastic modulus of an object is defined as the slope of its stress–strain curve in the elastic deformation region.

Experiment shows that exposure to Elmex geleé results in increase of both loading and unloading YS in both wire types in comparison to exposure to dH20 (Table 2). This effect is statistically significant in unloading YS for Ni-Ti wires ($p = 0.007$). Impact of differences among wire types is visible for dH2O, where regular Ni-Ti showed significantly lower unloading YS, in comparison to nitrified Ni-Ti ($p = 0.029$). MI Paste Plus does not significantly influence mechanical properties of both wires type. The yield strength of a material is defined as the stress at which a material begins to deform plastically. Prior to the yield point the material will deform elastically and will return to its original shape when the applied stress is removed. Higher values of YS say that this archwires are more resistant to plastic deformation.

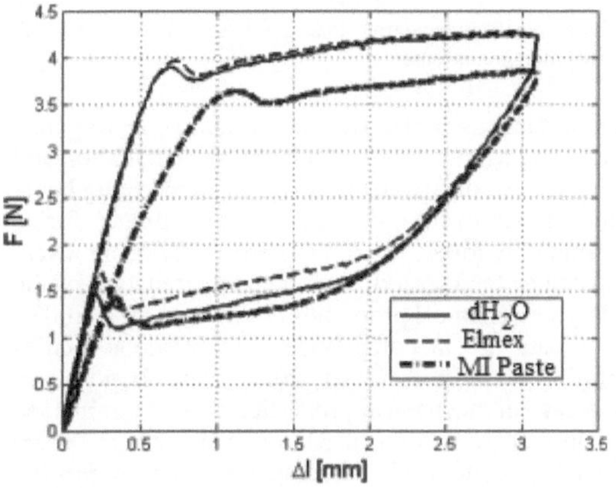

Figure 1. Representative load-defelction curves for nitrified Ni-Ti wires after treatments.

Force-deflection curves show the superelastic hysteresis characteristic for smart alloys, and it can be seen that in elastic area curve is horizontal. The hysteresis test shows an excellent elastic recovery and there is very little plastic strain.

For smart materials, it is characteristic that values for elastic modulus are similar, but yield strength is different (Es-Souni et al. 2002).

Results showed that nitrified Ni-Ti wires are more resistant to changes of mechanical properties due to exposure to aquatic media in comparison to Ni-Ti with untreated surface. Elastic modulus is less affected than YS (Fig. 1). Still, it appears that topical application of Elmex geleé during fixed orthodontic therapy can change chemical composition of the Ni-Ti wires so that it can in final affect on its mechanical properties (Fig. 2). With the same elasticity wire can have higher elastic range. Microstructure of wires results on phase transformation of shape memory alloy, and that transformation also influences on final mechanical properties of the samples.

3.3 *Surface corrosion*

Regular Ni-Ti wire has TiOx (Eliades & Athanasiou 2002), and nitrified Ni-Ti has titanium nitride (TiN)

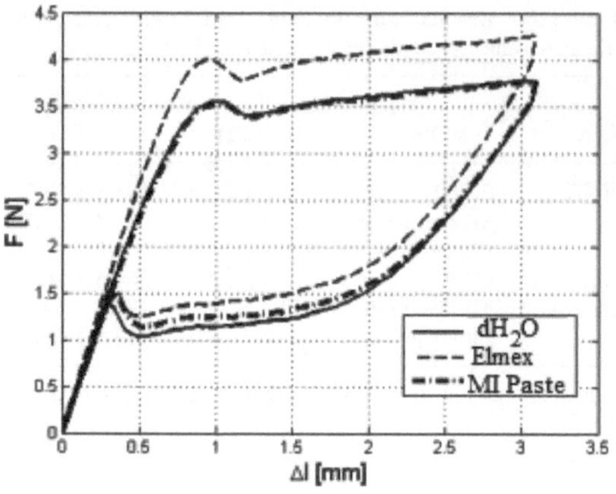

Figure 2. Representative load-defelction curves for Ni-Ti wires after treatments.

on surface, as protective surface component against corrosive agents. Fluoride ions cause degradation and loss of the oxide film, thus exposing underlying Ni-Ti alloy. High affinity of titanium with hydrogen forms titanium hydrides, which have been previously investigated as the cause of the related degradation of the alloy's mechanical properties (Yokoyama et al. 2003). Our data are in compliance with previous studies of Yokoyama et al. (2001, 2003), who found slight increase in mechanical properties of wires immersed in fluoride agent for up to 3 hours. Walker et al. (2005) found opposite result, decrease in mechanical properties after immersion period of 90 minutes. A laboratory study by Strietzel (1994) showed that the corrosion of titanium by fluoride containing gels occurred at pH of less than 4, and this also supports our findings, because none of the tested solutions had pH of 4 or less. In Elmex gelée larger part of fluoride is bind in aminfluoride molecules, from which fluoride ions are increasingly released in lower pH of dental plaque. Although MI Paste Plus had rather low fluoride content and somewhat higher pH, when compared to other tested fluoride agent, it also contained phosphates, which enhance release of fluoride ions. Study of Shabalovskaya (2002) showed that if the surface oxide layers are disrupted, the calcium phosphate deposits appear to significantly delay repassivation (i.e. recovery of a stable surface oxide layer), and similar was observed in a recent comparative study (McMahon et al. 2012). This should be taken into account in everyday work, as in-office manipulation can scratch the surface and damage surface coating. A number of studies used dH2O as negative control, and since it is strong solvent, it also causes hydrogen embrittlement of Ni-Ti alloys.

Surface changes in form of dark discolorations (i.e. corrosion) are visible in all tested groups.

Surface of Ni-Ti wires changes through nitration to titanium nitride (TiN), which improves wear resistance, surface hardness, resistance to chemical attack, and reduces friction (Liu et al. 2007). Our results are in agreement, nitrified Ni-Ti wire showed more consistent results, when exposed to various agents, and retained their superelasticity and shape memory (deflection and heath induced martensitic transformation) (Santoro et al. 2001).

4 CONCLUSIONS

Test results show that Elmex gelée affects significantly unloading mechanical properties of regular Ni-Ti wire with untreated surface, but has no significant influence on nitrified Ni-Ti wire.

MI Paste Plus has no significant effect on mechanical properties of tested wires.

Elmex gelée raises values of yield strength for both Ni-Ti and nitrified Ni-Ti wires, so wire immersed in Elmex gelée has bigger elastic filed, which is interesting for mechanical aspect of orthodontic therapy.

Nitrified Ni-Ti has better tribological properties and can be with similar efficiency used with different fluoridated agents. When using regular Ni-Ti with untreated surface better efficiency can be produced in corporation with Elmex gelée.

The transformation behavior and the ability to control or foresee transformation are of prime interest for the practical use of these alloys.

REFERENCES

American National Standard/American Dental Association. Specification No. 32. 2000. Orthodontic wires. American Dental Association, Council on Scientific Affairs, Chicago, Ill.

American Society for Testing and Materials. 2010. D790-10. Standard test methods for flexural properties of unreinforced and reinforced plastics and electrical insulating materials. American Society for Testing and Materials, West Conshohocken, Pa.

Eliades T, Athanasiou AE. 2002. In vivo aging of orthodontic alloys: implications for corrosion potential, nickel release, and biocompatibility. *Angle Orthodontist* 72: 222–237.

Es-Souni M, Es-Souni M, Fischer-Brandies H. 2002. On the properties of two binary NiTi shape memory alloys. Effects of surface finish on the corrosion behaviour and in vitro biocompatibility. *Biomaterials* 23: 2887–2894.

Gil FJ, Espinar E, Llamas JM, Manero JM, Ginebra MP, Variation of the superelastic properties and nickel release from original and reused NiTi orthodontic archwires. 2012. *Journal of the Mechanical Behaviour of Biomedical Materials* 6: 113–119.

Liu X, Wu S, Chan YL, Chu PK, Chung CY, Chu CL, Yeung KWK, Lu WW, Cheung KMC, Luk KDK. Structure and wear properties of NiTi modified by nitrogen plasma immersion ion implantation. 2007. *Materials Science and Engineering* A 444: 192–197.

Lucchese A, Gherlone E. 2012. Prevalence of white-spot lesions before and during orthodontic treatment with fixed appliances. *European Journal of Orthodontics* (Epub ahead of print).

McMahon RE, Ma J, Verkhoturov SV, Munoz-Pinto D, Karaman I, Rubitschek F, Maier HJ, Hahn MS. 2012. A comparative study of the cytotoxicity and corrosion resistance of nickel-titanium and titanium-niobium shape memory alloys. *Acta Biomaterialia* 8(7): 2863–2870.

Miura F, Mogi M, Ohura Y, Hamanaka H. 1986. The superelastic property of Japanese NiTi alloy use in orthodontics. *American Journal of Orthodontics and Dentofacial Orthopedics* 90: 1–10.

Robertson MA, Kau CH, English JD, Lee RP, Powers J, Nguyen JT. 2011. MI Paste Plus to prevent demineralization in orthodontic patients: a prospective randomized controlled trial. *American Journal of Orthodontics and Dentofacial Orthopedics* 140: 660–668.

Santoro M, Nicolay OF, Cangialosi TJ. 2001. Pseudoelasticity and thermoelasticity of nickeltitanium alloys: A clinically oriented review. Part I: Temperature transitional ranges. *American Journal of Orthodontics and Dentofacial Orthopedics* 119: 587–593.

Shabalovskaya SA. 2002. Surface corrosion and biocompatibility aspects of nitinol as an implant material. *Biomedical Materials and Engineering* 12: 69–109.

Strietzel R. 1994. Einfluss von fluoridhaltigen zahnpasten auf zahnoberflächen (Influence of fluoride-containing toothpastes on tooth surfaces). *Zahnärztliche Welt* 103: 82–84.

ten Cate JM. 1997. Review on fluoride, with special emphasis on calcium fluoride mechanisms in caries prevention. *European Journal of Oral Sciences* 105: 461–465.

Walker MP, White RJ, Kula KS. 2005. Effect of fluoride prophylactic agents on the mechanical properties of nickel-titanium-based orthodontic wires. *American Journal of Orthodontics and Dentofacial Orthopedics* 127: 662–669.

Yokoyama K, Hamada K, Moriyama K, Asaoka K. 2001. Degradation and fracture of Ni-Ti superelastic wire in an oral cavity. *Biomaterials* 22: 2257–2262.

Yokoyama K, Kaneko K, Moriyama K, Asaoka K, Sakai J, Nagumo M. 2003. Hydrogen embrittlement of NiTi superelastic alloy in fluoride solution. *Journal of Biomedical Materials Research* 65: 182–187.

Biodental Engineering II – Natal Jorge et al (Eds)
© 2014 Taylor & Francis Group, London, ISBN 978-1-138-00131-2

Use of a clinical decision-support system in implant-supported rehabilitations

V. Correia, A. Correia & J. Rocha
Master in Oral Rehabilitation, School of Dental Medicine, University of Porto, Porto, Portugal

ABSTRACT: SAC assessment tool is a Clinical Decision Support System (CDSS) used in the assessment of the potential difficulty of a rehabilitation with oral implants. The clinical cases can be classified as Straightfoward (low difficulty), Advanced (moderate difficulty) and Complex (high difficulty). The aim of this research was to characterize patients with indication for an implant-supported rehabilitation, by classifying the level of difficulty of the prosthetic rehabilitation. The study was conducted in the Master/Specialization Course in Oral Rehabilitation, from February to May of 2012, with a final sample of 41 individuals. To assess the difficulty level of the rehabilitation it has been used the CDSS Sac Assessment Tool, in its prosthetic perspective. The results indicated a larger number of cases of high complexity. A statistical relationship ($p < 0.05$) was observed between the scale and the number of appointments. Within the limitations of this research, mostly concerned with the sample size, it can be concluded that the SAC Assessment Tool may contribute to standardize the diagnosis of clinical rehabilitation with dental implants, and to promote a better approach to the treatment plan.

1 INTRODUCTION

1.1 *Clinical decision-support systems*

Decision support systems are a specific class of computerized information systems that support business and organizational decision making activities (Mendonca, 2004). In the health care industry, they are called by clinical decision-support systems. These systems are computer programs that are designed to provide expert support for health professionals making clinical decisions being used for diagnosis, prevention, treatment of health diseases and future evaluation of the patients. Examples of such systems can be found in several disciplines in health care: dentistry, medicine, and pharmacy, among others.

A 2005 systematic review of 100 studies concluded that CDSS improved practitioner performance in 64% of the studies (Garg et al. 2005). Another systematic review, (Kawamoto et al. 2003) evaluating the ability of CDSS to improve clinical practice and observed that 68% of CDSs improved clinical decision making.

Clinical decision support systems in dentistry may improve the oral status of the patient and may contribute to reduce errors in clinical practice (Newman, 2007). In addition they can provide easily clinical practice based on scientific evidence. Several sub-areas of dentistry have these systems, (White, 1996) like orofacial pain, dental emergencies and trauma, oral medicine, oral radiology, endodontics, orthodontics, oral surgery and oral implantology.

1.2 *Methodological basis of a CDSS*

There are many different methodologies that can be used by a CDSS in order to provide support to the health care professional. They can be classified into the following generic categories: algorithmic, neural networks, probabilistic, and logical/deductive (rule based) (Mendonca, 2004). There are also hybrid systems that use more than one methodological basis. Algorithmic systems use logical classification methods, represented as decision trees and flowcharts that lead the user to a desired end point (Mendonca, 2004). Neural networks are algorithmic that require training to create a set of solutions to a problem. After training these, these algorithms can make decisions on new problems with incomplete facts (Mendonca, 2004). Probabilistic systems incorporate rates of disease or problems in a population and the likelihood of various clinical findings in order to calculate the most likely explanation for a particular case. Probabilistic systems are also known as Bayesian systems (Vikram, 2009). Logical/deductive systems use branching logic – a collection of (if/than) rules to make decisions (Mendonca, 2004).

1.3 *SAC assessment tool*

The use of dental implants in oral prosthetic rehabilitation of edentulous patients has become a widely accept treatment. Although it is a treatment with good

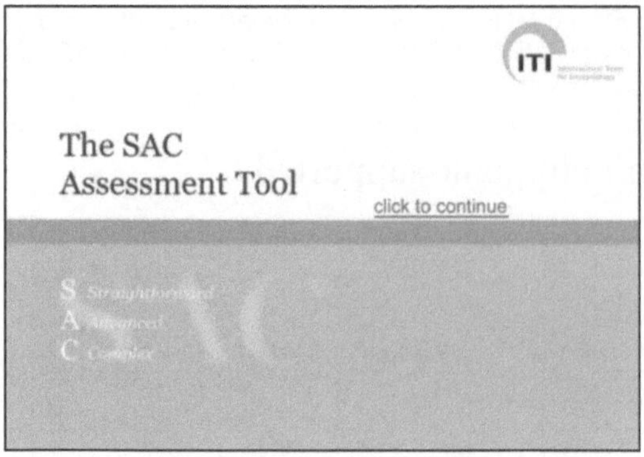

Figure 1. Image of the software SAC Assessment Tool.

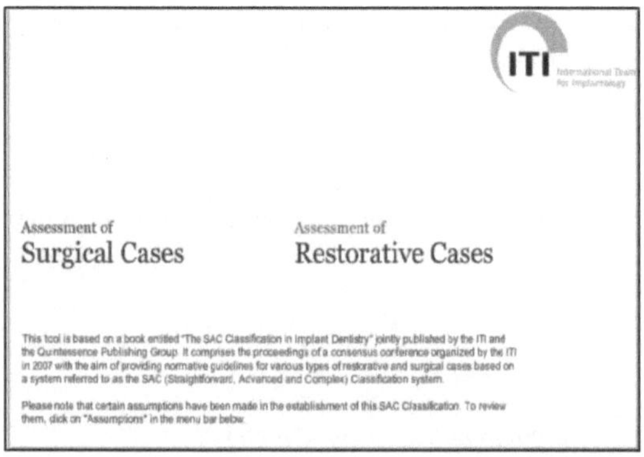

Figure 2. Image of the software SAC Assessment Tool. The two perspectives: Assessment of Restorative Cases and Assessment of Restorative Cases.

long-term prognosis, there are risks that must be identified (Buser et al. 1997).

In this sense, it has become important to develop tools to aid in the diagnosis of each clinical situation, enabling to identify the level of difficulty and associated risks of the rehabilitation. The SAC Classification is an instrument to access the potential difficulty and risk of a case and serves as a guide for clinicians in both case selection and treatment planning (Dawson et al. 2009).

The SAC assessment tool is a clinical decision-support system developed by the International Team for Implantology based on the SAC classification that classifies the difficulty and risk of a case in oral implantology. The clinical cases can be classified as Straightfoward, low difficulty, Advanced and Complex (high difficulty) in two perspectives: Surgical and Restorative (Dawson et al. 2009).

1.4 *Aim*

The aim of this research was to characterize patients with indication for implant supported rehabilitation, by classifying the level of difficulty of the prosthetic rehabilitation.

Table 1. Some of the factors assessed in a full arch removable prosthesis.

Edentulous Maxilla-Removable	Straightfoward Advanced	Complex
Inter-arch distance (bar/clip retained)	>10 mm	<10 mm = not indicated
Inter-arch distance (individuals elements)	>8 mm	<8 mm = not indicated
Loading protocol (bar/clip retained)	Early	Immediate (bar only)
Loading protocol (individuals elements)	Conventional/ Early	
Esthetic risk	Low	Moderate/high (unrealistic expectations)
Interim restorations during healing	Removable	
Oclusal parafunction	Absent	Present
Oclusal scheme/issues (fixed opposing arch)	Anterior guidance	No anterior guidance
Oclusal scheme/issues (Complete denture in opposing arch)	Balanced	Balanced is not possible

2 MATERIAL AND METHODS

The study was conducted at the Faculty of Dental Medicine of the University of Porto in the Master/Specialization Course in Oral Rehabilitation, from February to May of 2012. The study had a final sample of 41 individuals. All the individuals assign an informed consent and an explanation of the study.

To assess the difficulty level of the rehabilitation it has been used the Clinical Decision Support System SAC Assessment Tool, in its prosthetic perspective, Assessment of Restorative Cases.

The variables prosthesis type, number of appointments and difficulty level were analyzed using the Fisher exact test, the one-way ANOVA and the Tukey HSD test (SPSS®19.0).

3 RESULTS

3.1 *SAC classification*

The graphic 1 shows the level of difficulty distribution in the study. It was observed a majority of cases with difficulty Complex, followed by classification Advanced and Straightfoward.

3.2 *Prosthesis type*

The graphic 2 exhibit the distribution of prosthesis type observed in the study. The prosthesis type were divided

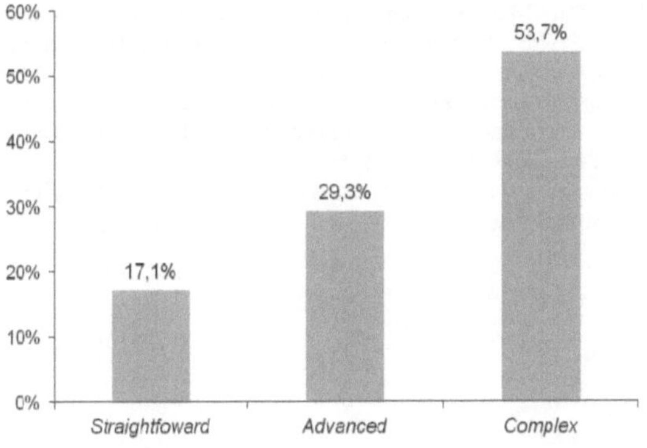

Graphic 1. Distribution of SAC Classification.

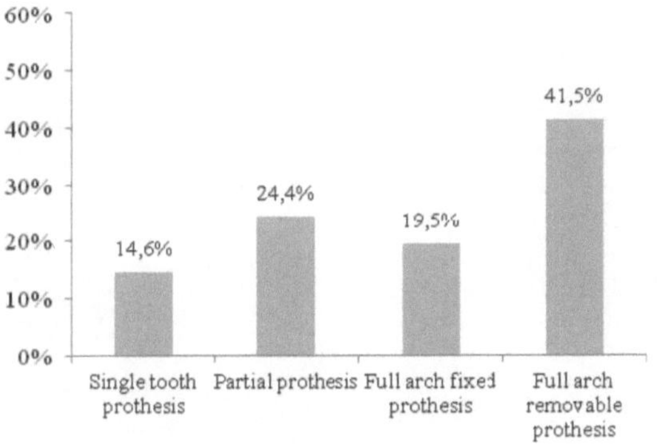

Graphic 2. Distribution of the Prosthesis type.

in four groups, single tooth, partial, full arch removable and full arch fixed prosthesis.

3.3 *Number of appointments*

The table 2 shows the distribution of appointments in the study, from the beginning of the prosthetic treatment until complete rehabilitation. The missing values were due to errors observed in the electronic oral health records and due to observed cases but not yet terminated at the end of the study. The majority of observed cases were concluded in five to ten appointments and the fewest cases were observed in more than fifteen appointments.

3.4 *Number of appointments and difficulty level of prosthetic rehabilitations*

The table 3 shows an ANOVA unilateral Tukey HSD test, comparing the means of appointments in the three groups of SAC Classification.

This ANOVA was used to test the hypothesis that the mean of appointments in the several groups were equal. It was observed a difference statistically significant between the group Complex and Straightfoward

Table 2. Number of appointments.

Number of appointments	Absolute frequency	Percentage
Missing values	9	22.0
[1–5]	6	14.6
[5–10]	19	46.3
[10–15]	4	9.8
[>15]	3	7.3
Total	41	100.0

Table 3. Number of appointments and Classification SAC.

SAC Classification	SAC Classification	Mean differences between the groups	Sig.
Straightfoward	*Advanced*	−1,600	.667
	Complex	−5,211	.011*
Advanced	*Straightfoward*	1,600	.667
	Complex	−3,611	.032*
Complex	*Straightfoward*	5,211	.011*
	Advanced	3,611	.032*

*Represents $p < 0.05$ (ANOVA unilateral Tukey HSD).

and Advanced groups. There was no statistically significant difference between the Straightfoward and Advanced groups.

4 CONCLUSION

Within the limitations of this research, mostly concerned with the sample size, it can be concluded that the SAC Assessment Tool may contribute to standardize the diagnosis of clinical rehabilitation with dental implants, and to promote a better approach to the treatment plan. It can also be concluded that the majority of the cases were classified as Complex and the cases classified as Complex, need more appointments regarding classifications Straightfoward and Advanced.

REFERENCES

Buser D, Mericske-Stern R, Bernard JP, Behneke A, Behneke N, Hirt HP, et al. Long-term evaluation of non-submerged ITI implants. Part 1: 8-year life table analysis of a prospective multi-center study with 2359 implants. Clin Oral Implants Res. 1997 Jun;8(3):161–72.

Dawson A, Chen S, Buser D, Cordaro L, Martin W, Belser U. An Introduction to the SAC Classification. In: Dawson A, Chen S, editors. The SAC Classification in Implant Dentistry. 1 ed. Berlin: Quintessence Publishing Ltd.; 2009. p. 2–4.

Garg AX, Adhikari NK, McDonald H, Rosas-Arellano MP, Devereaux PJ, Beyene J, et al. Effects of computerized

clinical decision support systems on practitioner performance and patient outcomes: a systematic review. JAMA. 2005 Mar 9;293(10):1223–38.
Kawamoto K, Houlihan CA, Balas EA, Lobach DF. Improving clinical practice using clinical decision support systems: a systematic review of trials to identify features critical to success. BMJ. 2005 Apr 2;330(7494):765.
Mendonca EA. Clinical decision support systems: perspectives in dentistry. J Dent Educ. 2004 Jun;68(6):589–97.
Newman MG. Clinical decision support complements evidence-based decision making in dental practice. J Evid Based Dent Pract. 2007 Mar;7(1):1–5.
Vikram K, Karjodkar FR. Decision support systems in dental decision making: an introduction. J Evid Based Dent Pract. 2009 Jun;9(2):73–6.
White SC. Decision-support systems in dentistry. J Dent Educ. 1996 Jan;60(1):47–63.

Biodental Engineering II – Natal Jorge et al (Eds)
© 2014 Taylor & Francis Group, London, ISBN 978-1-138-00131-2

Composite-reinforced glass fiber morphology

Sebastiana Arroyo Bote
Department of Odontostomatology, HUBc, University of Barcelona

Javier Martínez Arroyo
Nuclear Engineer

Javier Martínez Osorio
Department of Odontostomatology, HUBc, University of Barcelona

Patricia Carvalho Lobato & Mª Cristina Manzanares Céspedes
Human Anatomy and Embryology Unit, HUBc, University of Barcelona

ABSTRACT: We present the micromorphology of three materials developed using composite-reinforced glass fiber, GrandTEC, Ever stick and DEI® Experience Multi Fibers, and their integration with restorative materials. Observations were made under an Environmental Scanning Electron Microscope (ESEM), Quantac, images were taken at different magnifications. Observation of surfaces and sections of the samples allows observation of glass fiber sizes between 11 and 17 microns, coated with organic resin and its seamless integration with restorative materials, therefore we consider these materials must be taken into account in clinical situations in which an improvement of the fracture resistance of the treatment is desired.

1 INTRODUCTION

Fiberglass has been used in dentistry for years, due to the development of fiberglass tapes, which were especially suitable for prosthetic treatments made with composites providing greater hardness (Ganesh M. & S. Tandon 2006). However, the difficulty of handling fiberglass tapes did not popularizetheir use. With the development of composite-reinforced glass fiber (FRC) and the improvement of adhesive techniques that allow minimally invasive treatments (Bagis B. et al., 2010), the indications of these materials have increased, making them particularly suitable for conducting composite bridges (Gollner P. et al., 2009, Tayab T. et al., 2010) providing greater resistance to fracture. However, the increase of minimally-invasive treatments based on adhesive restorative techniques has significantly fostered the utilization of these materials, making them suitable for very different clinical treatments such as prosthetics, periodontics, orthodontics, trauma, restorative dentistry, endodontics, etc.

2 MATERIALS AND METHODS

Three different types of composite-reinforced glass fibers (FRC) have been chosen:

GrandTEC (VOCO)
Ever stick (GC)
DEI® Experience Multi Fibras (DEI Italia)

Table 1. Material compositions.

Material	% fiber weight	% fiber volume	Resin matrix	Inorganic filler	Nª of fibers
GrandTEC	55%		UDMA TEGDMA	no	4000–4500
Ever stick	67%	47%	BisGMA PMMA	no	4000
DEI® Experience	60%	40%	BisGMA, diuretano	Glass bario, dióxido de silicio	

These materials have been chosen because they represent the evolution of these kind of materials in the dentistry field. GrandTEC and Ever Stick are composed of unidirectional glass fibers, presented as malleable tape and developed primarily for treatments performed directly on the patient, glass fibers of both materials are impregnated or reinforced with resin. DEI® Experience is presented as malleable sheet and developed, mainly, for laboratory treatments.

All three materials are photopolymerizable and compatible with current adhesive systems and composites.

Samples are observed under the environmental scanning electron miscroscope Quantac 200 (FEI Co).

Selected materials were fixed to the miscroscope sample holder and observed without any sample coating. Images were taken at 50, 100, 750, 1000 and 5000 magnifications.

In order to observe the binding of these materials to composites GrandTEC FRC tape was used in an angle restoration of a superior incisor and Multi DEI® Experience was used in an onlay restoration of an inferior molar.

3 RESULTS

GrandTEC (VOCO) FRC tape has a flat section of approximately 1 mm, and a longitude of 5.5 mm. Glass fibers can be observed at the tip ends, unidirectional fibers of a size between 12–15 microns in diameter, embedded in methacrylate resins. Significant glass fiber density can be observed. The bonding between the fibers is labile making it possible to be easily separated, possibly due to the higher proportion of glass fiber when compared to the resin density.

Ever Stick FRC tape has a circular section of about 1.5 mm diameter, with unidirectional fibers of 15–17 mm diameter respectively, with a more compact

GrandTEC

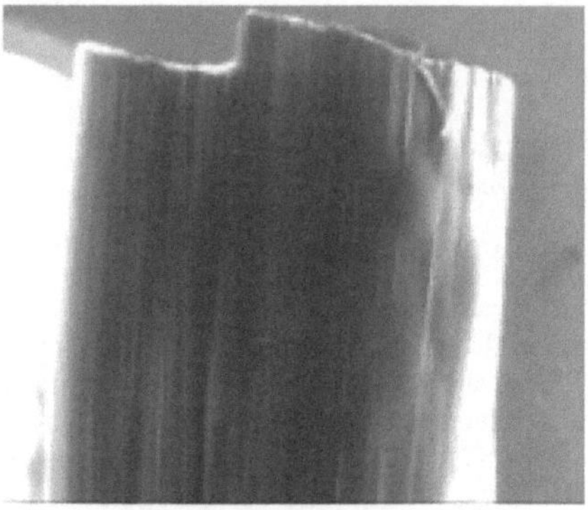

Figure 1. ×100.

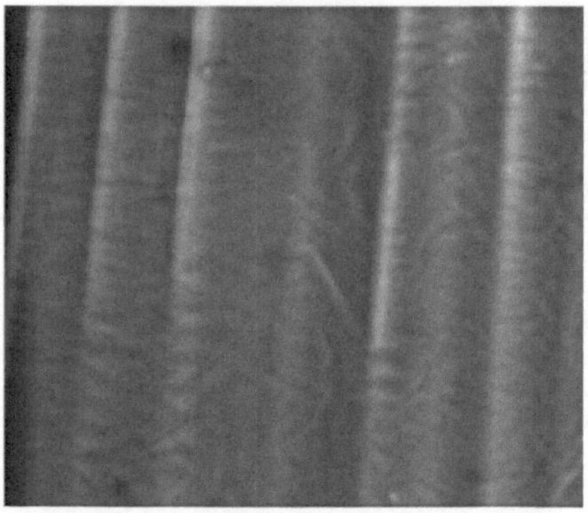

Figure 2. ×750.

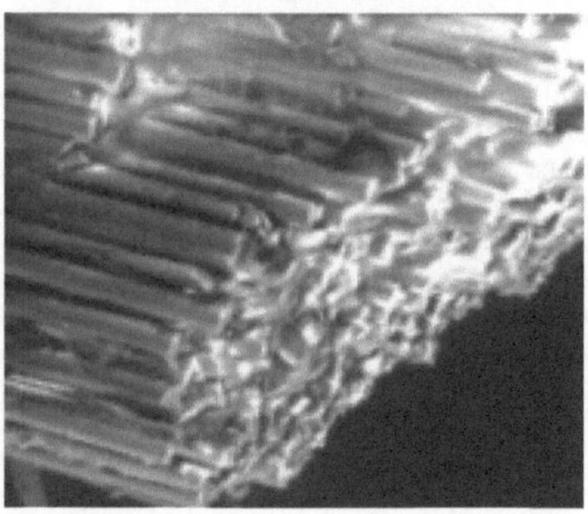

Figure 3. ×1000.

Ever stick

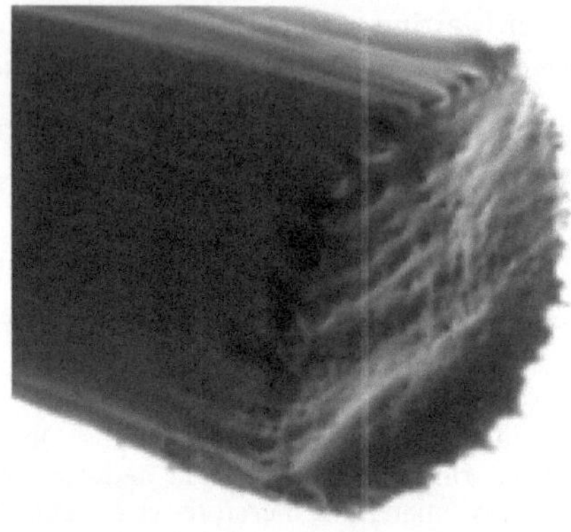

Figure 4. ×100.

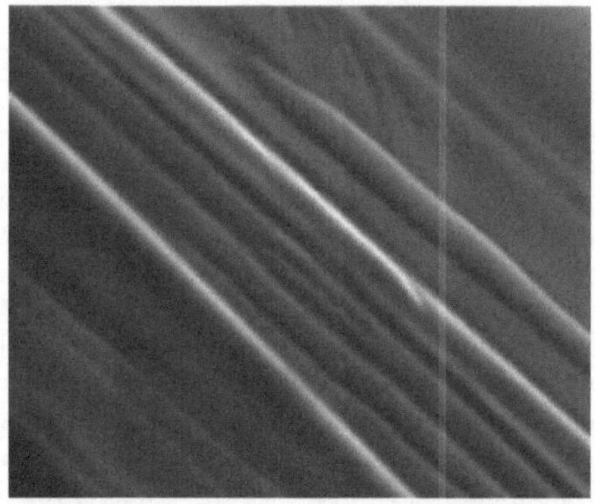

Figure 5. ×750.

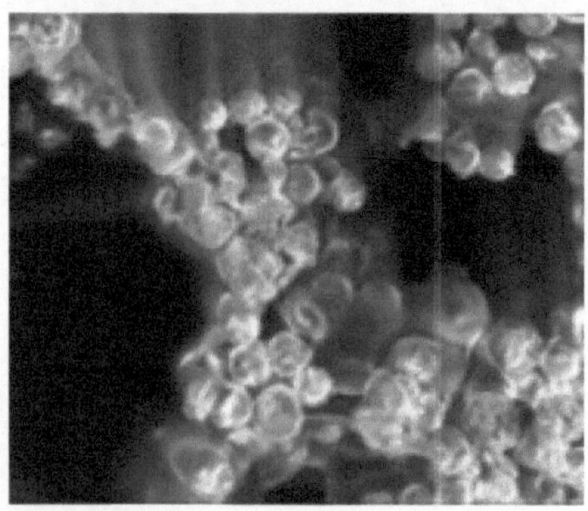

Figure 6. ×1000.

junction than GrandTEC. Glass fibers can also be separated in order to observe the grid created between them. Spaces between the grid points allow for the composite to penetrate into the tape when performing adhesive reconstructive treatments, creating a compact and strong joint between both materials.

The DEI® Experience Multi Fibras fiberglass sheet shows glass fibers of about 11 microns intersecting to form a three dimensional lattice. Each DEI® Experience sheet consists of 6 layers of intersecting fibers overlapping with each other. During restoration this particular disposition allows having longitudinal and perpendicular fibers, according to the restoration reference, which provides greater resistance to the compound material, therefore the main indication of these materials is indirect restoration inlays, onlays, crowns or bridges.

Figure 10 shows a central incisive (2.1) with an angle distal fracture. A GrandTec fiberglass tape has been adhered to the palatal surface of the incisor. The horizontal direction of the glass fibers, which will provide strength to the composite restoration ameliorating its resistance to fracture, can be clearly observed in the figure.

In Figure 11 perfect integration of the FRC tape with composite is observed, resulting in a homogeneous mass that joins glass fibers, organic resin and inorganic composite fill particles.

Figure 12 allows the observation of the longitudinal section of an onlay performed with DEI® Experience Multi Fibras and laboratory-hybrid composite Dei Experience. Parallel and perpendicular glass fibers integrated on the composite mass can be observed, some fill particles of the composite can be appreciated as well as perpendicular sections of the glass fibers and horizontal glass fibers arranged parallel to one another.

DEI® Experience Multi Fibras

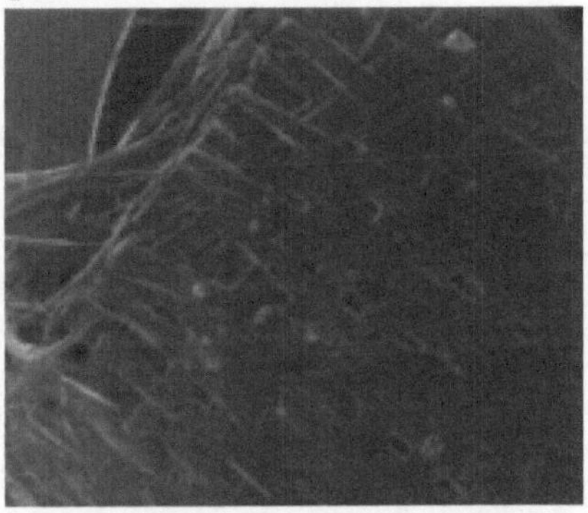

Figure 7. ×100.

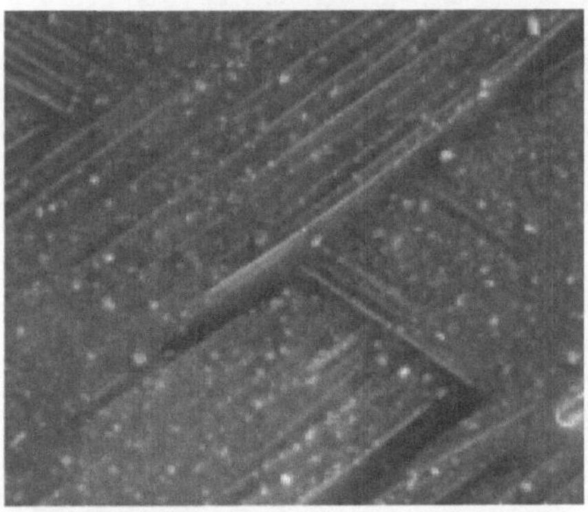

Figure 8. ×750.

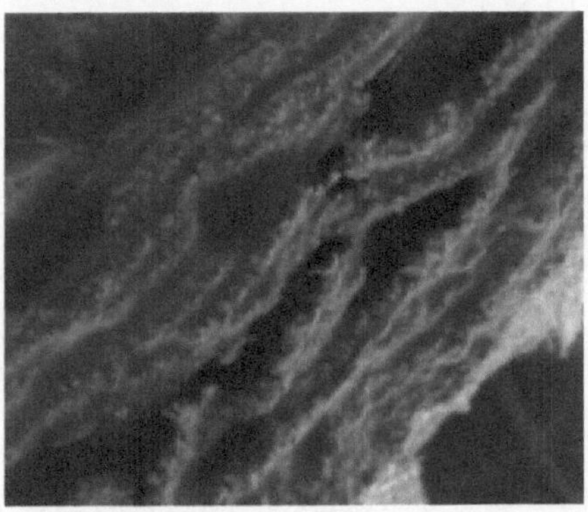

Figure 9. ×1000.

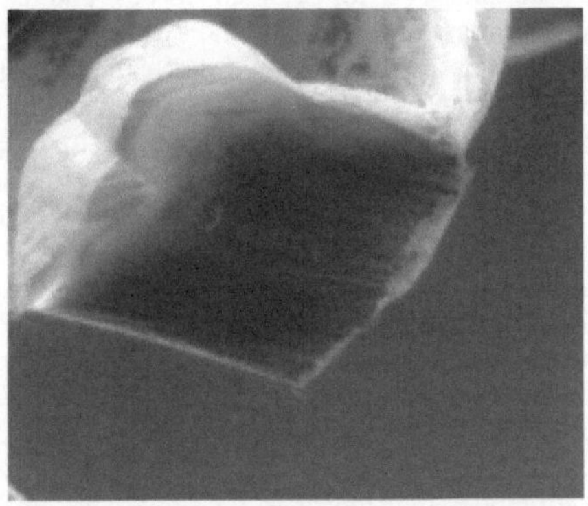

Figure 10. ×50.

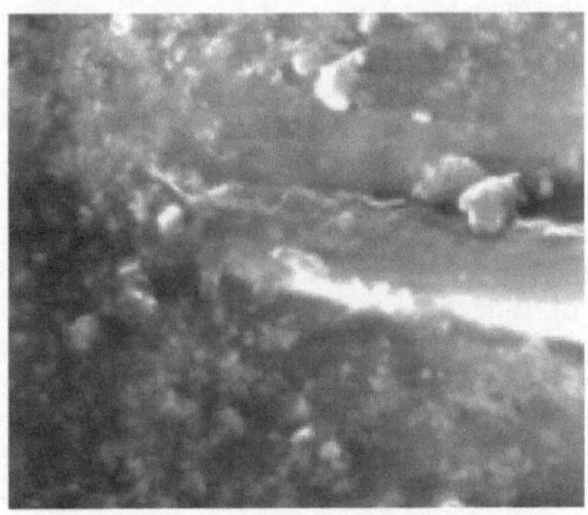

Figure 11. ×5000.

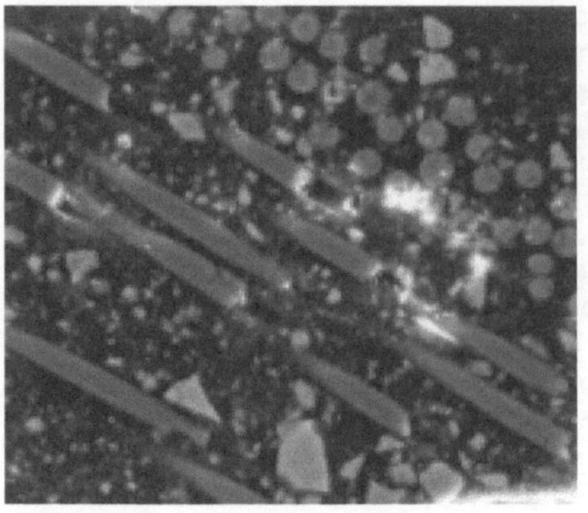

Figure 12. ×1000.

4 DISCUSSION

Increased fracture resistance of restorations made with composite materials and fiberglass has been proven by many researchers, especially in studies focused on the direct restoration of dental fractures caused by traumas, either using reconstruction composite materials (Şen B.H. et al., 2011) or with the same tooth fragment (Deepak S. et al., 2011).

Angle restorations performed with composite may suffer fractures due to occlusal forces and extrusive and protusive forces (Watanabe H. et al., 2008), and in many cases restored teeth suffer new injuries (Pissiotis A. et al., 2007), which results in the failure of the restorations. It is therefore important to give the highest possible strength to the primary restoration, using the best techniques and materials available to us (Deepak S. et al., 2011).

Studies by Abdulmajeeda (Abdulmajeeda et al., 2011) demonstrate that incorporation of unidirectional FRC improve some mechanical properties of the composites such as the hardness, following the law of proportionality between organic matrix and inorganic filler. Badakar (Badakar et al., 2011) in an in-vitro study concludes that the resistance to fracture of the angle restorations reinforced with glass fiber is similar to the original tooth. Fennis (Fennis et al., 2009), in an in vitro study in which the tooth fragment was replaced placing small fiberglass substrates, concluded that the use of glass fiber increases the resistance to fracture of these restorations. However, it is important to note that the position, orientation and adhesion of the fibers has a significant role in the resistance of these treatments (Ganesh M. et al., 2006) The use of these materials in the dental trauma reconstructive treatments can reduce index of re-fractures.

In indirect treatments, with either total or partial coverage on natural teeth or implants, these materials have advantages over ceramic because they have a lower rate of fractures. They are less rigid than ceramic. The modulus of elasticity of the glass fibers is very similar to that of dentin, and occlusal load received by the restorations exerts less force on the natural pillars or implants than ceramics, especially on patients with bruxism or other parafunctions.

The use of composite materials in indirect restorations has shown acceptable clinical success (Jongsma et al., 2012) being very relevant in the design of the preparations and their in-clinic indication, as evidenced by the work of Ausiello (Ausiello, et al., 2011).

The use of composites in prosthetic rehabilitation allows the reparation of fractures that can occur during the utilization and function time of the restoration, reaching binding forces between the old and new composite over 20–22 MPa (Maneenuta, et al., 2011), provided that the organic matrix is bisglycidyl dimethacrylate (BisGMA) and/or urethane di-methacrylate (UDMA). In fractured restorations where used materials are not known, we cannot apply a fully-effective surface treatment of old composite, but we can recommend the application of phosphoric acid or sandblasting with particles of 30 to 50 microns (Loomans, et al., 2011). The restoration repair made with composites and FRC tape can be performed directly (Wolff, et al., 2012), since there is a good spread of adhesive monomers within the fiber-reinforced composite, previously polymerized, ensuring the successful repair of the possible fractures in the material.

FRC has applications not only in the dental field but in other fields: bone implants with multilayer FRC tape for craniofacial surgery have shown, in vitro, the formation of calcium phosphate crystals within the porosities of the FRC (Nganga et al., 2012), which opens the door for the use of these materials in other medical specialties.

5 CONCLUSIONS

Micromorphology of the surface and section of the studied materials allows the observation of gassfibers from 11 to 17 microns, filled with resin and its perfect integration within the restorative materials.

REFERENCES

Abdulmajeeda AA, Närhia TO, Vallittu PK & Lassilab LV. 2011 The effect of high fiber fraction on some mechanical properties of unidirectional glass fiber-reinforced composite. Dental Materials 2 7: 313–321

Ausiello P, Franciosa P, Martorelli M & Watts D C. 2011Numerical fatigue 3D-FE modeling of indirect composite-restored posterior teeth. dental materials 2 7 423–430

Badakar C.M., Shashibhushan k k, Naik N.S. & Subba Reddy V.V. 2011 Fracture resistance of microhybrid composite, nano composite and fibre-reinforced composite used for incisal edge restoration Dental Traumatology 27: 225–229

Bagis B, Satiroglu I, Korkmaz FM & Ates SM. 2010. Rehabilitation of an extracted anterior tooth space using fiber-reinforced composite and the natural tooth. Dent Traumatol 26:191–4

Deepak S, Garg S, Sheoran N, Swami S & Singh G. 2011 Multidisciplinary approach to the rehabilitation of a tooth with two trauma episodes: systematic review and report of a case. Dental Traumatol 27: 321–326

Fennis WMM, Kreulen C.M., Wolke J.G.C., Fokkinga W.A., C. Machado C. & N.H.J. Creugers N.H.J. 2009 Fracture resistance of reattached incisor fragments with mini fibre-reinforced composite anchors. Journal of Dentistry 37: 462–467

Ganesh M &Tandon S. 2006 Versatility of Ribbond in contemporary dental practice trends biomater. Artif Organs 20:53–8.

Gollner P, Jung BA, Wehrbein H, Liechti T. New method of temporary rehabilitation after traumatic tooth loss in a juvenile patient: a case report. Dent Traumatol 2009;25:238–41.

Jongsma L.A., Kleverlaan C.J & Feilzer A.J. Clinical success and survival of indirect resin composite crowns: Results of a 3-year prospective study. Dental Materials 2012: 28 : 952–960

Loomans B.A.C., Cardoso M.V., Roeters F.J.M., Opdam N.J.M., De Munck J., Huysmans J.M. & Van Meerbeek B. Is there one optimal repair technique for all composites? Dental Materials 2011: 27: 701–709

Maneenuta C, Sakoolnamarkaa R & Tyasb MJ. 2011. The repair potential of resin composite materials. Dental Materials: 27: e20–e27

Nganga S, Zhang D, Moritz N, Vallittu P K & Hupa L. 2012. Multi-layer porous fiber-reinforced composites for implants: In vitro calcium phosphate formation in the presence of bioactive glass. Dental Materials 28: 1134–1145

Pissiotis A, Vanderas AP & Papagiannoulis L. 2007. Longitudinal study on types of injury, complications and treatment in permanent traumatized teeth with single and multiple dental trauma episodes. Dental Traumatology 23:222–5.

Şen B H, Özer S Y, Kaya S & Adıgüzel Ö. 2011 Influence of Fiber-reinforced Composites on the Resistance to Fracture of Vertically Fractured and Reattached Fragments. Journal of Endodontic 37: 549–53

Tayab T, Vizhi K & Srinivasan I. 2010 Space maintainer using fiber-reinforced composite and natural tooth – a non-invasive technique Dental Traumatology 27: 159–162.

Watanabe H, Khera SC, Vargas MA, Qian F. 2008 Fracture toughness comparison of six resin composites. Dental Materials 24:418–25.

Wolff D, Geiger S, Ding P, Staehle HJ & Frese C. 2012 Analysis of the interdiffusion of resin monomers into pre-polymerized fiber-reinforced composites. Dental Materials d 2 8: 541–547

Biodental Engineering II – Natal Jorge et al (Eds)
© 2014 Taylor & Francis Group, London, ISBN 978-1-138-00131-2

Biomaterials in critical-size bone defects: pointers for a standardized analysis

M.C. Manzanares & P. Carvalho
Human Anatomy and Embryology Unit, HUBc-Bellvitge, University of Barcelona

O. Torres
Escola de Medicina Dentària, Instituto Superior de Ciències da Saùde – Norte, CESPU, Portugal

B. González, A. Fuertes, S. Arroyo & J.J. Echeverría
Department of Odontostomatology, HUBc-Bellvitge, University of Barcelona

ABSTRACT: Critical size defects are frequently used to study the osteointegration of biomaterials. However, there is an enormous dispersion on the methods aplied both for its assessment. Critical-size bone defects in the internal surface of rabbit tibia are proposed as a standardized methodology for both a quantitative and a qualitative analysis of the osteointegration of biomaterials.

1 INTRODUCTION

Critical-size bone defects are a well-established method to analyze the resorption, the osteoconduction and the bone architecture in biomaterial science. However, the methodology used to quantitatively assess bone formation in the defects is very variable. The use of different species is reported: mice (Manassero et al, 2012; Zwingenberger et al, 2012), rat (An et al, 2012; Pisciotta et al, 2012), rabbit (Soffer et al, 2005; Savarino et al, 2007; Calvo-Guirado et al, 2011) and pig (López-López et al, 2009). The bones employed can be of mesenchymal origin, such as calvaria (An et al, 2012; Pisciotta et al, 2012; Gomes et al, 2012) and mandible (López-López et al, 2009) or endochondral bones, such as femur (Soffer et al, 2005; Savarino et al, 2007) and tibia (Calvo-Guirado et al, 2011). Moreover, the size itself of the osseous defect, and its position respect to the anatomical bone structure, as well as the observation technique and the quantification method applied differ for each study. Our group has devised a standardized procedure to assess both quantitatively and qualitatively the bone regeneration around biomaterials in critical-size defects in rabbit tibia.

2 MATERIAL AND METHODS

The study protocol was approved by the University of Barcelona Animal Experimentation Ethics Committee (Reference DMAH-4621, CEEA, UB).

2.1 *Experimental animals*

Two groups of New Zealand White adult rabbits, weighing 3.48+/−0.2 kg were submitted to an experimental surgery protocol. In the first group ($N = 8$), critical size defects were drilled in the internal surface of the right tibia. In the second group ($N = 12$), the defects were drilled alternatively in the right tibial or in the right femoral internal surface. The animals were kept in individual cages and were fed and watered *ad libitum*.

2.2 *Surgical procedure*

The animals received an intramuscular injection of Ketolar® (40 mg/kg) and Xilacina® (5 mg/kg). An intravenous access was opened via a 22G teflon cannula into the marginal auricular vein, in order to maintain the anesthesia with new dosis of Ketolar if needed. Moreover, 0.02 ml of Buprex® were injected subcutaneously (0.005 mg/kg) to obtain intra-operatory analgesia. The skin was shaved and washed with 1.5% aqueous chlorhexidine digluconate. The tibial defects, 6 mm in diameter, were created using trephine surgical drills at a low speed with constant serum irrigation. Two defects, separated by a standardized distance of 8 mm, were performed in the proximal diaphyseal internal surface, after carefully dissecting the skin and the periosteal layers to the animals of the first group (Fig. 1); only one defect was performed in the tibiae of the second group of animals. The femoral 6 mm diameter defects were performed in the distal internal femoral surface, near the femoral condyle, and

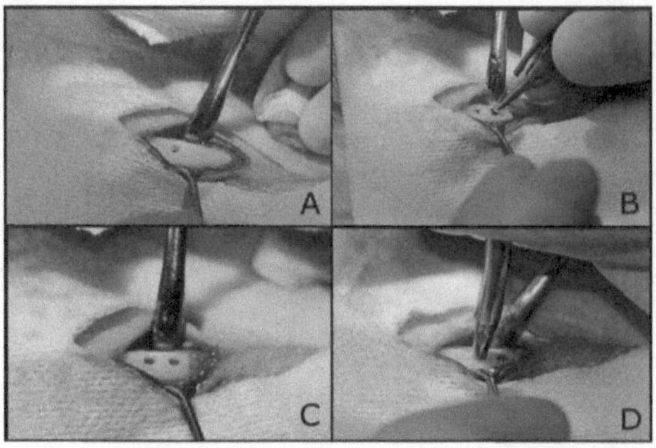

Figure 1. Surgical procedure in the rabbit tibia: A: drilling of the first defect; B: drilling of the control defect; C: assessment of the 8 mm distance between the defects; D: filling of the biomaterial.

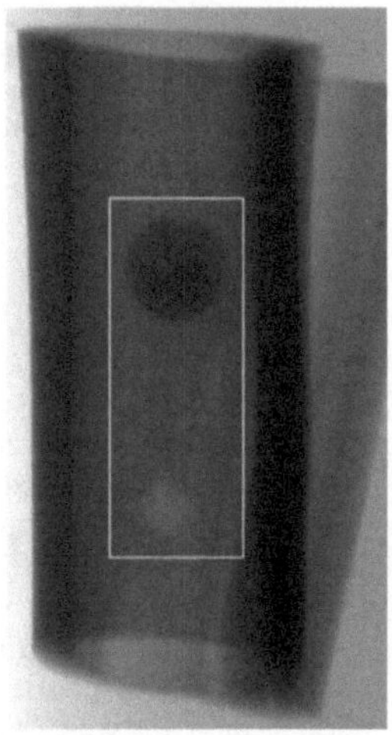

Figure 2. MicroCT of a tibial diaphysis: selection of the Region of Interest (ROI).

required the section of a muscular layer before the dissection of the periosteum. In the first group, the tibial proximal defect was filled with Mineral Trioxide Aggregate (MTA), while the distal did not receive any filling and was used as a control. In the second group, both the tibiial and the femoral defects were filled with a composite bone graft material (BoneC®).

2.3 *Imaging analysis*

The tibial diaphysis of the first group animals were fixed in 4% neutral formalin and submitted to microCT observation. After determining the Region of Interest (ROI) the tibial diaphysis (Fig. 2), were scanned individually in a Skyscan 1076®. The micro-CT settings for the images were 70 kV and 139 μA, with a rotation step of 180° and the image was voxel size 20 μm; the scan duration was approximately 28 min.

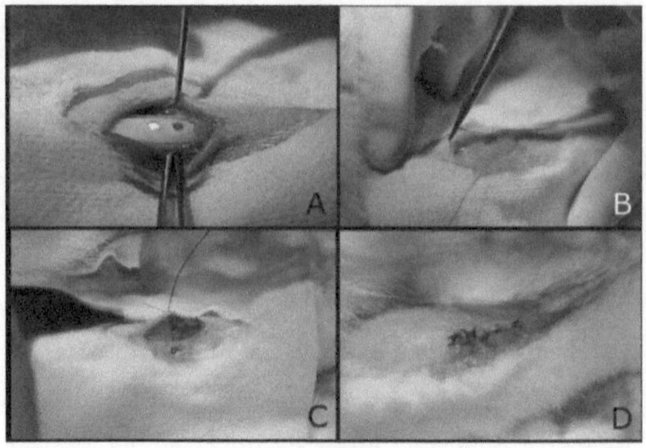

Figure 3. Surgical procedure in the rabbit tibia: A: assessment of the filling of the first defect; B: suture of the periosteal layer; C: suture of the skin; D: washing with antiseptic solution.

2.4 *Preparation of the specimens for backscattered electron microscopy (BSE-SEM)*

All the operated bones were included in ligth-cured resins without decalcification as described by López-López et al (2009) to obtain sections cut perpendicular to the long axis to be submitted to Backscattered Scanning Electron Microscopic (BS-SEM). The scanning electron microscope (LEO 200, LEO Electron Microscopy Ltd., Cambridge, England) was operated at 20 kV and 1 mA at a constant working distance (BSE Detector, Type 202, K.E. Developments Ltd., Cambridge, England) in line with our previous studies (Manresa et al, 2013).

3 RESULTS

The surgical procedure was simpler in the tibiae than in the femora due to the morphology of the bone surface, flat in the tibia, curved in the femur. Moreover, the femoral intervention required the incision of a muscular layer. The management and the loading of the biomaterials as well as the control of the diameter of the tibial defects and their distance were thus easier to assess (Fig. 3).

The Micro-CT analysis permits to assess the repair process in the control defect as compared with the operated one.

However, the information about the calcified tissues involved with the osteointegration of the biomaterials was not obtained by this method since it only permits to distinguish between the material-filled lesions from the control ones by means of the X-ray mode (Fig. 4) and the section mode (Fig. 5). The section mode is useful to assess the degree of refilling of the cortical defect, even if the exact nature of the tissues involved in not clearly distinguishable.

The most effective method to observe the osseous tissues involved in the recovering of a cortical defect, either with or without a regenerative material is the

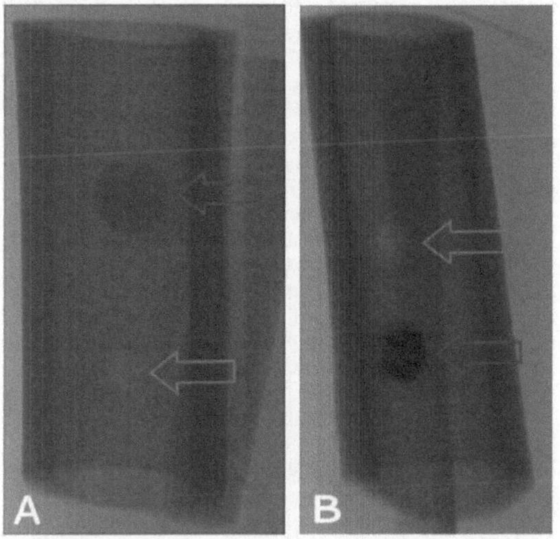

Figure 4. X-Ray mode of the MicroCT: A and B: assessment of the bone defects in the tibial dyaphysis. Red arrow: control lesion; Blue arrow: biomaterial-filled lesion.

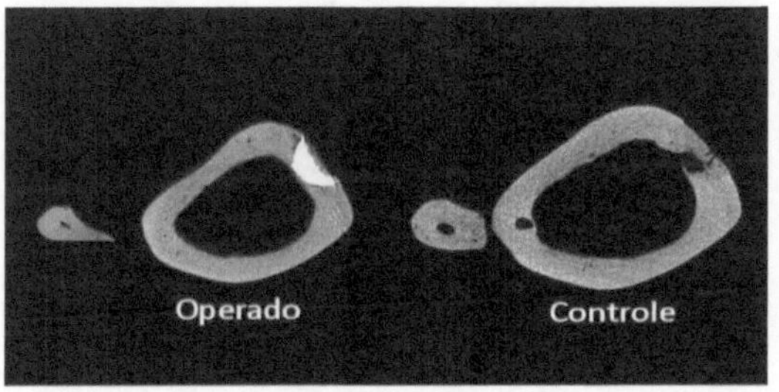

Figure 5. Sectionnal mode of the MicroCT: assessment of the bone defects in the tibial diaphysis. Operado: biomaterial-filled lesion; Controle: control lesion.

BS-SEM (Fig. 6) as suggested by López-Heredia et al (2012), because it offers a morphological observation added to a chemical characterization of the tissues involved by means of EDX microanalysis.

The differences of the femoral (Fig. 7A) and the tibial (Fig. 7B) anatomy explain the different localization of the biomaterial in their respective bone walls. The higher magnifications visible in Figure 8A and B illustrate the difficulties to apply to the BS-SEM femoral images an automatic quantification method such as the one described by Manresa et al (*in press*).

Those difficulties are due to the variations in the contact between the cortical osseous tissues and the biomaterial as visible in Figure 8. Moreover, the standardization of the morphometry parameters, such as the biomaterial particles size and number, requires the selection of a homogeneous Region of Interest (ROI).

The selection of the ROI and the morphometric study are easier in a regular, flat cortical wall such as the tibial one (Fig. 8A).

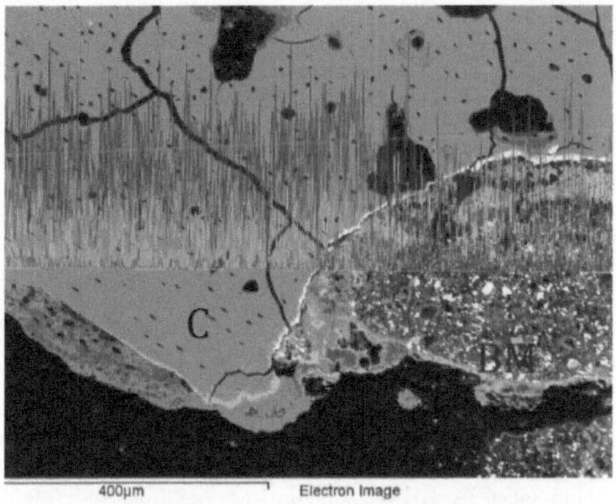

Figure 6. BS-SEM of a section of the tibial diaphysis. C: pre-existing cortical lamellar bone tissue; BM: biomaterial. The color lines correspond to the EDX analysis.

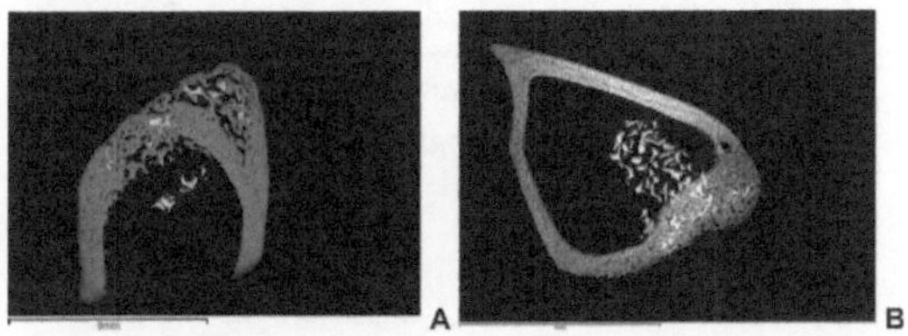

Figure 7. BS-SEM observation of an operated femur (A) compared with a tibia (B).

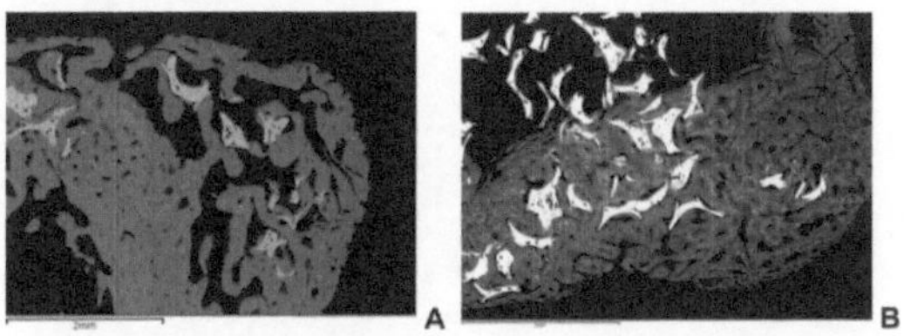

Figure 8. BS-SEM observation at a higher magnification tan in Figure 7. A: operated femur; B: operated tibia.

4 CONCLUSIONS

Critical-size defects in the tibial internal surface are an easily reproductible and fiable model for both a qualitative (MicroCT, BS-SEM, Histology) and quantitative assessment (Histomorphometry, Microanalysis) of the osteointegration of biomaterials when carried out in a standardized manner.

REFERENCES

An SH., Matsumoto, T., Miyajima, H., Nakahira, A., Kim K-H. & Imazato, S. 2012. Porous zirconia/hydroxyapatite scaffolds for bone reconstruction. *Dental Materials*, 28, 1221–1231.

Calvo-Guirado, J. L., Delgado-Ruız, R. A., Ramirez-Fernandez, M. P., Mate-Sanchez, J. E., Ortiz-Ruiz, A. & Marcus, A. 2011. Histomorphometric and mineral degradation study of Ossceram s: a novel biphasic B-tricalcium phosphate, in critical size defects in rabbits. *Clinical Oral Implant Research* 23: 667–675.

Gomes, S.P., Deliberador, T.P., Gonzaga, C.C., Klug, L.G., da Costa Oliveira, L., de Andrade Urban, C., Zielak, J.C. & Giovanini, A.F. 2012. *The Journal of Craniofacial Surgery*, 23, (5): 1239–1244.

Lopez-Heredia, M.A., Bongio, M., Cuijpers, V.M.J.I., van Dijk, N.W.M., van den Beucken, J.J.J.P., Wolke, J.G.C. & Jansen, J.A. 2012. Bone Formation Analysis: Effect of Quantification Procedures on the Study Outcome. *Tissue Engineering: Part C*. 18 (5) 369–373.

López-López, J., Chimenos-Küstner, E., Manzanares-Céspedes, M.C., Muñoz-Sánchez, J., Castañeda-Vega, P., Jané-Salas, E., Álvarez-López, J-M. & Gimeno-Sandig, A. 2009. Histomorphological study of the bone regeneration capacity of platelet-rich plasma, bone marrow and tricalcium phosphate Experimental study on pigs. *Medicina Oral Patologia Oral Cirugia Bucal*. Dec 1; 14 (12):e620–7.

Manassero, M., Viateau, V., Matthys, R., Deschepper, M., Vallefuoco, R., Bensidhoum M. & Petite, H. 2012. A Novel Murine Femoral Segmental Critical-Sized Defect Model Stabilized by Plate Osteosynthesis for Bone Tissue Engineering Purposes. *Tissue Engineering: Part C*. 19 (4) 1–10.

Manresa, C., Bosch, M., Manzanares, M.C., Carvalho, P. & Echeverria, J.J. 2013. A new standardized-automatic method for Bone-to-Implant-Contact histomorphometric analysis based on Backscattered Scanning Electron Microscopy images. *Clinical Oral Implants Research*, in press.

Pisciotta, A., Riccio, M., Carnevale, G., Beretti, F., Gibellini, L., Maraldi, T., Cavallini, G.M., Ferrari, A., Bruzzesi, G. & De Pol, A. 2012. Human Serum Promotes Osteogenic Differentiation of Human Dental Pulp Stem Cells In Vitro and In Vivo. *PLOS One*, 7 (11), e50542.

Savarino, L. Baldinia, N. Grecoa, M. Capitanic, O. Pinnac, S. Valentinic, S. Lombardo, B., Esposito, M.T., Pastore, L. Ambrosio, L., Battistab, S. Causab, F. Zeppetelli, S. Guarino, V., Netti, P.A. 2007. The performance of poly-e-caprolactone scaffolds in a rabbit femur model with and without autologous stromal cells and BMP4. *Biomaterials* 28 :3101–3109.

Soffer, E., Ouhayoun, J.P., Meunier, A. & Anagnostou, F. 2006. Effects of Autologous Platelet Lysates on Ceramic Particle Resorption and New Bone Formation in Critical Size Defects: The Role of Anatomical Sites. *Journal of Biomedical Materials Research Part B: Applied Biomaterials*. DOI: 10.1002/jbm.b.30516.

Zwingenberger, M., Niederlohmann, E., Vater, C., Rammelt, S., Matthys, R., Bernhardt, R., Valladares, R.D., Goodman, S.B. & Stiehler, M. 2012. Establishment of a femoral critical-size bone defect model in immunodeficient mice. *Journal of Surgical Research*, In press.

Biodental Engineering II – Natal Jorge et al (Eds)
© 2014 Taylor & Francis Group, London, ISBN 978-1-138-00131-2

Fluorescence *versus* confocal microscopy for the assessment of bone remodelling

P. Carvalho & B. Gallardo
Human Anatomy and Embryology Unit, HUBc-Bellvitge, University of Barcelona

M. Bosch
Scientific and Technological Centers, University of Barcelona

S. Arroyo
Department of Odontostomatology, HUBc-Bellvitge, University of Barcelona

M.C. Manzanares
Human Anatomy and Embryology Unit, HUBc-Bellvitge, University of Barcelona

ABSTRACT: The use of fluorochromes allows the assessment of the timing and the localization of the bone remodelling process. However, there is neither a standard procedure (dosage, timing, selection of the fluorochromes) nor a comparison between the results obtained with fluorescence and the ones obtained with confocal microscopy. The objective of our study is to establish an effective standard protocol of labelling injections and observation for the assessment of bone remodelling.

1 INTRODUCTION

The injection of calcium-binding fluorescent dyes is a well-established method to label the different stages of bone remodelling. The chelating fluorochromes and their dosages as well as their recommended sequence for *in vivo* administration were described by Rahn (1977). The methodology used to assess bone remodelling by fluorochrome labelling differs if the observation is carried out by fluorescence (Lee et al, 2003; O'Brien et al, 2007; Pautke et al, 2005, 2010; Lee et al, 2010; Cacchioli et al, 2011) or by confocal microscopy (Jones et al, 2005; Maggiano et al, 2006; Smith et al, 2006; Pilloli et al, 2008, Manresa et al, 2013). However, as reported by Van Gaalen et al (2010), despite the fact that this labelling technique has been used for years in bone tissue studies, it lacks a standardized protocol. Moreover no studies have been carried out to compare both observation methods.

The objective of our study is to establish an effective standard protocol of fluorochrom injection and observation for the assessment of bone remodelling by comparing the fluorescence and the confocal microscopy observation in the same sample series.

2 MATERIAL AND METHODS

2.1 *Experimental animal*

An adult female wistar rat, weighing 828 gr was submitted to an experimental surgery protocol. The study protocol was approved by the University of Barcelona Animal Experimentation Ethics Committee (Reference DAAM-6470, CEEA, UB).

2.2 *Surgical procedure*

An experimental lesion was made in the internal surface of the right tibia. Afterwards, the periosteum and the fascial and skin planes were repaired with resorbable sutures. The protocol for intraperitoneal injections of the fluorochromes started on day 0, with 7-days intervals, by using successively Doxycyclin® (1 mgr/kg), Xylenol Orange (1.5 mgr/kg), GreenCalcein (5 mgr/kg), a second dosis of Doxycyclin® (15 mgr/kg) and finally BlueCalcein (2 mgr/kg). The animal was kept in an individual cage and was fed and watered *ad libitum*. The animal was sacrificed by anesthetic overdose six weeks after the surgery.

2.3 *Preparation and observation of the specimens*

Both tibiae were recovered and included in ligth-cured resins without decalcification as described by López-López et al (2009) to obtain sections cut perpendicular to the tibial long axis, to be submitted successively to fluorescence and confocal microscopy observation, following the excitation and emission curves described by Lee et al (2010).

3 RESULTS

The first observation series showed that all the markers were visible with both fuorescence microscopy (Fig. 1) and confocal microscopy (Figs 2 and 3). The first labelling signal, however, was very feeble, probably due to the low dose of doxycyclin injected in the postoperatory period.

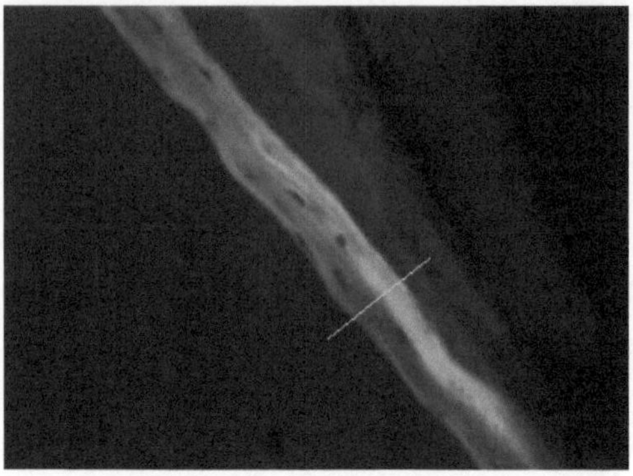

Figure 1. Fluorescence microscopy image of the operated tibial wall (×50). The first visible marker in the table is orange, followed by green calcein, and two blue markers (calcein and doxyciclin). White line: measurement line for the plot in Table 1.

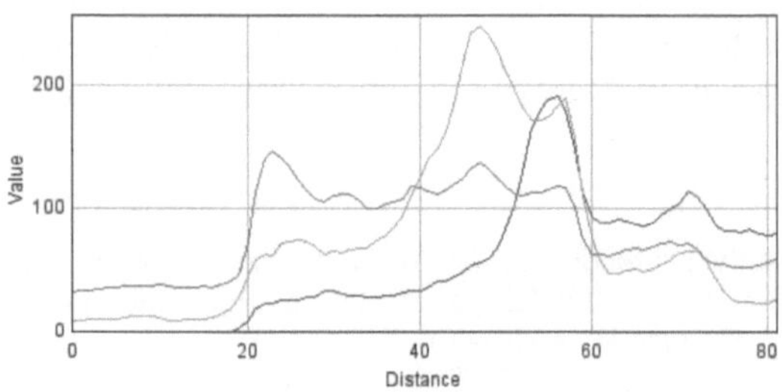

Table 1. Plot of signals along the line (right) of the operated tibial wall in Figure 1.

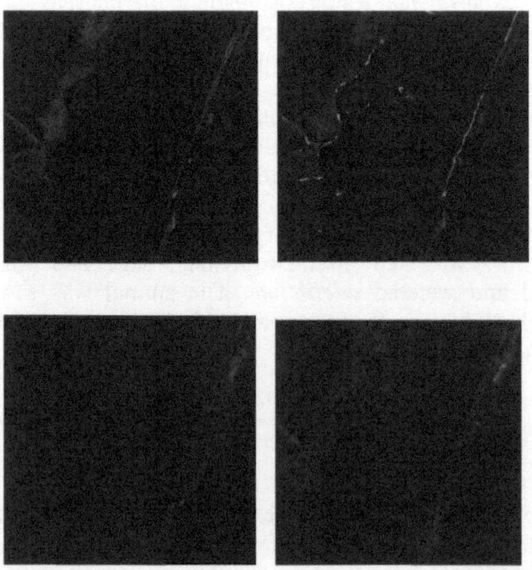

Figure 2. Confocal microscopy images of the operated tibial wall (×50) Isolated labels. The first visible marker in the table is orange, followed by green calcein, and the two blue markers (blue calcein and doxyciclin).

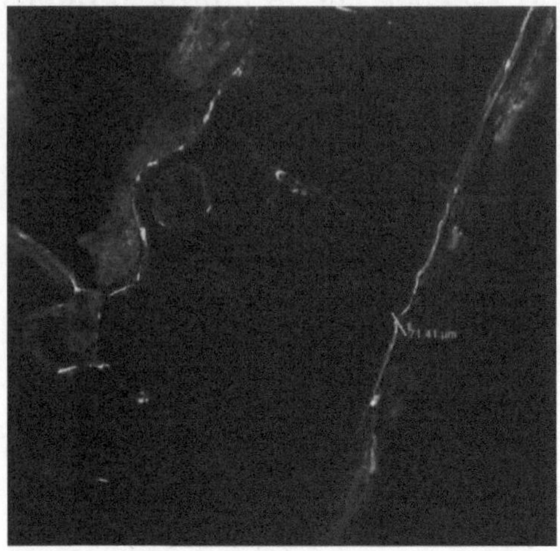

Figure 3. Snapshot of all the successive markers reproduced in Figure 2. Operated tibial wall (×50).

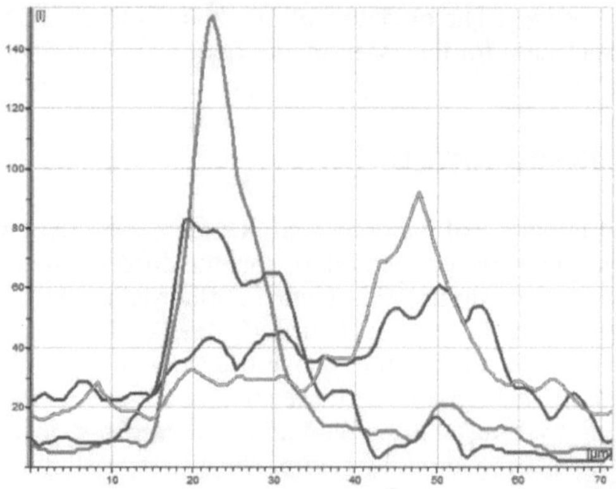

Table 2. Plot of signals along the line (left = 71.41 μm) of the operated tibial wall in Figure 3.

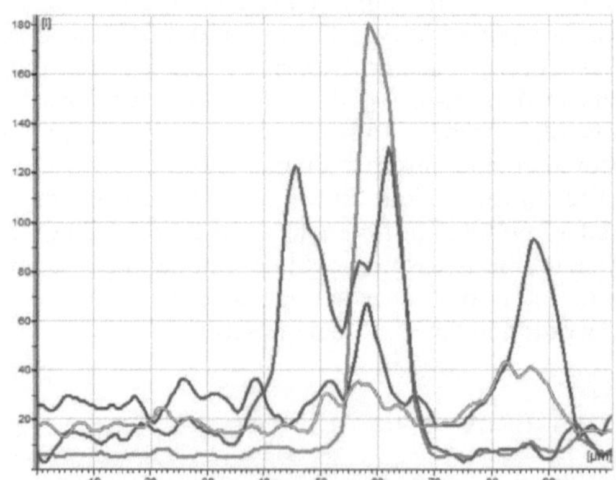

Table 3. Plot of signals along the line (right = 100.08 μm) of the operated tibial wall in Figure 3.

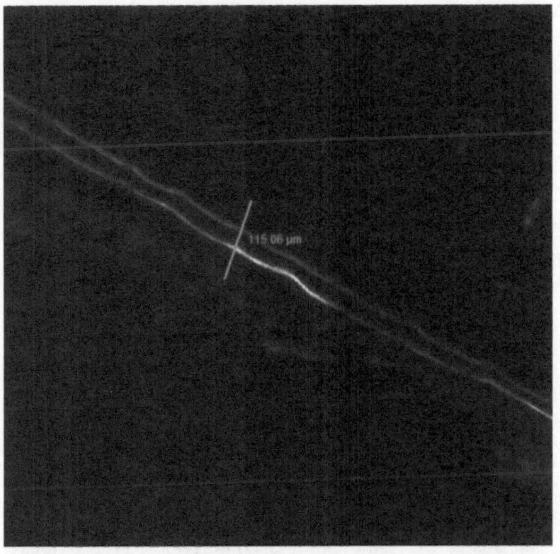

Figure 4. Confocal microscopy image of the non-operated tibial cortical. The lines corresponding to the first and the last visible markers show the difference in the bone apposition between the surgery and the sacrifice.

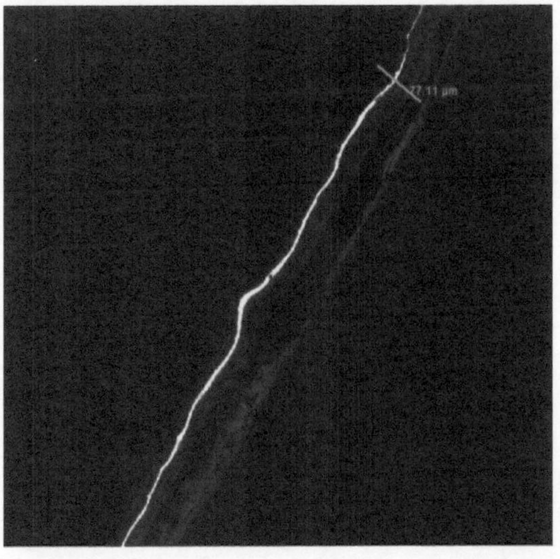

Figure 5. Confocal microscopy image of the operated tibial cortical. The lines corresponding to the first and the last visible markers show the difference in the bone apposition between the surgery and the sacrifice.

Confocal microscopy detects only the light emitted from the focal plane of the sample (Figs 2 and 3), thus increasing the accuracy and the fiability of the measurements.

Consequently, the lines corresponding to a particular marker can be selected and their distances measured with a higher degree of precision.

The possibility of selecting each labelling fluorochrome emission line in confocal microcopy can be useful to compare the bone remodellation in two samples. When comparing the concentric lines of bone remodelling of the tibial diaphysis in the operated respect to the non-operated side, an obvious difference was observed.

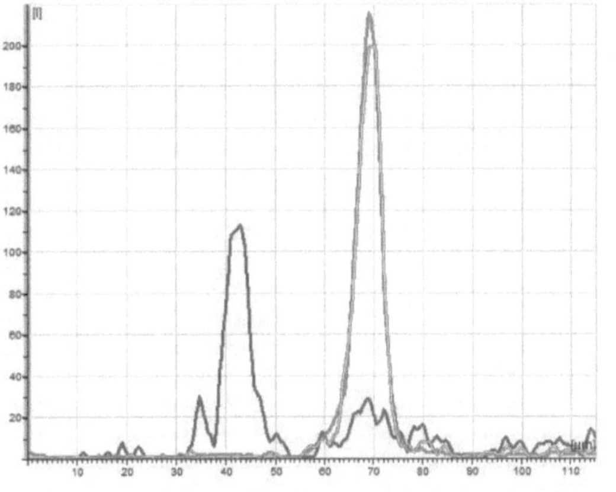

Table 4. Plot of the operated tibia corresponding to the confocal image in Fig. 4. The peaks of the first and the last visible markers show the difference in the bone apposition between the surgery and the sacrifice.

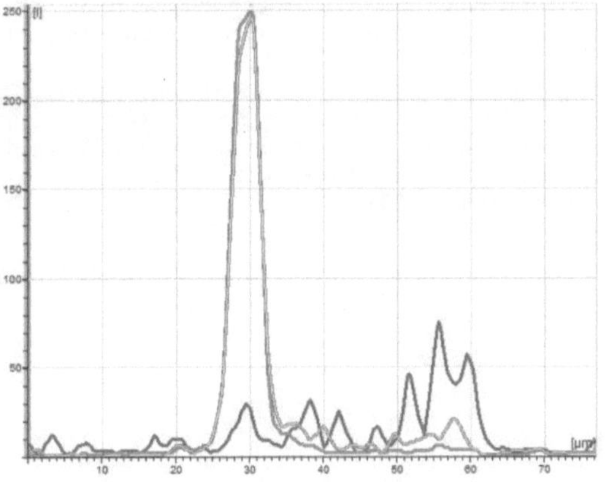

Table 5. Plot of the non-operated tibia corresponding to the confocal image in Fig. 5. The peaks of the first and the last visible markers show the difference in the bone apposition between the surgery and the sacrifice.

The distance between the first and the last labelling line is higher in the non-operated side, when measured by the plots representing the selected fluorochrome lines (Tables 4 and 5).

4 CONCLUSIONS

The standardized method of fluorochrome staining together with confocal microscopy observation permits a more precise assessment of the bone remodelling in undecalcified samples.

REFERENCES

Cacchioli, A., Ravanetti, F., Soliani, L. & Borghetti P. 2011. Preliminary Study on the Mineral Apposition Rate in distal femoral epiphysis of New Zealand White Rabbit at Skeletal Maturity. An*atomy Histology Embryology*. 41:163–169.

Jones CW, Smolinski D, Keogh A, et al. (2005) Confocal laser scanning microscopy in orthopaedic research. *Progress Histochemistry Cytochemistry* 40, 1–71.

Lee, T. C., Mohsin, S., Taylor, D., Parkesh, R., Gunnlaugsson, T., O'Brien, F. J., Giehl, M. & Gowin, W. 2003. Detecting microdamage in bone. *Journal of Anatomy*, 203: 161–172.

Lee J, Decker JF, Polimeni G, Cortella CA, Rohrer MD, Wozney JM, Hall J, Susin C, Wikesjö UME. 2010. Evaluation of implants coated with rhBMP-2 using two different coating strategies: a critical-size supraalveolar peri-implant defect study in dogs. *Journal of Clinical Periodontology*.37: 582–590.

López-López, J., Chimenos-Küstner, E., Manzanares-Céspedes, M.C., Muñoz-Sánchez, J., Castañeda-Vega, P., Jané-Salas, E., Álvarez-López, J-M. & Gimeno-Sandig, A. 2009. Histomorphological study of the bone regeneration capacity of platelet-rich plasma, bone marrow and tricalcium phosphate Experimental study on pigs. *Medicina Oral Patologia Oral Cirugia Bucal*. Dec 1;14 (12):e620–7.

Maggiano, C., Dupras, T., Schultz, M., and Biggerstaff, J. Spectral and photobleaching analysis using confocal laser scanning microscopy: a comparison of modern and archaeological bone fluorescence. *Molecular and Cell Probes* 20, 154, 2006.

Manresa, C., Bosch, M., Manzanares, M.C., Carvalho, P. & Echeverria, J.J. 2013. A new standardized-automatic method for Bone-to-Implant-Contact histomorphometric analysis based on Backscattered Scanning Electron Microscopy images. *Clinical Oral Implants Research*, in press.

O'Brien, F.J., Taylor, D. & Lee, T.C. 2007. Bone as a composite material: The role of osteons as barriers to crack growth in compact bone. *International Journal of Fatigue* 29: 1051–1056.

Pautke, C., Vogt, S., Tischer, T., Wexel, G., Deppe, H., Milz, S., Schieker, M. & Kolk, A. 2005. Polychrome labeling of bone with seven different fluorochromes: Enhancing fluorochrome discrimination by spectral image analysis. *Bone* 37: 441–445.

Pautke, C., Vogt, S., Kreutzer, K, Hackzek, C., Wexel, G., Kolk, A., Imhoff A., Zitzelsberger, H., Milz, S., & Tischer, T. 2010. Characterization of eight different tetracyclines: advances in fluorescence bone labeling. *Journal of Anatomy* 217: 76–82.

Pilolli GP, Lucchese A, Maiorano E, et al. 2008. New approach for static bone histomorphometry: confocal laser scanning microscopy of maxillo-facial normal bone. *Ultrastructural Pathology* 32, 189–192.

Rahn B. 1976. Die polychrome Sequenzmarkierung Intravitale Zeitmarkierung zur tierexperimentellen Analyse der Knochenund Dentinbildung. Freiburg: Habilitationsschrift.

van Gaalen, S.M., Kruy, M. C., Geuze, R. E., de Bruijn, J.D., Alblas J, & Dhert, W. J.A. 2010. Use of Fluorochrome Labels in In Vivo Bone Tissue Engineering Research *Tissue Engineering: Part B*, 16 (2) 209–217.

Biodental Engineering II – Natal Jorge et al (Eds)
© 2014 Taylor & Francis Group, London, ISBN 978-1-138-00131-2

Evaluation of the mechanical environment of the median palatine suture during rapid maxillary expansion

Larissa Carvalho Trojan Serpe & Libardo Andrés González-Torres
Departamento de Engenharia de Estruturas, Universidade Federal de Minas Gerais, Brazil

Ricardo Luiz Utsch
Departamento de Engenharia Mecânica, Universidade Federal de Minas Gerais, Brazil

Ana Claudia Moreira Melo
Instituto Latino Americano de Pesquisa e Ensino Odontológico – Curitiba/PR, Brazil

Estevam Barbosa de Las Casas
Departamento de Engenharia de Estruturas, Universidade Federal de Minas Gerais, Brazil

ABSTRACT: Rapid Maxillary Expansion (RME) is a common procedure in the dental practice, indicated to increase the perimeter of the dental arch by means of opening the Median Palatine Suture (MPS). The manner how the separation of MPS occurs depends on the level of resistance that it presents along its length. Due to the loads the sutures have to support during RME, they experience a remodelling process also present in the maxillary and alveolar bone. In this work we study the mechanical environment generated in the MPS under orthopaedic and normal loads using a computational approach; our objective is to evaluate the mechanical environment generated inside MPS during RME. With this study we want to improve in the understanding of the role of the stiffness of cranial sutures connected to maxilla in RME and to examine the significance of orthopaedic and normal loads experienced by the maxilla during the treatment. Two different three-dimensional models have been considered for tests, one simplified and another with realistic (obtained from CT images) geometries. Some similar results were obtained for the simplified and the realistic geometries of the maxilla. We obtained the typical inverted V shape of MPS and also observed that the two kinds of loads applied to maxilla affected importantly the mechanical environment in the MPS. Finally, we concluded that during the REM, sutures connected to maxilla have an important role for the opening of the maxilla and also for the mechanical environment generated in the MPS. The changes in mechanical environment generated in the MPS during expansion and mastication were significant, for this reason, both forces have to be considered to study the MPS during the RME.

Keywords: Rapid Maxillary Expansion, Structural Analyses, Finite Element Model, Median Palatine Suture, Palatal Expander

1 INTRODUCTION

Rapid maxillary expansion (RME) is a common procedure in dental practice since the mid 1960s (Lagravere et al. 2006). This approach provides an increase in bone mass of the upper dental arch (Byrum Jr. 1971, Gardner and Kronman 1971, Haas 1973, Haas 1970, Wertz 1970) and increases the dental arch perimeter by applying lateral forces on superior posterior tooth (Townend 1980). The main recommendation to apply RME is an atresic upper dental arch (with triangular shape) associated to an incorrect buccolingual position of the posterior teeth (Fig. 1), which generally results in a posterior cross-bite malocclusion (Capelozza-Filho & Silva-Filho 1997).

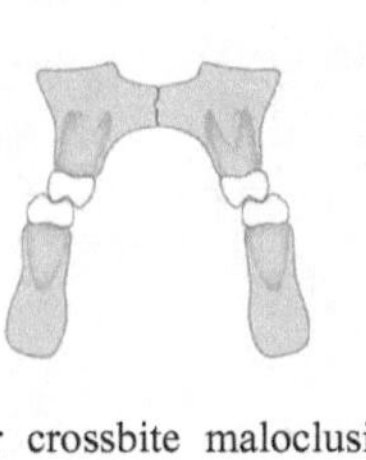

Figure 1. Posterior crossbite maloclusion (Lock et al., 2008).

The bone perimeter gain helps to correct the bone-tooth negative discrepancy or tooth crowding in the maxillary arch, irregularity frequently diagnosed in clinical practice and commonly associated with atresia of the upper dental arch. The RME corrects this situation by means of opening the junction between the two parts of the maxilla (Fig. 2), the median palatine suture (MPS). The manner

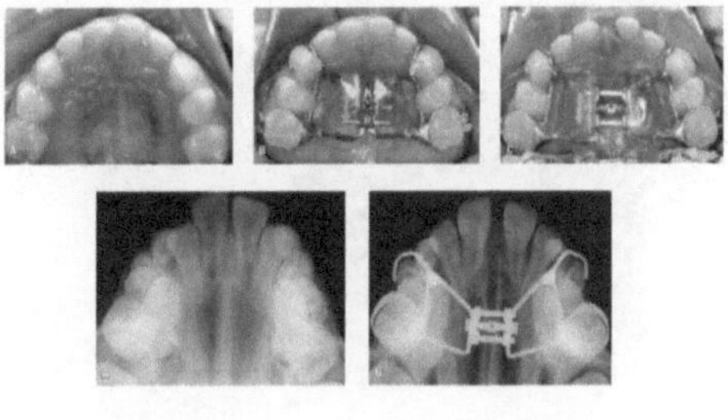

Figure 2. Rapid maxillary expansion (Silva et al., 2007).

how the separation occurs depends on the level of resistance experienced by the maxilla and MPS during opening.

The effects of RME on alveolar bone and teeth have been constantly subjected to animal studies and clinical research (Haas 1961, Haas 1970, Da Silva et al. 1991, Garib et al. 2006, Sun et al. 2011). It has been observed that the MPS itself may not be considered as the unique resistant element during RME because its obliteration rate (level of mineralization) is very low, even in elderly people (N'Guyen et al. 2007, Korbmacher et al. 2007). In clinical experiences with patients over 25 years of age, conventional RME is often difficult to achieve even when the MPS presents a small obliteration. Other factors such as a high inter-digitation of the midpalatal suture, as well as an increase of rigidity of the other maxillary sutures with age, may be the reasons for the observed resistance (Issacson & Ingram 1964, Wertz 1970). At this regard it is important to note that, during initial stages of ERM, the frontonasal, zygomaticotemporal and zygomaticomaxillary sutures show increased cellular activity (Starnbach et al. 1966). Furthermore, according to other study (Provatidis et al. 2008) the frontal part (composed of transseptal fibres) and the ossification degree of the MPS, the zygomaticomaxillary sutures and the zygomatic arch influence importantly the resistance to MPS expansion (Provatidis et al. 2008).

The suture is a fibrous joint, characterized by the union of two motionless bones, with opposing joint surfaces firmly bonded by fibrous connective tissue (Johnson & Moore 1985). Due to their slow growth, these surfaces become interdigitated and serrated, increasing the joint disjunction resistance (Melsen 1975).

Sutures are adapted to support tension loads (Enlow 1993), and absorb and transmit loads generated in natural activities (e.g. mastication) and external forces (e.g. orthopaedic forces) (Mao 2002). During RME, cranial sutures experience a remodelling process also observed in the maxillary and the alveolar bone (Ghoneima et al. 2011). Considering the MPS during growth, it is observed that maxillary bones are separated by a membrane with osteogenic activity and bone apposition. Cell death is observed mainly in the central area of the suture, which is relatively avascular and is generally associated with discrete ossification points (Ten Cate et al. 1977). The main elements that make up the sutures are osteocytic cells, fibroblasts, fibers and blood vessels (Wagemans et al. 1988).

In the simulation area, multiple studies have been performed and obtained consistent results with the tissue differentiation observed during tissues regeneration and remodelling (Isaksson et al. 2006, Lacroix & Prendergast 2002, Gomez-Benito et al. 2005). These studies correlated the new tissue that appeared with different levels of hydrostatic stress and tensile strain during the regeneration process. Thus, the use of mechanoregulatory models has increased the quantitative and qualitative understanding of how tissue remodelling and regeneration is influenced by mechanical loading (Isaksson et al. 2006), based on mechanoregulatory theories (Pauwels 1960, Perren 1979, Perren & Cordey 1980) that correlate tissue differentiation to mechanical loading. Prendergast et al. (1997) proposed a mechanoregulatory model for tissue differentiation, based on a poroelastic material model for the tissues. According to this model, the stimuli that control the differentiation process are the maximal distortional strain and the relative fluid velocity. High values of both solid strain and fluid velocity favor fibrous tissue formation, while intermediate values lead to cartilaginous tissue. Bone can be formed only if the values are sufficiently low (Geris et al. 2009).

Given the observed influence of mechanical factors on tissue regeneration and remodelling, came the need of a structural study of the maxilla to evaluate the role of mechanics in the mechanism of tissue formation. In this work we qualitatively study the MPS, to evaluate the mechanical environment present inside it during the treatment for the RME, and study if it could have some influence on the tissue formation. This study intends to improve the understanding of the role of cranial sutures connected to maxilla during RME, and other factors that generate resistance to expansion.

2 MATERIALS AND METHODS

In order to evaluate the mechanical environment (magnitude of displacements, stresses and strains) generated in the MPS under orthopaedic and normal loads, we developed computational models for two geometries representing the maxilla: the first (Fig. 3) is a simplified geometry considering the general shape and dimensions of the maxilla and its components, and just two materials (one for bone and teeth and another one for the MPS); and the second (Fig. 4) considers the real bone shape and dimensions.

The more realistic model was obtained using computed tomography (CT) images of a young man with normal occlusion. In order to develop a FE model, CT

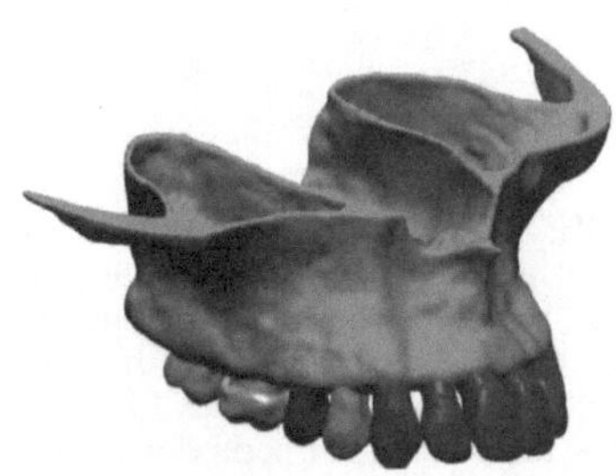

Figure 4. Realistic 3D model of maxilla.

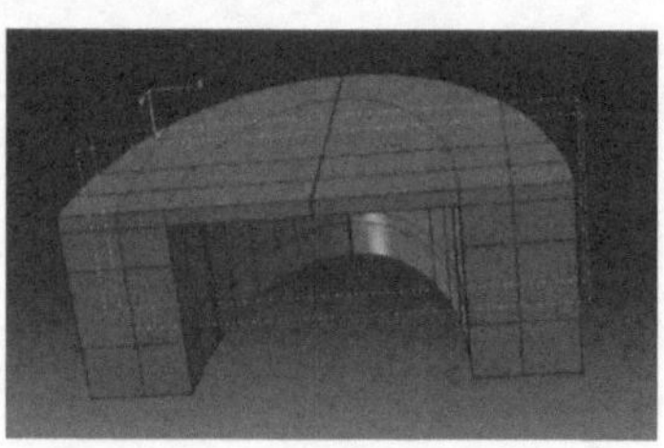

Figure 3. Simplified 3D geometry of maxilla.

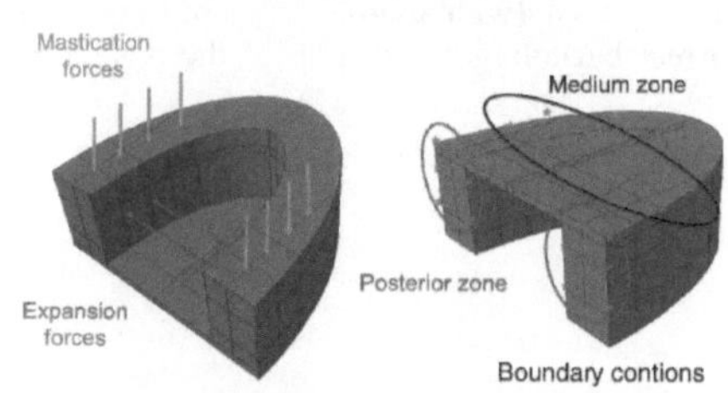

Figure 5. Boundary condition and forces applied on simplified 3D geometry of maxilla.

images in Dicom format were segmented in the software Simpleware® (Innovation Centre, Exerter, United Kingdom) to extract the 3D geometry of the maxilla in STL format. Then, this geometry was processed in the computer aided design (CAD) software SolidWorks® v19.4 (Concord, Massachusetts, USA, 1993), to correct some defects, soften the surfaces and add new features to the geometrical model. Finally, after the geometry was defined, the mesh for the finite element model was created in Ansys ICEM v11.0 (Ansys Inc., Canonsburg, PA, USA) and then imported in the computer aided engineering (CAE) software Abaqus v6.12 (Providence, Rhode Island, 1978). The whole FE model (Fig. 6) was composed of 9.450.114 tetrahedral elements and 1.653.710 nodes.

We considered isotropic homogeneous linear elastic materials for all parts. The mechanical properties considered were respectively, for elastic modulus and Poisson's ratio: stainless steel parts, 200 GPa and 0.33; bone, 10000 MPa and 0.3 (a value between trabecular and cortical bone properties); enamel, 84100 MPa and 0.33 (Jones et al. 2001); dentin, 18600 MPa and 0.3 (Jones et al. 2001); and periodontal ligament, 0.69 MPa and 0.49 (Yoshida et al. 2001).

For both models, some aspects were tested by computational analysis. Different boundary conditions were tested, considering fixed or free boundary conditions in different zones of the models (Figs. 5 and 6). These conditions represent high or low levels of constraint of maxilla due to cranial sutures, in zones fixed or free, respectively.

Regarding loading, the external (expansion) force was considered to be of approximately 36 N (Issacson & Ingram 1964) and the internal (mastication) forces of approximately 311.4 N (Widmork et al. 1995) (Figs. 5 and 6). We considered these two loading conditions because they both are present during the RME treatment and could influence the tissue remodeling in maxillary bone and suture, similarly to the remodeling process in long bones (Cowin 2001).

To take into account different states of the midpalatal suture (MPS), its elastic modulus was changed similarly to the computational study of Provatidis et al. (2008). Table 1 resumes all performed tests.

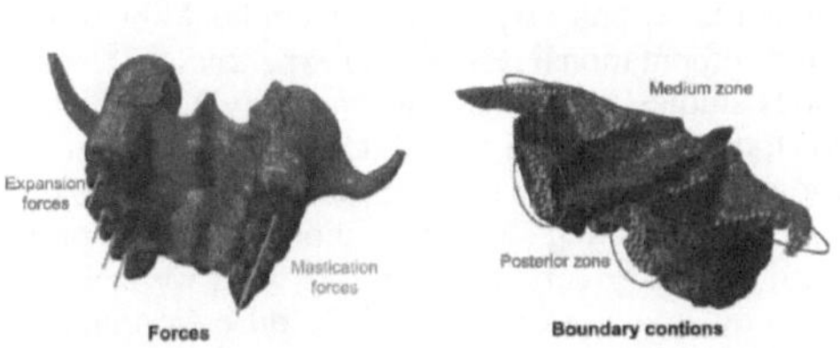

Figure 6. Boundary condition and forces applied on realistic 3D model of maxilla.

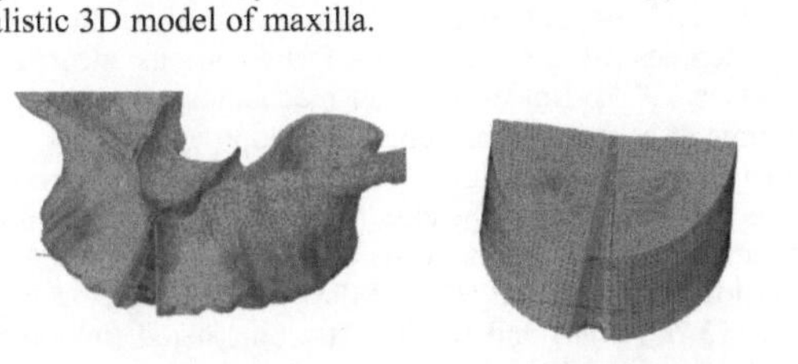

Figure 7. MPS opening with realistic and simplified 3D models. Maxilla fixed in posterior and medium zones, and MPS of 1 MPa.

3 RESULTS

The results for the simplified and the realistic geometries were computed using the FE program. We observed for both models the opening of MPS in a triangular fashion formed by the two parts of the maxilla (Fig. 7). We also observed that masticatory and expander loads applied to the maxilla affected importantly the mechanical environment of the MPS and the maxillary bone (Figs. 8 to 12).

In the case of the maxillary bone under expansion forces, we observed the stiffness of MPS affected the experienced stresses. With the least stiff suture (E = 1 Mpa), the maximum stresses in maxilla appeared at the medium zone and near to the supporting teeth, the values of the stresses at mentioned locations were above 4 MPa (Fig. 8). For the stiffest suture (E = 500 MPa), the value of maximum stresses was reduced to approximately a half of the values (above 2 MPa, Fig. 9) compared to the values for the least stiff suture. Apart from that, the posterior part of maxilla showed high levels of stresses, comparable with the maximum stresses in this second case.

The medium palatine suture was affected differently along its length by expansion forces. In general terms, the MPS was most deformed in anterior and oral zones during expansion.

For the maxilla only fixed at the posterior part, the maximum strains in flexible suture (E = 1 MPa) were above 5% at the zone anterior and oral, compared to 0.4% at the posterior zone of the suture (Fig. 10). For the stiffest suture (E = 500 MPa), the qualitative results were similar, but the value of strains was reduced to less than a half compared to the values for flexible suture. In the case of the maxilla fixed in the medium and the posterior zone, the results were similar to the maxilla only fixed at the posterior part, but the values of strains were reduced to above a half of the values of the first case (Fig. 11).

When mastication forces were considered, maximum strains were in the same order of magnitude that the ones obtained with only the expansion force. Maximum values of strains were above 9% at the anterior and nasal part of the suture and 0.8% at the anterior and oral region (Fig. 12).

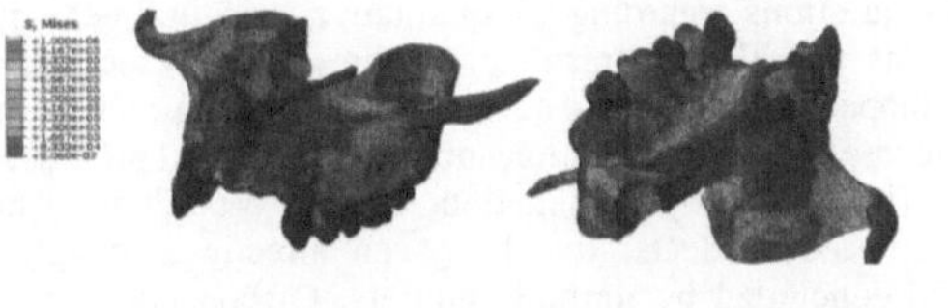

Figure 8. Von Misses stresses (in MPa) for the expanded maxilla, considering E = 1 MPa for the MPS.

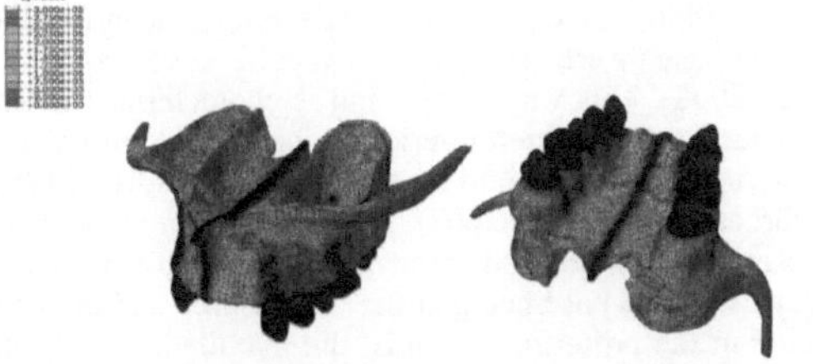

Figure 9. Von Mises stresses (in MPa) for the expanded maxilla, considering E = 500 MPa for the MPS.

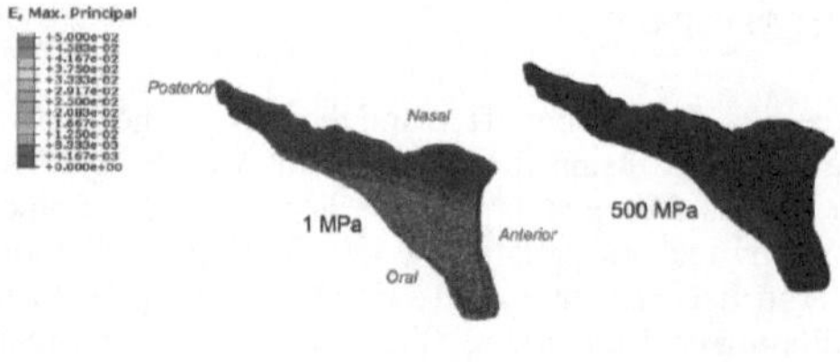

Figure 10. Maximum strains in midpalatal suture submitted to the expansion force. Maxilla only fixed in posterior zone.

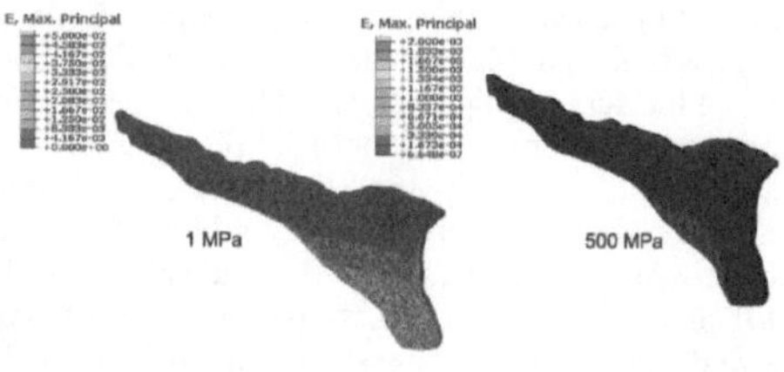

Figure 11. Maximum strains in midpalatal suture submitted to the expansion force. Maxilla fixed in posterior and medium zones.

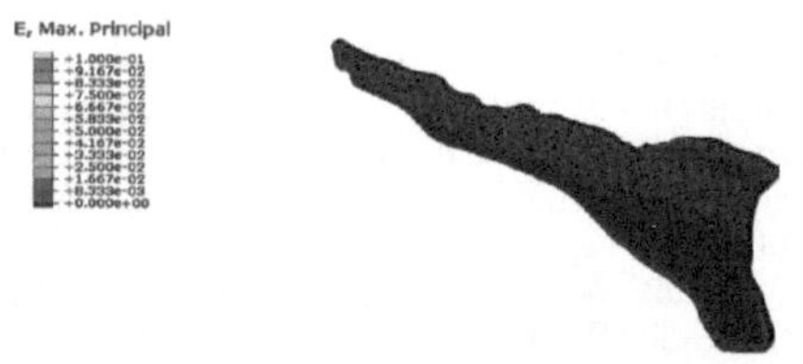

Figure 12. Maximum strains in midpalatal suture submitted to the mastication force. Maxilla fixed in posterior and medium zones, and MPS of 1 MPa.

4 DISCUSSION

This study was based on a computational analysis of a 3D finite element model of maxillary bone. The study was conducted to investigate the biomechanical effects generated on the MPS during RME. This section is aimed at discussing the questions regarding the qualitative structural behavior of the maxilla as a result of application of orthodontic-orthopaedic loads and to comment their interaction with the process of suture separation and some biological processes.

The maxillary disjunction causes orthodontic and orthopaedic effects; this has been already investigated and concluded by multiple authors. Orthopaedic effects improve the perimeter of the upper arch when MPS is opened. The triangular shape of MPS observed during expansion both anteroposteriorly and vertically may be justified because the maxilla articulates with ten different bones within the facial structure and the anterior and middle cranial base (Wertz 1970, Da Silva et al. 1995, Provatidis et al. 2008). This way of opening is characterized by the base turned to the anteroinferior region and fulcrum placed posterior superiorly (Gardner & Kronman 1971, Hass 1961, Jafari et al. 2003, Mao 2002). The results obtained with the present analysis showed the maxilla opened in a triangular shape with the base being at the incisor area and the apex being in the posterior region of the maxillae. The results corroborated those described by Jafari et al. (2003) that measured maximum displacements at the maxilla below the hard palate on the region of central incisors to the second

Table 1. Cases simulated.

Nr.	EMPS (Mpa)	Posterior BCs	Medium BCs	Anterior BCs	Mastication force (N)	Expansion force (N)	Model
1	1	Fixed	Fixed	–	0	36	Simple
2	500	Fixed	Fixed	–	0	36	Simple
3	500	Fixed	–	–	0	36	Simple
4	1	Fixed	Fixed	Fixed	311.4	0	Simple
5	1	Fixed	Fixed	–	0	36	Complex
6	500	Fixed	Fixed	–	0	36	Complex
7	500	Fixed	–	–	0	36	Complex
8	1	Fixed	Fixed	–	311.4	0	Complex
9	1	Fixed	–	–	0	36	Complex

premolars. Minimum strains were observed at the pterygoid plates close to the cranial base.

The literature suggests that posterior sutures are the main resistance for RME. The pterygoid plates of the sphenoid limited the ability of the palatine bones to separate (Haas 1961, Bishara & Staley 1987, Kudlick 1973). As the sphenoid is a single structure bilaterally placed, the pterygoid plates can only bend under the pressure of the expansion forces (Jafari et al. 2003, Holberg & Rudzki-Janson 2006). But, according to Provatidis et al. (2008) the maxillolacrymal, frontomaxillary, nasomaxillary, the transverse palatal sutures, and the suture between the maxilla and the pterygoid process of the sphenoid bone do not influence the outcome of RME. On the contrary, the zygomatico-maxillary sutures at the level of the zygomatic arch influence the response of the craniofacial complex to the expansion forces. Starnbach et al. (1966) demonstrated that, during the early phases of RME, the frontonasal, zygomaticotemporal, and zygomatico-maxillary sutures all showed signs of increased cellular activity. In the present study, the presence of pterygomaxillary sutures (on the posterior zone of maxilla) contributed to the triangular shape of MPS observed in children, and when the zygomatic sutures resistance was simulated, the triangular shape was attenuated.

The precision of the simulation depends on the accuracy with which the finite element model represents the real case. To evaluate this, the model validation should be addressed in several ways, one of them could be to compare the computational results with experimental results of previous studies, additionally a sensitivity analyses could be performed to determine which parameters are more important in the model. Different cases should be studied considering the acting loading conditions, material properties and boundary conditions. In this work we began this analysis by studying cases under the different conditions presented in Table 1.

The degree of ossification of the circummaxillary sutures of the craniofacial complex resulted in varying degrees of displacement of the various structures (Melsen 1975). Since the exact mechanical properties of sutures at each stage of human development are not well defined in the literature, Provatidis et al. (2008) compared the results with the circummaxillary sutures at three stages: when all sutures of the craniofacial complex were considered unossified ($E = 1$ MPa), when totally ossified ($E = 13\,700$ MPa) and when partly unossified (hypothetically $E = 500$ MPa). Based on this study, we considered two different stages of suture development: the first, as an unossified ($E = 1$ MPa) and the second with an intermediate ossification degree ($E = 500$ MPa). The MPS totally ossified was not considered because this stage only occurs in adults and this is not the objective on this study.

The expansion forces considered here were measured by Isaacson & Ingram (1964) using an expansion appliance with a force-measuring dynamometer between the expansion screw and the bands placed on two maxillary teeth. They measured the force for a single activation (0.25 mm of displacement for the appliance acrylic bases), which generated forces of about 3 to 10 pounds. This variation of magnitude may be affected by the resistance of the facial skeleton to expansion. After the appliance installation, with three activations applied in an interval of few minutes a force of 16 pounds could be achieved. Nevertheless, all activations produced forces that decay 10 per cent in 5–10 minutes. Based on the graphics presented by Isaacson & Ingram (1964), we estimated the forces present after one hour of the first activation and considered it in the model.

Our results showed that strains in the MPS when applied expansion forces were higher when the elastic moduli was 1 MPa (Fig. 10) for the maxilla fixed only on the posterior zone. When the fixation also included the medium zone (suggesting the participation of zygomatic sutures) the strain rate reduces (Fig. 11). But the strains concentrated in anterior and oral part of the MPS for both cases. This could explain the fact that the anterior region is related on the literature as the last region to finish the remodelling process. The new formation occurs on the bordering bones to the mid line, beginning on the posterior past of the MPS (Chang et al. 1997, Cleall et al. 1965, Melsen 1975, Ennes 2002, Werbein & Yildizhan 2001).

The masticatory forces produced strains in the same order of magnitude of the strains generated with expansion forces, but they were more concentrated in anterior and nasal part of the suture. Masticatory forces are cyclical and could be associated to the stimulus of regeneration process as occurs in long bones fractures (Gomez-Benito et al. 2005). Once the stimulus controls the tissue differentiation process, high values of both strain in the tissues and interstitial fluid velocity favor fibrous tissue formation, while intermediate values lead to cartilaginous tissue. Bone is formed only if the values are sufficiently low (Geris et al. 2009). The simplified model of maxilla was used to determine some qualitative effects of RME (Fig. 5), like shape of opening. This model may help to study this regeneration process with lower computational costs compared to more realistic models.

According to some authors (Hilton 1988, Katsaros et al. 1994, Behrents et al. 1978) the suture appears to be exceptionally sensitive in its response to mechanotransduction. As little as a change in the amount of solid food consumed or incisor extractions in animal studies led to significant changes in morphology and metabolism suture. Relation between form and function of the cranial sutures and masticatory muscles were confirmed by many authors in animal studies (Byron et al. 2004, Katsaros et al. 2006, Sun et al. 2004). Some justify their results in animal experiments in the reduction of strains in sutures caused by mechanical forces exerted by masticatory muscles.

The most significant contribution of finite element models in dental biomechanics consists in the possibility simulate real processes and try to improve in the understanding of biological processes, which is in many cases impossible in living organisms. This approach is limited because of the many variables involved, but it could importantly contribute to achieve a deeper knowledge of real biological processes with simplified models, helping to improve the clinical practice.

5 CONCLUSIONS

- A simplified model of maxilla allows to determine some qualitative effects of RME on maxilla and SPM (like shape of opening), and may help to study other factors with lower computational costs than with more realistic models.
- The mechanical changes in strain and stresses generated in the MPS during expansion and mastication are significant. For this reason, both forces should be considered to study the progress of MPS during RME.
- During REM, sutures connected to the maxilla have an important role. The presence of pterygomaxillary sutures (on the posterior zone of maxilla) contributes to the "V" shape of SPM observed in children. In addition, the stiffness of MPS affects importantly the shape and the deformation of the MPS and the level of stresses experienced in bone.
- The anterior and oral zone of MPS experiences the highest level of strains. It could explain the later regeneration of this zone during RME.
- Future studies should consider: the existence of cortical and trabecular bone in maxilla; the suture model as a more complex material (e.g. hyperelatic), considering it is formed of fibrous; the estimation of the real stiffness of cranial sutures on the mechanical environment of maxilla. The inclusion of these elements may allow estimating more realistically the mechanical environment in the MPS.

ACKNOWLEDGMENT

The authors want to thank to the Brazilian funding agency CAPES for supporting the development of the present work.

REFERENCES

Behrents, R.G. et al. 1978. In vivo analysis of bone strain about the sagittal suture in macaca mulatta during masticatory movements. *Journal of Dental Research* 57:904–908.

Bishara, S.E. & Staley, R.N. 1987. Maxillary expansion: clinical implications. *American Journal of Orthodontics and Dentofacial Orthopedics* 91:3–14.

Byron, C.D. et al. 2004. Effects of increased muscle mass on mouse sagittal suture morphology and mechanics. *The anatomical record. Part A, Discoveries in molecular, cellular, and evolutionary biology* 279:676–84.

Byrum Jr., A.G. 1971. Evaluation of anteriorposterior and vertical skeletal changes vs. dental changes in rapid palatal expansion cases as studies by lateral cephalograms. *American Journal of Orthodontics and Dentofacial Orthopedics* 60(4):419. (abstract)

Capelozza-Filho, L. & Silva-Filho, O.G. 1997. Expansão Rápida da Maxila: Considerações Gerais e Aplicação Clínica. Parte I. *Revista Dental Press de Ortodontia* e *Ortopedia Facial* 2(3):88–102.

Chang, H. et al. Angiogenesis and expanded suture osteogenesis in an orthopedically. 1997. *American Journal of Orthodontics and Dentofacial Orthopedics* 111(4): 382–90.

Cleall, J.F. et al. 1965. Expansion of the midpalatal suture in the monkey. *Angle Orthodontics* 35(1):23–35.

Cowin, S.C. 2001. *Bone Mechanics Handbook*. Boca Raton: CRC Press.
Da Silva Filho, O.G. et al. 1991. Rapid maxillary expansion in the primary and mixed dentitions: a cephalometric evaluation. *American Journal of Orthodontics and Dentofacial Orthopedics* 100:171–179.
Enlow, D.H. *Crescimento Facial*. Porto Alegre: Artes Médicas.
Ennes, J.P. 2002. *Análise morfológica da sutura palatina mediana de ratos, de coelhos, de macacos e de homens em diferentes fases do desenvolvimento cronológico*. (BR). University of São Paulo. Dentistry School of Bauru. (Phd tesis).
Gardner, G.E. & Kronman, J.H. 1971. Cranioskeletal displacements caused by rapid palatal expansion in the Rhesus Monky. *American Journal of Orthodontics and Dentofacial Orthopedics* 59(2):146–55.
Garib, D.G. et al. 2006. Periodontal effects of rapid maxillary expansion with tooth-tissue-borne and tooth-borne expanders: A computed tomography evaluation. *American Journal of Orthodontics and Dentofacial Orthopedics* 129(6):749–758.
Geris, L. et al. 2009. In silico biology of bone modelling and remodelling: regeneration. *Philosophical Transactions of the Royal Society A* 367: 2031–2053.
Ghoneima, A. et al. 2011. Effects of rapid maxillary expansion on the cranial and circummaxillary sutures. *American Journal of Orthodontics and Dentofacial Orthopedics* 140:510–519.
Gomez-Benito, M.J. et al. 2005. Influence of fracture gap size on the pattern of long bone healing: a computational study. *Journal of Theoretical Biology* 235(1):105–119.
Haas, A.J. 1961. Rapid expansion of the maxillary dental arch and nasal cavity by opening the midpalatal suture. *Angle Orthodontics* 31(2):73–90.
Haas, A.J. 1973. Rapid paladal expansion: recommended pre requisite to class III treatment. *Transactions of the European Orthodontic Society* 1:311–318.
Hinton, R.J. 1988. Response of the intermaxillary suture cartilage to alterations in masticatory function. *The Anatomical Record* 220:376–387.
Holberg, C. & Rudzki-Janson, I. 2006. Stresses at the cranial base induced by rapid maxillary expansion. *Angle Orthodontics* 76:543–550.
Isaacson, R.J. & Ingram, A.H. 1964. Forces produced by rapid maxillary expansion. II. Forces present during treatment. *Angle Orthodontics* 34:261–270.
Isaksson, H. et al. 2006. Corroboration of mechanoregulatory algorithms for tissue differentiation during fracture healing: comparison with in vivo results. *Journal of Orthopaedic Research* 24:898–907.
Jafari, A. et al. 2003. Study on stress distribution and displacement of various craniofacial structures following application of transverse orthopedic forces—a three-dimensional FEM study. *Angle Orthodontics* 73:12–20.
Johnson, D.R. & Moore, W.J. 1985. *Anatomy for dental students*. London: Oxford.
Jones, M.L. et al. 2001. A validated finite element method study of orthodontic tooth movement in the humam subject. *Journal of Orthodontics* 28:29–38.
Katsaros, C. et al. 1994. Functional influence on sutural growth. A morphometric study in the anterior facial skeleton of the growing rat. *European Journal Orthodontics* 16:353–360.
Katsaros, C. et al. 2006. Functional influence on sutural bone apposition in the growing rat. *American Journal of Orthodontics and Dentofacial Orthopedics* 129:352–357.
Korbmacher, H. et al. 2007. Age-dependent Three-dimensional Microcomputed Tomography Analysis of the Human Midpalatal Suture. *Journal of Orofacial Orthopedics* 68(5):364–376.
Kudlick, E.M. 1973. A study utilizing direct human skulls as models to determine how bones of the craniofacial complex are displaced under the influence of mid-palatal expansion (Master's thesis). Fairleigh Dickinson University, Rutherford, New Jersey.
Lacroix, D. & Prendergast, P.J. 2002. A mechano-regulation model for tissue differentiation during fracture healing: analysis of gap size and loading. *Journal of Biomechanics* 35(9):1163–1171.
Lagravere, M.O. et al. 2006. Metaanalysis of immediate changes with rapid maxillary expansion treatment. *Journal of the American Dental Association* 137:44–53.
Mao, J. 2002. Mechanobiology of craniofacial sutures. *Journal Dental Research* 81(12):810–816.
Melsen, B. 1975. Palatal growth studied on human autopsy material. A histologic microradiographic study. *American Journal of Orthodontics* 68(1):42–54.
N'Guyen, T. et al.. 2007. Anatomical modifications of the mid palatal suture during ageing: a radiographic study. *Surgical and Radiologic Anatomy* 29:253–259.
Pauwels, F. 1960. Eine neue Theorie über den Einfluβ mechanischer Reize auf die Differenzierung der Stützgewebe. *Zeitschrift fur Anatomie und Entwicklungsgeschichte* 121:478–515.
Perren, S. M. 1979. Physical and biological aspects of fracture healing with special reference to internal fixation. *Clinical Orthopaedics and Related Research* 138:175–195.
Perren, S. M. & Cordey, J. 1980. Concepts of interfragmentary strain. In *Current concepts of internal fixation of fractures*. New York: Springer.
Provatidis, C. et al. 2008. Evaluation of craniofacial effects during rapid maxillary expansion through combined in vivo/in vitro and finite element studies. *European Journal of Orthodontics* 30:437–448.
Starnbach, H. et al. 1966. Facioskeletal and dental changes resulting from rapid maxillary expansion. *Angle Orthodontics* 36(2):152–164.
Sun, Z. 2011. Mechanical strain at alveolar bone and circummaxillary sutures during acute rapid palatal expansion. *American Journal of Orthodontics and Dentofacial Orthopedics* 139(3):e219–e228.
Sun, Z. et al. 2004. Cranial sutures and bones: growth and fusion in relation to masticatory strain. *The anatomical record. Part A, Discoveries in molecular, cellular, and evolutionary biology* 276:150–161.
Ten Cate, A.R. 1977. Sutural development: structure and its response to rapid expansion. *American Journal of Orthodontics* 71(6):622–36.
Townend, P.I. 1980. Technique of rapid expansion in patients with cleft lip and palate. *British Journal of Orthodontics*7(2):65–67.
Wagemans, P.A. et al. 1988. Sutures and forces: a review. *American Journal of Orthodontics and Dentofacial Orthopedics* 94(2):129–141.
Wertz, R.A. 1970. Skeletal and dental changes accompanying rapid midpalatal suture opening. *American Journal of Orthodontics and Dentofacial Orthopedics* 58(1): 41–66.
Widmork, G. et al. 1995. Functional evaluation after T.M.J. surgery. *Journal of Oral Rehabilitation* 22(8):589–593.
Yoshida, N. et al. 2001. In vivo measurement of the elastic modulus of the human periodontal ligament. *Medical Engineering and Physics* 23:567–572.

Biodental Engineering II – Natal Jorge et al (Eds)
© 2014 Taylor & Francis Group, London, ISBN 978-1-138-00131-2

Numerical model of thermal necrosis due a dental drilling process

E.M.M. Fonseca, K. Magalhães & M.G. Fernandes
Polytechnic Institute of Bragança, Bragança, Portugal

M.P. Barbosa & G. Sousa
University of Minas Gerais, Belo Horizonte, Brasil

ABSTRACT: The main goal of this paper is to present a numerical model for studying the thermal necrosis due a dental drilling process. The finite element method was used with Ansys program for the transient thermal analysis. Also an experimental process is explained to determine the thermal occurrence in a pork mandible. The increase of temperature produced during the drilling is compared using the two different methodologies. According the obtained results, the numerical model could be a technique to induce appropriated results without using in-vivo models.

1 INTRODUCTION

When cutting tools, as drills, are used to cut a material, heat is produced and temperature increases of both the tool and material. The drilling parameters (drill speed, drill depth, drill diameter, applied load and feed rate) are important to determine the effect on thermal necrosis. When the irrigation is possible, the effect is decreasing the temperature rise in bone (Davidson, 1999). Bone is a poor conductor of heat, and heat generation is a common problem during any type of drilling (Hillery, 1999). The value on the threshold of temperature above which cell necrosis occurs have been presented by different researchers. The literature shows that if the temperature rises above 55°C for a period of longer than 30s, serious bone damage will be done (Hillery, 1999).

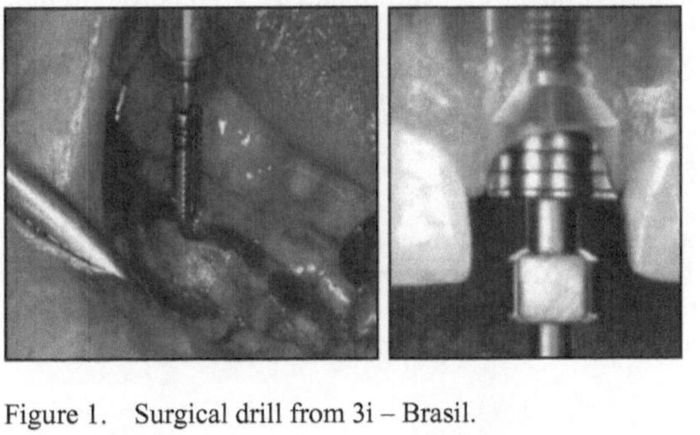

Figure 1. Surgical drill from 3i – Brasil.

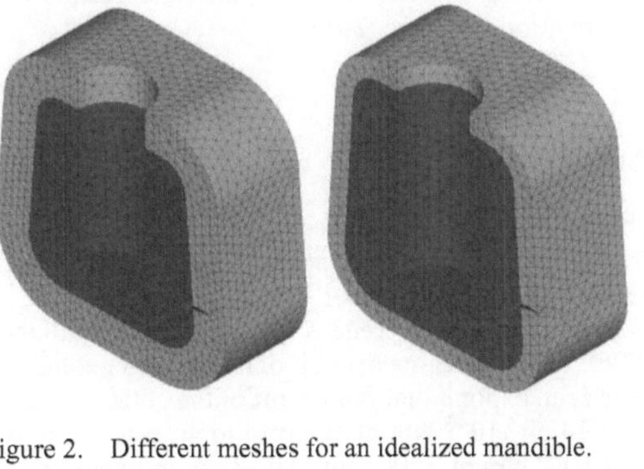

Figure 2. Different meshes for an idealized mandible.

2 MATERIALS AND METHODS

In order to model the thermal necrosis due a dental drilling process, a finite element method was used with Ansys program and a comparison with an experimental methodology using a pork mandible. The numerical analysis was conducted with transient heat conduction by modelling the heat flux from the drill process, as represented in figure 1.

The finite element mesh constituted by cortical and trabecular dental bone has a hole with diameter equal to the cylindrical part of the drill, figure 2. A solid finite element (Solid90) with 20 nodes was used in Ansys program. A typical mesh with an element length equal to 0.5 mm was chosen. An initial-boundary condition with a temperature $T0 = 37°C$ was considered in all dental bone model.

For experimental process, a pork mandible was submitted to a drilling with a conic drill bit and a rotational speed equal to 750 rpm. The initial temperature of the pork mandible is equal to 20°C.

Figure 3 shows the experimental setup used during the drilling. The experimental results are obtained with a Flir infrared thermography camera.

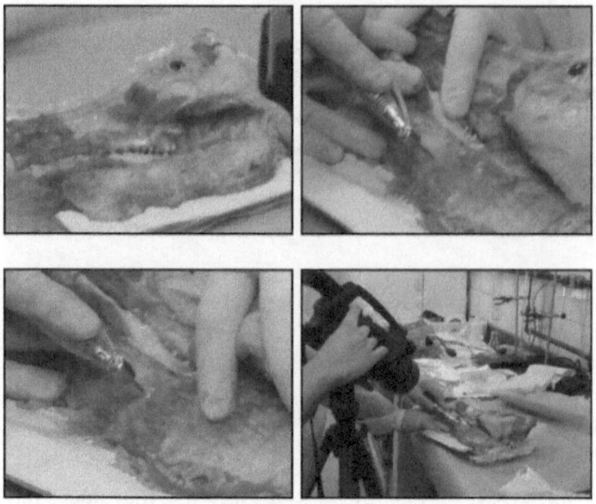

Figure 3. Experimental setup.

3 NUMERICAL MODEL

3.1 *Drilling parameters*

The modelling of heat propagation from drill process was described by a heat flux density q received in the bone surface.

The heat flux density is according the following equation (Basiaga, 2011):

$$q=P_c/S \quad (\mathrm{W/m^2}) \tag{1}$$

where P_c = total cutting power, and S = surface area. The total cutting power is a combination between the power derived from the feed component (P_f) and the power derived from the cutting torque (P_M).

$$P_c=P_f+P_M \quad (\mathrm{W}) \tag{2}$$

The following expressions give particular results for each relation (Basiaga, 2011):

$$P_f=V_f \times F_{fw} \quad (\mathrm{W}) \tag{3}$$

$$P_M=M_W \times n \times 2\pi/60 \quad (\mathrm{W}) \tag{4}$$

where V_f = feed ratio speed (m/s), F_{fw} = axial cutting force (N), M_w = cutting torque (Nm), and n = rotational speed (rpm).

According the references (Hillery, 1999; Hillery, 1996), using the same drill bit diameter and geometry there is an exponential falling-off of the cutting torque from 14.5×10^{-3} Nm at 400 rpm to an asymptote of 10×10^{-3} Nm at 2000 rpm. And also an exponential falling-off of the thrust force from 48 N at 400 rpm to an asymptote of 23 N at 2000 rpm.

In the surgical process used in ***3i - Brasil*** different steps for dental drilling are considered, always with a speed rotation equal to 750 rpm during 10 s:

- 1st step: initial perforation with a spherical round drill to punch the position;
- 2nd step: specific drill with a diameter d = 2 mm;
- 3rd step: conic drill with d = 3.2 mm and length l = 10 mm;
- 4th step: conic drill with d = 4.1 mm and l = 10 mm.

Table 1. The drilling parameters.

Final conic drill bit	
d	4.1 mm
l	10 mm
V_f	50 mm/min
n	750 rpm
M_W	12.5×10^{-3} Nm
F_{fw}	37.5 N
q	7.14 kW/m^2

Table 2. Bone thermal properties.

Properties	Bone	C1	C2	C3	C4
Density, kg/m^3	Cortical		2100		
	Trabecular	2200	1100	2200	1100
Conductivity, W/mK	Cortical		0.4		
	Trabecular		0.5		
Specific heat, J/kgK	Cortical		1260		
	Trabecular		1490		
Cortical thickness, mm		2	2	1	1

This standard drill for the last step is always the most used. According this situation the parameters used in the numerical simulation corresponds to this surgical drill with straight shank, 4.1 × 10 and a rotational speed equal to 750 rpm.

The feed rate speed varies according the surgeon, and it was chosen a value equal to 50 mm/min.

Table 1 shows the parameters used in the numerical simulation.

3.2 *Geometries and material properties*

The geometry considered in all numerical simulations represents a part of a dental bone with a hollow cavity equal to the drill bit diameter and a depth equal to 10 mm.

Four different idealized mandibular cross sections were used. Cortical bone of 2 mm thickness with medium density (C1) or low density trabecular bone (C2), and cortical bone of 1 mm thickness with medium density (C3) or low density trabecular bone (C4).

Based in the literature (Davidson, 1999; Hillery, 1996; Mazzullo, 1991; Lin, 2007) the thermal properties for cortical and trabecular bone are presented in table 2.

A solid mandibular cross-section with different nodal positions, neighbourhood to the drill hole (t = 0 mm) and at a distance t = 0.5 mm, is presented in figure 4.

Six different positions are considered to measure the thermal necrosis, two nodal locations in cortical

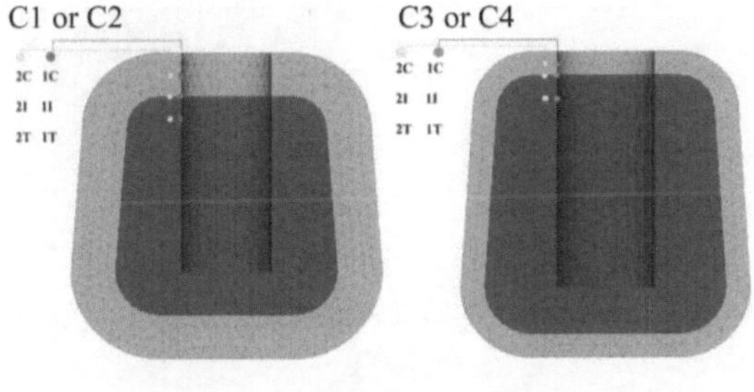

Figure 4. Nodal positions for each model.

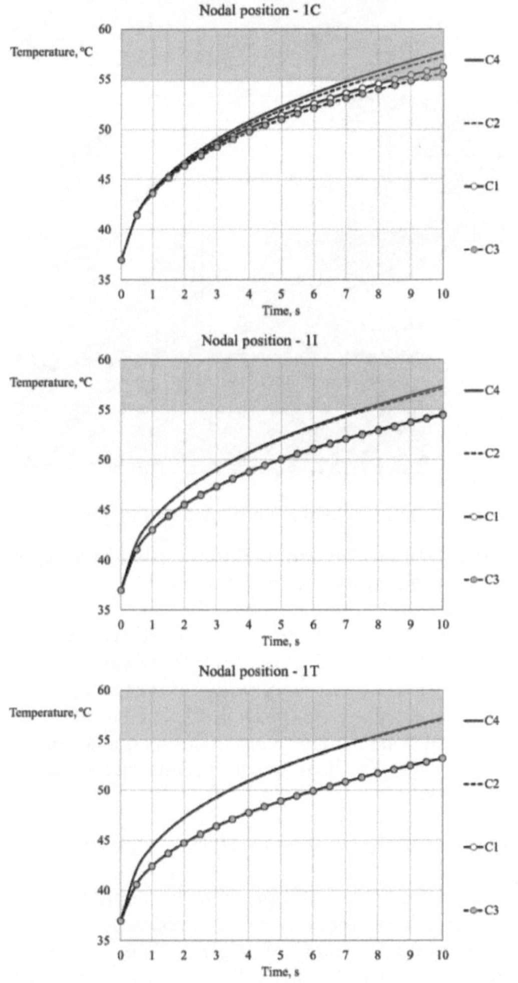

Figure 5. Time-temperature history for 1C, 1I, 1T.

(1C, 2C), trabecular (1T, 2T) and intermediate zone (1I, 2I).

3.3 *Numerical results*

Figure 5 and 6 show different graphics with all time-temperature history for all nodal positions. The grey zone represents the bone damage on the threshold of 55°C. Figure 5 represents the numerical results obtained in the neighbourhood of the drilling process. The numerical results are obtained for each nodal position (1C, 1I, 1T) and for all studied cases.

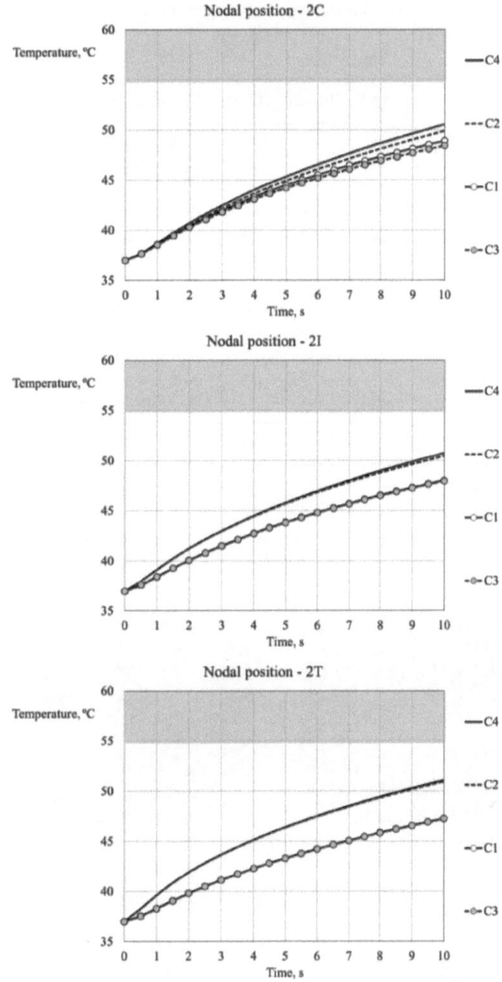

Figure 6. Time-temperature history for 2C, 2I, 2T.

The nodal positions in the models C4 and C2 get the threshold value of damage after 7s. These models have an increase of temperature equal to 20°C. In the models C1 and C3 only the cortical zone gets the threshold value of bone damage after 9s. And they have an increase of temperature equal to 15°C–17°C.

Figure 6 represents the second position of the nodal temperatures in all studied cases.

Studied cases C1 and C3 have a different behaviour in trabecular and intermediate zone with lesser temperatures.

The effect of the cortical thickness doesn't affect with relevance the obtained numerical values. But the density in trabecular bone interferes in all studied cases.

The medium density of the trabecular bone (C1 and C3) offers more thermal resistance than the lower bone density (C2 and C4).

Table 3. Thermal necrosis occurrence, time s.

	Nodal position					
	In the hole t = 0 mm			Distance t = 0.5 mm		
Studied case	1C	1I	1T	2C	2I	2T
C1 or C3	9.0	10.0	–	–	–	–
C2 or C4	7.0	7.5	7.5	–	–	–

Table 4. Bone damage (%) at 1s of exposure 55°C heat.

	Nodal position					
	In the hole t = 0 mm			Distance t = 0.5 mm		
Studied case	1C	1I	1T	2C	2I	2T
C1 or C3	11.1	10.0	–	–	–	–
C2 or C4	14.3	13.3	13.3	–	–	–

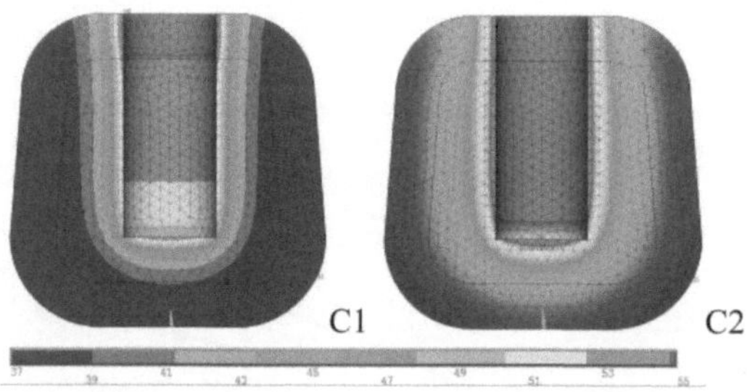

Figure 7. Bone damage (t = 0.25 mm) for cases C1 and C2.

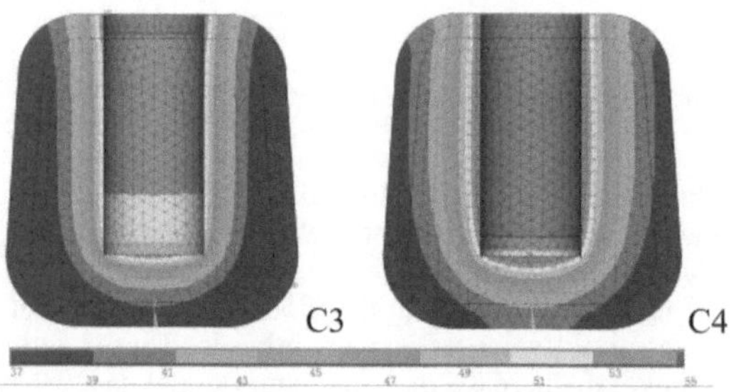

Figure 8. Bone damage (t = 0.25 mm) for cases C3 and C4.

At 0.5 mm in front of the drill there is no bone damage. The increase of temperature is equal of 13°C for models C4 and C2 and 11°C for C1 and C3.

Based in figures 5 and 6, table 3 represents the time instant that thermal necrosis occurs for each study case.

Due the drilling process, the surrounding bone is heated, and the temperature around the drilled bone hole exceeds the critical imposed limit and it is equal to 55°C. The result is the irreversible death of cells, representing the thermal necrosis. Bone cell necrosis or damage, happens when receives heat during a period of time. The temperature threshold levels, for heat induced injury, are time-dependent.

In this work, the damage could be calculated as a percentage of bone damage when receives heat, as proposed by (Fukushima, 2007). Bone cell necrosis, or damage at 100%, occurs when it receives 55°C of heat. Consequently, it is possible to conclude about the amount of bone damage, caused during one-second of exposure to 55°C heat, according an equation as the following:

$$Damage\ (55^{\circ}C) = (1/time) \times 100\% \qquad (5)$$

In our study, table 4 represents the amount of bone damage, at one second of exposure 55°C heat.

The worst positions are neighbourhood to the drill hole and for cases C2 or C4. For one exposure at 55°C of heat, the amount of bone damage is equal to 14.3%. The nodal positions at 0.5 mm, don't present any bone damage. Figures 7 and 8 represent the extension of bone damage, (ash zone) at the end of a drilling process (10s) for all studied cases.

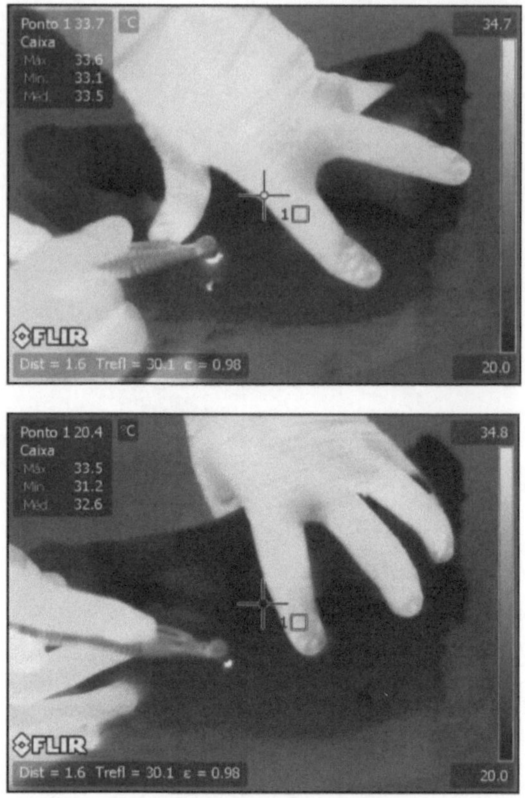

Figure 9. Infrared thermal images without irrigation.

4 EXPERIMENTAL PROCESS

4.1 *Infrared thermal images*

The results obtained with the experimental process are show in figures 9 and 10.

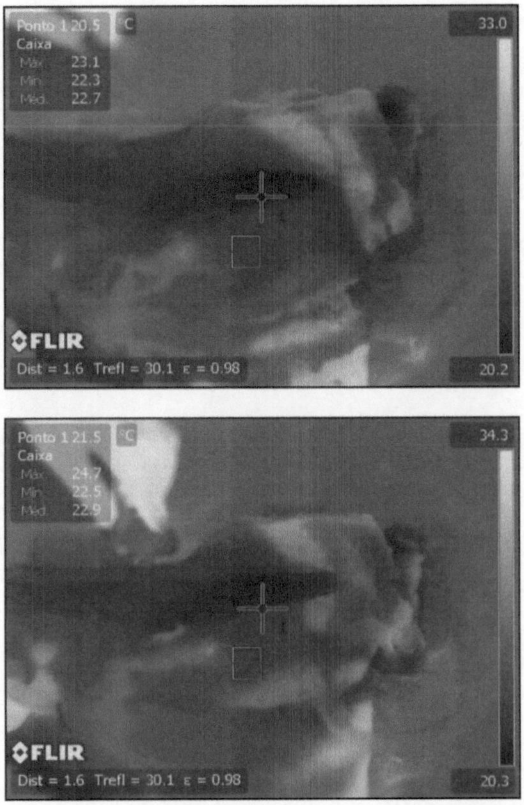

Figure 10. Infrared thermal images with irrigation.

Two different types of tests were produced using irrigation during the drilling process and without irrigation. The recorded temperatures are in the surface of the pork mandible during the drilling process.

Figure 9 represents the infrared thermal images obtained during the drilling process without irrigation.

Figure 10 represents two images obtained during the drilling process with irrigation.

4.2 *Experimental results*

The increase of temperature is equal to almost 14°C, relative to the initial temperature (20°C) when the experimental test is without irrigation. With irrigation, the increase of temperature is almost equal to 5°C, relative to the initial temperature (20°C) of the pork mandible. Comparing the increase of the temperature obtained in the experimental process without irrigation, the range is similar to the obtained results from numerical analysis.

5 CONCLUSIONS

In this work two different methodologies are presented to assess the thermal necrosis due a dental drilling process.

The numerical model presents a methodology to calculate the amount of bone damage. The parameters selection (drill diameter and rotational speed) are important to increase a surgical planning definition and the prevention of the thermal necrosis.

An experimental methodology could be used, as recording the thermal images.

Comparing the increase of temperature between all methodologies, the range is similar when using the numerical model with higher bone density (C1 or C3) and the drilling without irrigation in the experimental process.

In conclusion, the numerical methodology could be a technique to induce appropriate results, without using in-vivo models.

ACKNOWLEDGEMENTS

The authors gratefully acknowledge to the companies that made possible this work, Implantec, Dmc group and 3i-implants innovation incorporation.

REFERENCES

Basiaga, M., Paszenda, Z., Szewczenko, J., Kaczmarek, M. 2011. Numerical and experimental analyses of drills used in osteosynthesis. *Acta of Bioengineering and Biomechanics* 13(4): 29–36.

Davidson, S.R.H. 1999. *Heat transfer in bone during drilling. Applied Science Master Degree*, University of Toronto, Canada.

Fukushima, H., Hashimoto, Y., Yoshiya, S., Kurosaka, M., Matsuda, M., Kawamura, S., Iwatsubo, T. 2002. Conduction Analysis of Cement Interface Temperature in Total Knee Arthroplasty. *Kobe J. Med. Sci.*, 48: 63–72.

Hillery, M.T., Shuaib, I. 1999. Temperature effects in the drilling of human and bovine bone. *Journal of Materials Processing Technology* 92–93: 302–308.

Hillery *et al*, IMC-13:33–42, Ireland, 1996.

Lin, D., Li, Q., Li, W., Ichim, I., Swain, M. 2007. *Evaluation of dental implant induced bone remodelling by using a 2D Finite Element model. 5th Australian Congress on Applied Mechanics*, ACAM, 2007, Brisbane, Australia.

Mazzullo, S., Paolini, M. Verdi, C. 1991. Numerical simulation of thermal bone necrosis during cementation of femoral prostheses. *Journal of Mathematical Biology*, 29: 475–494.

Biodental Engineering II – Natal Jorge et al (Eds)
 ISBN 978-1-138-00131-2

The occlusion in total prosthesis

P. Fonseca & M.H. Figueiral
FMDUP, Porto, Portugal

M. Vaz
FEUP – INEGI, Porto, Portugal

ABSTRACT: Total denture occlusion still remains a very demanding work to the clinician and to the technician in order to obtain bi-balanced interdental contacts. To define the importance of posterior occlusion determinants in complete denture, were defined as main aims of this work: 1 – to develop systems that can identify interdental contacts; 2 – to test the ability to simulate the 3D mandibular movement; 3 – to evaluate the impact of sagital condylar guidance changes in occlusal contacts. It was been proved that the new technologies created are useful to obtain the primary goal of total oral rehabilitation that is the functional harmony between teeth and the dynamic of temporomandibular joint.

1 INTRODUTION

In a total edentulous patient the only relationship that exists between the upper and lower jaw occurs in the temporomandibular joint (TMJ). Although some authors consider important individualize the condylar sagital guidance (SCG) to a correct preparation of a bimaxilar denture (Gennari Filho 2007, Kubrak 1998), others claim that the reference values must be used, making the whole process simpler and without great clinical damage (Carlsson 2006). Therefore total denture manufacture still remains a very demanding work.

Over the last few years, it is possible to combine engineering techniques and computer-aided-design systems (CAD) to dental medicine (Drago 2007, Valente *et al.* 2009, Neto *et al.* 2010, Frisardi 2011). The main aims of this work are: 1 – to develop systems that can identify interdental contacts without the interference of any registration material; 2 – to test the ability to simulate the three-dimensional mandibular movement for the construction of total dentures; 3 – to evaluate the impact of sagital condylar guidance changes in occlusal contacts.

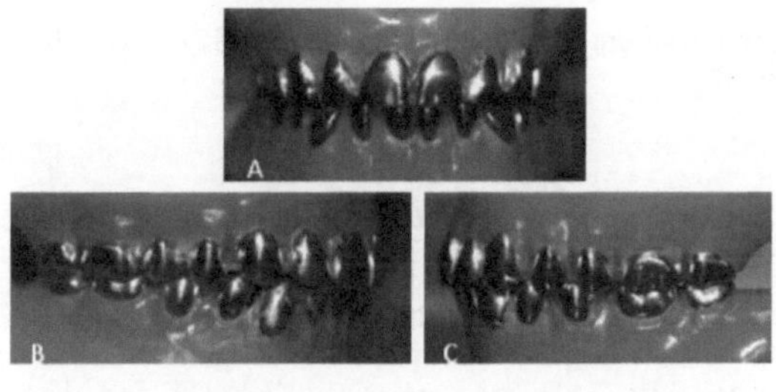

Figure 1. Replica of the prosthesis with CoCrMo alloy teeth. A. Anterior view; B. Lateral right view; C. Lateral left view.

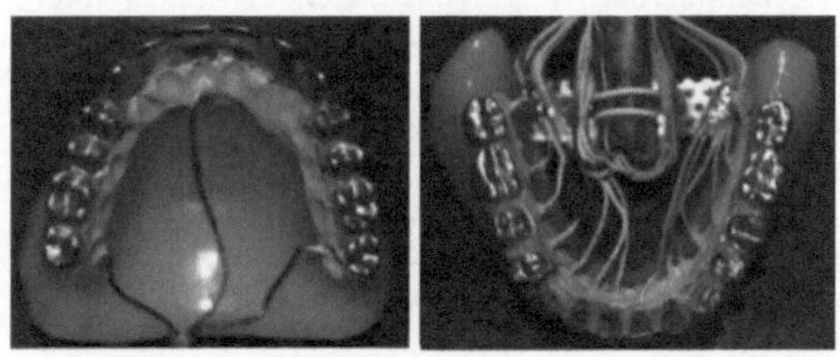

Figure 2. Electrification of the teeth: A. Maxilar; B. Mandibular.

2 MATERIAL AND METHODS

Total bimaxilar prosthesis is fabricated in a semi-adjustable articulator (A7 bioart Plus) with bi-balanced occlusion to 30° of SCG.

2.1 *Occlusal contacts evaluation in articulator*

A replica of the prosthesis was made with CoCrMo alloy teeth – Remannium GM 800 + Dentaurum® – conductor of electric current (Figure 1). This was followed by the electrification of the teeth, in the LOME-FEUP (Figure 2).

To each mandibular tooth corresponds a light-emitting diode (LED) and whenever there was contact of a maxilar tooth with a mandibular the corresponding LED lights up. To allow a rapid identification of the mandibular teeth into contact, LEDs were arranged according to the position of teeth in the arch (Figure 3). Contacts between the maxilar and mandibular teeth were evaluated for the position of protrusion and right

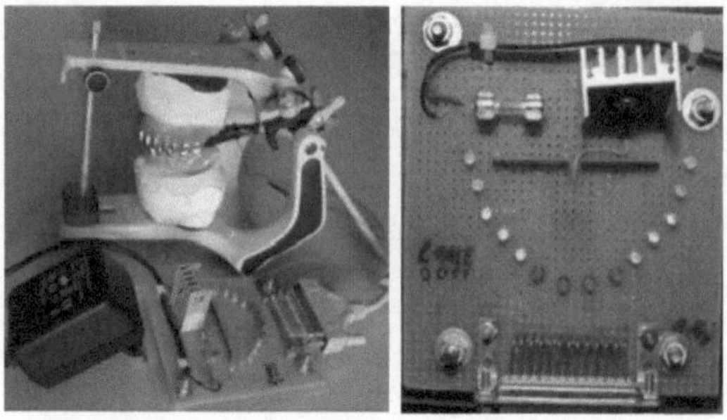

Figure 3. Electric circuit that allows the identification of interdental contacts.

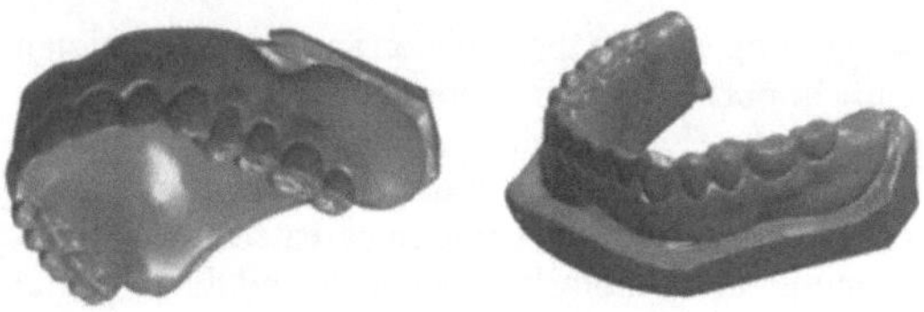

Figure 4. Geometry of maxilar and mandibular plaster model.

and left lateral movements to bilateral SCG from 20° to 50°.

2.2 *3D Occlusal contacts evaluation*

To determinate the geometry of plaster models of the prosthesis was used a 3Shape D250 3D dental scanner (Materialise®). The point cloud generated was inserted in CAD software, SolidWorks®, and then processed to have the final geometry of the models (Figure 4).

Bilateral condylar guidance, Bennett angles, intercondylar distance and condylar axis of rotation were determinate in patient and then transferred to the computer. By this way the solids were oriented in space and movements were simulated (Figure 5).

Contacts between the maxilar and mandibular teeth were evaluated for the position of protrusion and right and left lateral movements to bilateral SCG from 20° to 50° (Figure 6 and 7).

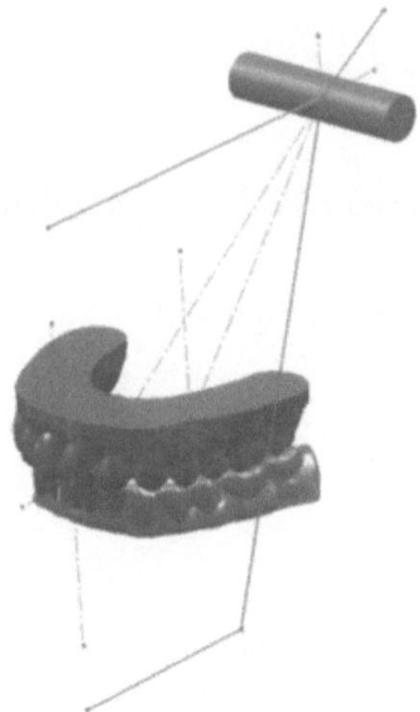

Figure 5. Spatial orientation of the solids.

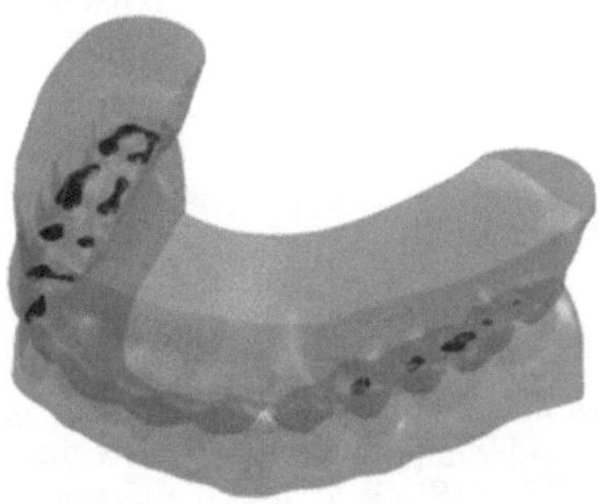

Figure 6. Contacts evaluation during left lateral movement.

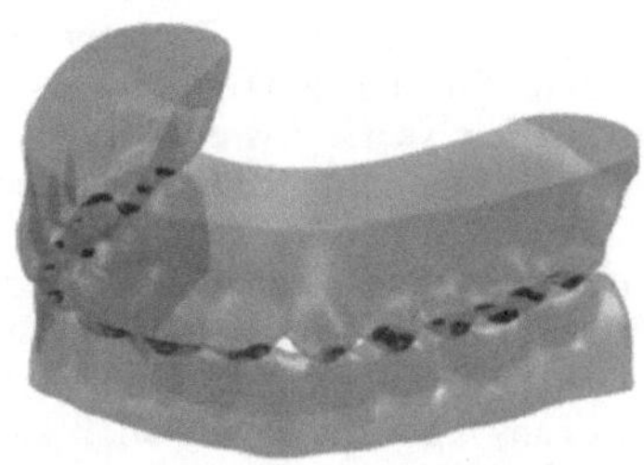

Figure 7. Contacts evaluation during protrusive movement.

3 RESULTS

The systems created proved to be able to simulate the three-dimensional mandibular movement in the construction of total dentures. The results achieved with two systems were similar. For 30° of SCG inclination all mandibular teeth had contacts in the final protrusion position. In the lateral movements there were total contacts on the work side and lack of contacts in the 1st premolar, canine and lateral incisor on the not working side. The movements were controlled by the TMJ and by the teeth in harmony. We found that, for values less than 30°, we had dental contacts similar to those exposed to the reference value. Despite of not losing the balanced occlusion, the teeth dictated the moves and not the TMJ. For values greater than 30°, we verified changes in interdental contacts and in the balance occlusion. With the progressive increase of SCG inclination there was loss of contacts on working and non-working side, losing the balance occlusion to values equal or greater than 45°. Like the observed for the protrusive movement, lateral movements also became progressively greater oriented by the TMJ instead of teeth.

4 DISCUSSION AND CONCLUSIONS

Although we cannot make a qualitative assessment of the contacts, we can evaluate them quantitatively without interference from any inter-arches registration material. Our results are consistent with Santos (Santos *et al.* 2003) which defines the molar region as the most affected by variation of the inclination of the SCG.

The systems created proved to be able to determinate dental interferences during mandibular function and failure of the bilateral balanced occlusion when SCG are individualized. This can help the clinician to choose the most indicate teeth to use in the fabrication of complete dentures. This way it is possible to promote better functional mandibular movements according to the posterior determinants of occlusion in order to obtain bilateral balanced contacts. This means that using a system that simulates the real patient's mandibular movement, enables the clinician/technician to see more clearly the premature contacts and interferences generated during physiologic movements.

REFERENCES

Carlsson, G.E. 2006. Facts and fallacies: an evidence base for complete dentures. *Dent Update* 33(3):134–6, 138–40, 142.

Drago, C. F. & Peterson, T. 2007. Treatment of an edentulous patient with CAD/CAM technology: a clinical report. *J Prosthodont* 16(3):200–8.

Frisardi, G., Chessa, G., Barone, S., Paoli, A., Razionale, A. & Frisardi, F. 2011. Integration of 3D anatomical data obtained by CT imaging and 3D optical scanning for computer aided implant surgery. *BMC Medical Image* 11:5.

Gennari Filho, H. 2007. Articulators. *Rev Odontol Araçatuba* 28(3):46–56.

Kubrak J. 1998. Comparative analysis of edentulous patients treated traditionally and with the use of a face-bow Quick Master articulator. *Ann Acad Med Stetin* 44:237–49.

Neto, A. F., Junior, W. M. & Carreiro, A. F. P. 2010. Masticatory efficiency in denture wearers with bilateral balanced occlusion and canine guidance. *Braz Dent J* 21(2):165–9.

Santos, J., Nelson, S. & Nowlin, T. 2003. Comparison of condylar guidance setting obtained from a wax record versus an extraoral tracing: A pilot study. *J Prosthet Dent* 89:54–9.

Valente, F., Schiroli, G. & Sbrenna, A. 2009. Accuracy of computer-aided oral implant surgery: a clinical and radiographic study. *Int J Oral Maxillofac Implants* 24(2): 234–42.

Biodental Engineering II – Natal Jorge et al (Eds)
© 2014 Taylor & Francis Group, London, ISBN 978-1-138-00131-2

Implant-abutment geometry and its role in bone level preservation

J. Ferreira
DMD, Biomedical Engineering, FEUP, INEGI

M. França
DVM, Biomedical Engineering, FEUP, INEGI

A. Correia
DMD, FMDUP, INEGI Researcher

A. Reis
FEUP, CETECOP (INEGI) Director

ABSTRACT: Once osteointegration is an established fact, the challenge, nowadays, is to keep the osteointegration over time, particularly when some risk factors can be identified. It is stated that, among other factors, the biological width formation could be influenced by the implant-connection geometry. The aim of this review is to identify, from the existent connections, which could be the most favorable to the biological width formation. The results described on the analyzed papers point to the internal connections, cone Morse type, with platform shifting as being the most bone crestal preserving.

1 INTRODUCTION

1.1 *Osteointegration*

Prior to the studies developed by Branemark (1) and Schroeder (2), there were no surgical protocols that could avoid the protein denaturation and the necrosis of many osteoblasts. That event forced the inflammatory response to take the fibrotic pathway (3). So, osteointegration was thought to be an impossible achievement. The development of surgical protocols had the ability to influence the inflammatory reaction towards tissue regeneration. The last decades had shown that the oral rehabilitation with osteointegrated implants is a valuable alternative, with high and predictable success rates (4).

Nowadays, the challenge is to keep the osteointegration over time, particularly when some risk factors can be identified (5).

1.2 *Biological width and peri-implantitis*

When a dental implant is exposed in the oral cavity, through the epithelial tissue, either when a supporting or a healing abutment is placed, a biological reaction resulting in the biological width formation takes place (Fig. 1).

The existent space in the implant-abutment interface, known as microgap, is colonized by bacteria and micromovements can be found at this level (6). The biological width formation is characterized by the soft and hard tissue remodelling around the implant, creating a distance of 1.5 to 2 mm from the bone crest to the implant-abutment connection, functioning as a biological barrier for the bacteria present in the microgap (7, 8). This distance barrier is necessary because, unlike what occurs with teeth, the epithelial union to the implant is very weak (8, 9) and the connective tissue fibers orientation, circumferentially and in parallel, around the implants, makes bone more vulnerable to bacterial contamination, creating conditions for the development of a peri-implantitis in sensitive patients.

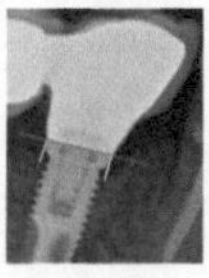

Figure 1. Biological width (yellow line) formation from the implant-abutment connection (red line) to the bone level.

Peri-implantitis is a multifactorial pathology. The presence of risk factors, inherent to the patient and factors related to the implant, as its surface, geometry or the type of abutment connection are considered important factors (10–12). The implant-abutment connection technology appears to have a significant impact on peri-implant crestal bone level (13).

2 MATERIALS AND METHODS

With the goal of finding the answers to the questions "what are the existing connections?", "does the implant-connection geometry have some influence in the biological width formation?" and, in case of a positive answer, "which connection could play the most positive role in reducing the marginal bone loss?", a bibliographic review was performed. The keywords used were "internal connection", "external connection", "cone Morse" and "platform shifting" and the

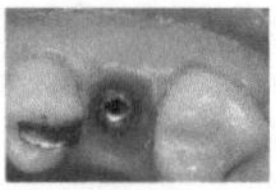

Figure 2. Clinical image of an external hexagon.

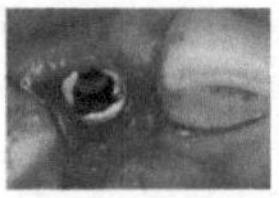

Figure 3. Clinical image of an internal connection trilobe.

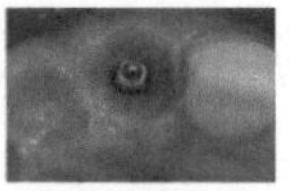

Figure 4. Clinical image of an internal connection cone Morse type.

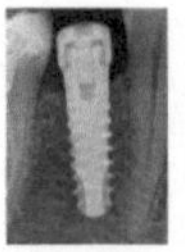

Figure 5. Radiografic image of an external hexagon.

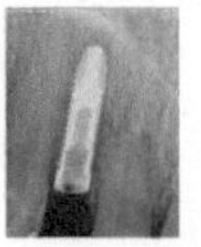

Figure 6. Radiographic image of an internal trilobe connection.

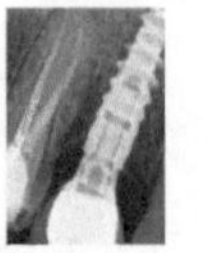

Figure 7. Image of an internal connection cone Morse type, platform shifting.

search was performed on the PubMed database. The articles published in the last five years were analyzed, as well as the relevant references indicated in those papers. The papers that, even referring to the issue under review, had, as main goal, the comparison of materials or methods of retention, or had, as critical factor for analysis, other concept, such as implant neck geometry or surface, were excluded from the present review.

A total of 81 papers were considered. Of these, 13 referred to *in vitro* studies, including 6 fatigue analysis and 7 bacterial contamination analysis. Twenty-one were finite element studies and 6 were photoelastic analysis. Eight papers described animal experimentation and 3 referred to histomorphometric studies in humans. Clinical studies included 10 papers reported randomized controlled trials, 3 radiographic studies, 2 retrospective clinical trials and 6 prospective clinical trials. Six systematic reviews and 3 reviews complete the total of the papers considered.

3 RESULTS

3.1 *What are the existing connections?*

The connection between implant and abutment may display two types: the external connection, when the implant penetrates the abutment or the internal connection when the abutment penetrates the implant.

The external connections are constituted by an external hexagon (Fig. 2 and 5). On the contrary, internal connections configurations adopted by different companies are not alike. When analyzing the implant-abutment coupling of internal connections, some different systems have been described, such as cylindrical connection, internal hexagon, internal octagon, trilobe (Figs 3 and 6), spline and a combination of screwed and friction systems, among which, due to its importance in bibliography, the cone Morse connection (Figs 4 and 7) must be emphasized (14).

These connections can exist in two different concepts: the platform matching and platform shifting or switching were described. The platform matching concept is the classical concept where the diameter of the implant is the same as the abutment. The platform switching concept refers to the use of an abutment of smaller diameter connected to an implant neck of larger diameter. This connection shifts the perimeter of the implant-abutment junction inwards towards the central axis of the implant (Fig. 7).

3.2 *Does the implant-connection geometry have some influence in the biological width formation?*

All the papers included in the present review showed different results for the different connections analyzed, indicating that is plays an important role on the biological width formation.

3.3 *Which connection could play the most positive role in reducing the marginal bone loss?*

The articles concerning to *in vitro* studies examining the fatigue resistance of the complex implant-abutment, showed that, when compared with external connections, the internal connections do not exhibit any strength advantage (15), appearing to have a poorer load fatigue performance (16). However, that result is not valid for all internal connections: long internal tube-in-tube connections and cam–slot fixation show advantages regarding to longevity and fracture strength (17); the existence of friction-locking mechanics and solid design provided greater resistance to deformation when compared to the internal hexagon abutments (18). Sabet et al (19), stated the unfavorable strain distribution in mandibular overdentures, when platform switching abutments were used.

The studies that focus the attention on the bacterial leakage formation along the implant-abutment interface, showed that the internal connections, under no-loading conditions have a perfect sealing (20). The results also indicated that the cone Morse connection exhibit less bacteria contamination than the other connections (21–25). Despite, the qualitative analysis had not shown differences in the peri-implant microbiota (26).

The photoelastic analysis evaluates the bone stress distribution with different implant-abutment connections. The results showed that the internal connections (27), especially when using platform switch abutments (28, 29), decrease stress concentrations in the cervical region. The Rossi (30) experiences strongly suggest that the use of platform switching design can prevent bone loss around the implant-abutment platform, which is also supported by Pellizer (29). A different result was obtained when analyzing three-unit crowns where lower stress levels were found with external hexagon platforms (28, 31).

The finite elements studies investigated the influence of connections on three different aspects: 1) on peri-implant bone stress; 2) on stress distribution at the connection components; 3) on abutment micromovements.

Analyzing the effect of the different connections on peri-implant bone stress, a large variety of finite element studies can be found. The results point to a reduced stress when internal connections are used (32–34) and when the platform shifting is present, either with internal or external connection (17, 35–43). The use of wide diameter platform implants was also correlated with reduced bone stress (44–46). Only three studies did not find any advantage to the biomechanical environment of implants in using circumferential horizontal mismatch between the abutment and the implant (45–47).

Pellizzer et al (44), Çimen et al (36) and Tabata et al (48), studies with external connections, reported higher levels of stress concentration in the retention screw when abutments of small diameter than the fixture were used. Freitas Jr. et al (49) reported the same results but, when using internal connections, higher levels of stress at the abutment screw were not found. Canay et al (45) also reported that platform switch affect the mechanical properties of the implant-abutment connection. Saidin (50) analyzing different types of internal connections with platform shifting, showed that non-cylindrical abutments, such as cone Morse and trilobe, provided a stable locking mechanism that reduced micromotion, However, as stress tends to concentrate at the vertices of the abutment, microfractures may occur.

Even though Becker et al (51, 52) have not found significant differences when using platform matching or platform shifting abutments, five studies (53–57) with animal experimentation evidenced that bone loss was significantly less when the abutment had a smaller diameter than the fixture. Cochran (54) considered that the bone remodeling could be five- to six-folds less with this implant-abutment connections.

Some histomorphometric analyses in humans indicate that the internal cone Morse connection with platform shifting may preserve the peri-implant tissues (58–60).

One review (61) and one systematic review (62) indicate that there is no sufficient evidence that could lead to affirm the better performance of one type of connection over another. Nevertheless, looking to reviews (63, 64) and systematic reviews (65–68) on the effect of platform switch on the bone level preservation, all affirm that its use has advantages over the other connections.

The randomized clinical trials indicated different results. Comparing internal matching connections to internal platform shift connections, Pieri (69) found that the crestal bone was very stable with both types. Two more trials, comparing matching to switched external platforms did not confirm that the peri-implant bone loss was reduced when switched platforms were used (70, 71). However, a significant number of studies comparing matching platforms with shifted platforms, found better results with the platform switch type (72–77). Canullo et al (78) indicated a possible relation with individual factors, in particular the TNF-α. Other clinical studies, including radiological analysis, prospective and retrospective studies, stated the worst performance in maintaining the crestal bone levels by the external connections (13, 79). All the papers included in this section, showed that platform switching seems to reduce peri-implant crestal bone resorption and increase the long-term predictability of implant therapy (80–87), with results considered proven over five years (88).

4 DISCUSSION

This review includes a large range of clinical situations and simulations, from single unit to full-arch rehabilitations. Also includes studies *in vitro, in silico*, animal experimentation, human histology, clinical trials and reviews. A large consensus can be observed. When we consider the stress transmission to bone crest by the different implant-abutment connections, it is possible to conclude that the internal connections are more favorable than the external ones (27). The same conclusion can be drawn considering the platform shift concept. This could be one fact that contributes for the reduced bone loss when internal connections with platform shift are used, as the papers relative to clinical trials, animal experimentation, histomorphometric studies in humans and reviews state.

Another contribution for the reduced bone loss found with platform switch may be the different organization of the biological width as a result of the inward shift of the inflammatory connective tissue zone at the implant-abutment junction (59) that is located in a more central position, protecting the peri-implant tissues (89).

On the other hand, the internal connections present a higher strain concentration within the implant-abutment joint and in the fixation screw, when compared with the external connections. This fact can lead to fractures that will enlarge the microgap (18, 45). To minimize this problem the recourse to cone Morse connections appears to be the most valuable option (18).

5 CONCLUSIONS

Although there is no unanimity, exists a large consensus on the advantages in bone crest preservation when implants with internal connection, cone Morse type and with the platform shifting concept are used.

This has an important clinical relevance because, if risk factors are identified in the anamnesis and clinical history, the selection of the implant and the implant-abutment connection can have a positive impact on the biological width formation and on the bone remodeling.

Notwithstanding, more independent studies are necessary, as some doubts still persist. In the same way, some problems were not eliminated, showing the need of continuous research to obtain new concepts.

REFERENCES

[1] Brånemark P-I, Zarb GA, Albrektsson T. Tissue Integrated Prostheses: Osseointegration in Clinical Dentistry. Chicago: Quintessence Publ Co.; 1985.

[2] Schroeder A, van der Zypen E, Stich H, Sutter F. The reactions of bone, connective tissue, and epithelium to endosteal implants with titanium-sprayed surfaces. J Maxillofac Surg. 1981;9:15–25.

[3] Ratner D, Hoffman A, Schoen F, Lemons J. Biomaterials Science – An Introduction to Materials in Medicine. London2004.

[4] Adell R, Lekholm U, Rockler B, Brånemark PI. A 15-year study of osseointegrated implants in the treatment of the edentulous jaw. International Journal of Oral Surgery. 1981;10(6):387–416.

[5] Lindhe J, Meyle J, on behalf of Group DotEWoP. Peri-implant diseases: Consensus Report of the Sixth European Workshop on Periodontology. Journal of Clinical Periodontology. 2008;35:282–5.

[6] Scarano A, Assenza B, Piattelli M, Iezzi G, Leghissa GC, Quaranta A, et al. A 16-year Study of the Microgap Between 272 Human Titanium Implants and Their Abutments. Journal of Oral Implantology. 2005;31(6):269–75.

[7] Ferreira J. Espaco biológico e conexões em implantologia. Maxilaris. 2011:54–6.

[8] Sorní-Bröker M, Peñarrocha-Diago M. Factors that influence the position of the peri-implant soft tissues: A review. Med Oral Patol Oral Cir Bucal. 2009;14(9):e475–9.

[9] Mª Ángeles Sánchez Garcés CGE. Periimplantitis. Patol Oral Cir Buca. 2004;9:63–74.

[10] Sánchez-Garcés M, Gay-Escoda C. Periimplantitis. Med Oral Patol Oral Cir Bucal. 2004;9(Suppl:S): 63–74.

[11] Heitz-Mayfield LJA. Diagnosis and management of peri-implant diseases. Australian Dental Journal. 2008;53:S43-S8.

[12] Algraffee H, Borumandi F, Cascarini L. Peri-implantitis. British Journal of Oral and Maxillofacial Surgery. 2012;50(8):689–94.

[13] Koo K, Lee E, Kim J, Seol Y, Han J, Kim T, et al. The effect of internal versus external abutment connection modes on crestal bone changes around dental implants: a radiographic analysis. J Periodontol. 2012 Sep;83(9):1104–9.

[14] Gracis S, Michalakis K, Vigolo P, Vult von Steyern P, Zwahlen M, Sailer I. Internal vs. external connections for abutments/reconstructions: a systematic review. Clinical Oral Implants Research. 2012;23:202–16.

[15] Ribeiro CG, Maia MLC, Scherrer SS, Cardoso AC, Wiskott HWA. Resistance of three implant-abutment interfaces to fatigue testing. Journal of Applied Oral Science. 2011;19:413–20.

[16] Seetoh Y, Tan K, Chua E, Quek H, Nicholls J. Load fatigue performance of conical implant-abutment connections. Int J Oral Maxillofac Implants. 2011 Jul–Aug;26(4):797–806.

[17] Steinebrunner L, Wolfart S, Ludwig K, Kern M. Implant-abutment interface design affects fatigue and fracture strength of implants. Clinical Oral Implants Research. 2008;19(12):1276–84.

[18] Coppedê A, Bersani E, Mattos MG, Rodrigues R, Sartori I, Ribeiro R. Fracture resistance of the implant-abutment connection in implants with internal hex and internal conical connections under oblique compressive loading: an in vitro study. Int J Prosthodont. 2009 May–Jun;22(3):283–6.

[19] Sabet M, El-Korashy D, El-Mahrouky N. Effect of platform switching on strain developed around implants supporting mandibular overdenture. Implant Dent. 2009 Aug;18(4):362–70.

[20] Sumi T, Braian M, Shimada A, Shibata N, Takeshita K, Vandeweghe S, et al. Characteristics of implant-CAD/CAM abutment connections of two different internal connection systems. Journal of Oral Rehabilitation. 2012;39(5):391–8.

[21] D'Ercole S, Scarano A, perrotti V, Mulatinho J, Piattelli A, Iezzi G, et al. Implants with external hexagon and conical implant-abutment connections: an in vitro study of the bacterial contamination. Journal of Oral Implantology. 2011.

[22] Assenza B, Tripodi D, Scarano A, Perrotti V, Piattelli A, Iezzi G, et al. Bacterial leakage in implants with different implant-abutment connections: an in vitro study. J Periodontol. 2012 Apr;83(4):491–7.

[23] Canullo L, Iannello G, Netuschil L, Jepsen S. Platform switching and matrix metalloproteinase-8 levels in peri-implant sulcular fluid. Clin Oral Implants Res. 2012 May;23(5):556–9.

[24] Nascimento C, Miani P, Pedrazzi V, Gonçalves R, Ribeiro R, Faria A, et al. Leakage of saliva through the implant-abutment interface: in vitro evaluation of three different implant connections under unloaded and loaded conditions. Int J Oral Maxillofac Implants. 2012 May–Jun;27(3):551–60.

[25] Tripodi D, Vantaggiato G, Scarano A, Perrotti V, Piattelli A, Iezzi G, et al. An in vitro investigation concerning the bacterial leakage at implants with internal hexagon and Morse taper implant-abutment connections. Implant Dent. 2012 Aug;21(4):335–9.

[26] Canullo L, Quaranta A, Teles R. The microbiota associated with implants restored with platform switching: a preliminary report. J Periodontol. 2010 Mar;81(3):403–11.

[27] Asvanund P, Morgano SM. Photoelastic stress analysis of external versus internal implant-abutment connections. The Journal of Prosthetic Dentistry. 2011;106(4):266–71.

[28] Coelho Goiato M, Pesqueira AA, Falcón-Antenucci RM, dos Santos DM, Haddad MF, Bannwart LC, et al. Stress distribution in implant-supported prosthesis with external and internal implant-abutment connections. Acta Odontologica Scandinavica.0(0):1–6.

[29] Pellizzer EP, Falcón-Antenucci RM, de Carvalho PSP, Santiago JF, de Moraes SLD, de Carvalho BM. Photoelastic Analysis of the Influence of Platform Switching on Stress Distribution in Implants. Journal of Oral Implantology. 2010;36(6):419–24.

[30] Rossi F, Zavanelli AC, Zavanelli RA. Photoelastic comparison of single tooth implant-abutment bone of platform switching vs conventional implant designs. The journal of contemporary dental practice. 2011;12(2):124–30.

[31] Tonella B, Pellizzer E, Falcón-Antenucci R, Ferraço R, Almeida D. Photoelastic analysis of biomechanical behavior of single and multiple fixed partial prostheses with different prosthetic connections. J Craniofac Surg. 2011 Nov;22(6):2060–3.

[32] Yamanishi Y, Yamaguchi S, Imazato S, Nakano T, Yatani H. Influences of implant neck design and implant–abutment joint type on peri-implant bone stress and abutment micromovement: Three-dimensional finite element analysis. Dental Materials. 2012;28(11):1126–33.

[33] Baggi L, Cappelloni I, Di Girolamo M, Maceri F, Vairo G. The influence of implant diameter and length

on stress distribution of osseointegrated implants related to crestal bone geometry: A three-dimensional finite element analysis. The Journal of Prosthetic Dentistry. 2008;100(6):422–31.

[34] Rodríguez-Ciurana X, Vela-Nebot X, Segalà-Torres M, Rodado-Alonso C, Méndez-Blanco V, Mata-Bugueroles M. Biomechanical repercussions of bone resorption related to biologic width: a finite element analysis of three implant-abutment configurations. Int J Periodontics Restorative Dent. 2009 Oct;29(5): 479–87.

[35] Martini AP, Barros Rosália M, Freitas Júnior Amilcar C, Rocha Eduardo P, Almeida Erika O, Ferraz Cacilda C, et al. Influence of patform and abutment angulation on peri-implant bone. A three-dimensional finite element stress analysis. Journal of Oral Implantology. 2012.

[36] Çimen H, Yengin E. Analyzing the Effects of the Platform-Switching Procedure on Stresses in the Bone and Implant-Abutment Complex by 3-Dimensional Fem Analysis. Journal of Oral Implantology. 2010;38(1):21–6.

[37] Khurana P, Sharma A, Sodhi Kiranmeet K. Influence of fine threads and platform-switching on crestal bone stress around implant – A three dimensional finite element analysis. Journal of Oral Implantology. 2011.

[38] Ferraz CC, Anchieta RB, de Almeida EO, Freitas Júnior AC, Ferraz FC, Machado LS, et al. Influence of microthreads and platform switching on stress distribution in bone using angled abutments. Journal of Prosthodontic Research. 2012; 56(4):256–63.

[39] Carvalho N, Almeida E, Rocha E, Freitas AJ, Anchieta R, Kina S. Short implant to support maxillary restorations: bone stress analysis using regular and switching platform. J Craniofac Surg. 2012 May;23(3):678–81.

[40] Tabata L, Assunção W, Barão A, Sousa E, Gomes E, Delben J. Implant platform switching: biomechanical approach using two-dimensional finite element analysis. J Craniofac Surg. 2010 Jan;21(1):182–7.

[41] Vargas L, Almeida E, Rocha E, Freitas Jr A, Anchieta R, Kina S, et al. Regular and platform switching. Bone stress analysis with varying implant diameters. J Oral Implantol. 2011 Jan;13. [Epub ahead of print].

[42] Chang C, Chen C, Hsu M. Biomechanical effect of platform switching in implant dentistry: a three-dimensional finite element analysis. Int J Oral Maxillofac Implants. 2010 Mar-Apr;25(2):295–304.

[43] Liu X, Li Z, Xia H. Influence of implant-abutment connection mode on stress distribution in peri-implant bone. Zhonghua Kou Qiang Yi Xue Za Zhi. 2008 Jan;43(1):50–3.

[44] Pellizzer EP, Verri FR, Falcón-Antenucci RM, Júnior JFS, de Carvalho PSP, de Moraes SLD, et al. Stress Analysis in Platform-Switching Implants: A 3-Dimensional Finite Element Study. Journal of Oral Implantology. 2010;38(5):587–94.

[45] Canay S, Akça K. Biomechanical aspects of bone-level diameter shifting at implant-abutment interface. Implant Dent. 2009 Jun;18(3):239–48.

[46] Hsu J, Fuh L, Lin D, Shen Y, HL H. Bone strain and interfacial sliding analyses of platform switching and implant diameter on an immediately loaded implant: experimental and three-dimensional finite element analyses. J Periodontol. 2009 Jul;80(7):1125–32.

[47] Pessoa RS, Vaz LG, Marcantonio E, Vander Sloten J, Duyck J, Jaecques SV. Biomechanical evaluation of platform switching in different implant protocols: computed tomography-based three-dimensional finite element analysis. The International journal of oral & maxillofacial implants. 2010;25(5):911–9.

[48] Tabata L, Rocha E, Barão V, Assunção W. Platform switching: biomechanical evaluation using three-dimensional finite element analysis. Int J Oral Maxillofac Implants. 2011 May-Jun;26(3):482–91.

[49] Freitas-Júnior AC, Rocha EP, Bonfante EA, Almeida EO, Anchieta RB, Martini AP, et al. Biomechanical evaluation of internal and external hexagon platform switched implant-abutment connections: An in vitro laboratory and three-dimensional finite element analysis. Dental Materials. 2012;28(10):e218-e28.

[50] Saidin S, Abdul Kadir MR, Sulaiman E, Abu Kasim NH. Effects of different implant–abutment connections on micromotion and stress distribution: Prediction of microgap formation. Journal of Dentistry. 2012;40(6):467–74.

[51] Becker J, Ferrari D, Herten M, Kirsch A, Schaer A, Schwarz F. Influence of platform switching on crestal bone changes at non-submerged titanium implants: a histomorphometrical study in dogs. Journal of Clinical Periodontology. 2007;34(12):1089–96.

[52] Becker J, Ferrari D, Mihatovic I, Sahm N, Schaer A, Schwarz F. Stability of crestal bone level at platform-switched non-submerged titanium implants: a histomorphometrical study in dogs. Journal of Clinical Periodontology. 2009;36(6):532–9.

[53] Oliveira R, Novaes AJ, Taba MJ, Papalexiou V, Muglia V. Bone remodeling adjacent to Morse cone-connection implants with platform switch: a fluorescence study in the dog mandible. Int J Oral Maxillofac Implants. 2009 Mar-Apr;24(2):257–66.

[54] Cochran D, Bosshardt D, Grize L, Higginbottom F, Jones A, Jung R, et al. Bone response to loaded implants with non-matching implant-abutment diameters in the canine mandible. J Periodontol. 2009 Apr;80(4):609–17.

[55] Xu P, Tan S, Xing L, Mao X, Yang X, Huang H. Histological observation of implant-bone interface in immediate loading implant with platform switching. Zhonghua Kou Qiang Yi Xue Za Zhi. 2011 Dec;46(12):759–61.

[56] Farronato D, Santoro G, Canullo L, Botticelli D, Maiorana C, Lang N. Establishment of the epithelial attachment and connective tissue adaptation to implants installed under the concept of "platform switching": a histologic study in minipigs. Clin Oral Implants Res. 2012 Jan;23(1):90–4.

[57] Rodriquez X, Vela X, Calvo-Guirado J, Nart J, Stappert C. Effect of platform switching on collagen fiber orientation and bone resorption around dental implants: a preliminary histologic animal study. Int J Oral Maxillofac Implants. 2012 Sep;27(5):1116–22.

[58] Degidi M, Iezzi G, Scarano A, Piattelli A. Immediately loaded titanium implant with a tissue-stabilizing/maintaining design ('beyond platform switch') retrieved from man after 4 weeks: a histological and histomorphometrical evaluation. A case report. Clinical Oral Implants Research. 2008;19(3): 276–82.

[59] Luongo R, Traini T, Guidone P, Bianco G, Cocchetto R, Celletti R. Hard and soft tissue responses to the platform-switching technique. Int J Periodontics Restorative Dent. 2008 Dec;28(6):551–7.

[60] Canullo L, Pellegrini G, Allievi C, Trombelli L, Annibali S, Dellavia C. Soft tissues around long-term platform switching implant restorations: a histological human evaluation. Preliminary results. J Clin Periodontol. 2011 Jan;38(1):86–94.

[61] Rompen E. The impact of the type and configuration of abutments and their (repeated) removal on the attachment level and marginal bone. Eur J Oral Implantol. 2012;5 Suppl:S83–90.
[62] Bateli M, Att W, Strub J. Implant neck configurations for preservation of marginal bone level: a systematic review. Int J Oral Maxillofac Implants. 2011 Mar–Apr;26(2):290–303.
[63] López-Marí L, Calvo-Guirado J, Martín-Castellote B, Gomez-Moreno G, López-Marí M. Implant platform switching concept: an updated review. Med Oral Patol Oral Cir Bucal. 2009 Sep;1;14(9):e450–4.
[64] Serrano-Sánchez P, Calvo-Guirado J, Manzanera-Pastor E, Lorrio-Castro C, Bretones-López P, Pérez-Llanes J. The influence of platform switching in dental implants. A literature review. Med Oral Patol Oral Cir Bucal. 2011 May;1;16(3):e400–5.
[65] Atieh M, Ibrahim H, Atieh A. Platform switching for marginal bone preservation around dental implants: a systematic review and meta-analysis. J Periodontol. 2010 Oct;81(10):1350–66.
[66] Al-Nsour M, Chan H, HL W. Effect of the platform-switching technique on preservation of peri-implant marginal bone: a systematic review. Int J Oral Maxillofac Implants. 2012 Jan–Feb;27(1):138–45.
[67] Annibali S, Bignozzi I, Cristalli MP, Graziani F, La Monaca G, Polimeni A. Peri-implant marginal bone level: a systematic review and meta-analysis of studies comparing platform switching versus conventionally restored implants. Journal of Clinical Periodontology. 2012;39(11):1097–113.
[68] Byrne G. Platform switching reduces peri-implant bone loss. The Journal of the American Dental Association. 2012;143(7):787–8.
[69] Pieri F, Aldini N, Marchetti C, Corinaldesi G. Influence of implant-abutment interface design on bone and soft tissue levels around immediately placed and restored single-tooth implants: a randomized controlled clinical trial. Int J Oral Maxillofac Implants. 2011 Jan–Feb;26(1):169–78.
[70] Crespi R, Capparè P, Gherlone E. Radiographic evaluation of marginal bone levels around platform-switched and non-platform-switched implants used in an immediate loading protocol. Int J Oral Maxillofac Implants. 2009 Sep–Oct;24(5):920–6.
[71] Enkling N, Jöhren P, Klimberg V, Bayer S, Mericske-Stern R, Jepsen S. Effect of platform switching on peri-implant bone levels: a randomized clinical trial. Clin Oral Implants Res. 2011 Oct;22(10):1185–92.
[72] Canullo L, Iurlaro G, Iannello G. Double-blind randomized controlled trial study on post-extraction immediately restored implants using the switching platform concept: soft tissue response. Preliminary report. Clinical Oral Implants Research. 2009;20(4):414–20.
[73] Prosper L, Redaelli S, Pasi M, Zarone F, Radaelli G, Gherlone E. A randomized prospective multicenter trial evaluating the platform-switching technique for the prevention of postrestorative crestal bone loss. Int J Oral Maxillofac Implants. 2009 Mar–Apr;24(2): 299–308.
[74] Trammell K, Geurs N, O'Neal S, Liu P, Haigh S, McNeal S, et al. A prospective, randomized, controlled comparison of platform-switched and matched-abutment implants in short-span partial denture situations. Int J Periodontics Restorative Dent. 2009 Dec;29(6):599–605.
[75] Canullo L, Fedele GR, Iannello G, Jepsen S. Platform switching and marginal bone-level alterations: the results of a randomized-controlled trial. Clinical Oral Implants Research. 2010;21(1):115–21.
[76] Telleman G, Raghoebar G, Vissink A, Meijer H. Impact of platform switching on inter-proximal bone levels around short implants in the posterior region; 1-year results from a randomized clinical trial. J Clin Periodontol. 2012 Jul;39(7):688–97.
[77] Vandeweghe S, De Bruyn H. A within-implant comparison to evaluate the concept of platform switching: a randomised controlled trial. Eur J Oral Implantol. 2012 Autumn;5(3):253–62.
[78] Canullo L, Iannello G, Götz W. The influence of individual bone patterns on peri-implant bone loss: preliminary report from a 3-year randomized clinical and histologic trial in patients treated with implants restored with matching-diameter abutments or the platform-switching concept. Int J Oral Maxillofac Implants. 2011 May–Jun;26(3):618–30.
[79] Peñarrocha-Diago M, Flichy-Fernández A, Alonso-González R, Peñarrocha-Oltra D, Balaguer-Martínez J, Peñarrocha-Diago M. Influence of implant neck design and implant-abutment connection type on peri-implant health. Radiological study. Clin Oral Implants Res. 2012 Aug;28.
[80] Cappiello M, Luongo R, Di lorio D, Bugea C, Cocchetto R, Celletti R. Evaluation of peri-implant bone loss around platform-switched implants. Int J Periodontics Restorative Dent. 2008 Aug;28(4): 347–55.
[81] Almeida F, Carvalho A, Fontes M, Pedrosa A, Costa R, Noleto J, et al. Radiographic evaluation of marginal bone level around internal-hex implants with switched platform: a clinical case report series. Int J Oral Maxillofac Implants. 2011 May–Jun;26(3):587–92.
[82] Cocchetto R, Traini T, Caddeo F, Celletti R. Evaluation of hard tissue response around wider platform-switched implants. Int J Periodontics Restorative Dent. 2010 Apr;30(2):163–71.
[83] Wagenberg B, Froum S. Prospective study of 94 platform-switched implants observed from 1992 to 2006. Int J Periodontics Restorative Dent. 2010 Feb;30(1):9–17.
[84] Canullo L, Goglia G, Iurlaro G, Iannello G. Short-term bone level observations associated with platform switching in immediately placed and restored single maxillary implants: a preliminary report. Int J Prosthodont. 2009 May–Jun;22(3):277–82.
[85] Li Q, Lin Y, Qiu L, Hu X, Li J, DI P. Clinical study of application of platform switching to dental implant treatment in esthetic zone. Zhonghua Kou Qiang Yi Xue Za Zhi. 2008 Sep;43(9):537–41.
[86] Fickl S, Zuhr O, Stein J, Hürzeler M. Peri-implant bone level around implants with platform-switched abutments. Int J Oral Maxillofac Implants. 2010 May–Jun;25(3):577–81.
[87] Bilhan H, Mumcu E, Erol S, Kutay O. Influence of platform-switching on marginal bone levels for implants with mandibular overdentures: a retrospective clinical study. Implant Dent. 2010 Jun;19(3):250–8.
[88] Calvo-Guirado J, Gómez-Moreno G, López-Marí L, Guardia J, Negri B, Martínez-González J. Crestal bone loss evaluation in osseotite expanded platform implants: a 5-year study. Clin Oral Implants Res. 2011 Dec;22(12):1409–14.
[89] Degidi M, Piattelli A, Scarano A, Shibli J, Iezzi G. Peri-implant collagen fibers around human cone Morse connection implants under polarized light: a report of three cases. Int J Periodontics Restorative Dent. 2012 Jun;32(3):323–8.

Biodental Engineering II – Natal Jorge et al (Eds)
© 2014 Taylor & Francis Group, London, ISBN 978-1-138-00131-2

Risk factors for implant treatment failure: a case-control study

C. Sedarat
University Bordeaux 2, Dental Unit, Bordeaux, France

S. de Chalvron
University Montpellier 3, Laboratory Epsylon, Montpellier, France
Environnemental Medicine Institute, Psychology and Neurosciences Laboratory, Paris, France

B. Ella
University Bordeaux 2, Laboratory of Anatomy Medical-Surgical, Bordeaux, France

M. Mesnard
Institute of Mechanics and Engineering, CNRS UMR 5295, Bordeaux, France

A. Ramos
University of Aveiro, Biomechanics Research Group, Department of Mechanical Engineering, Aveiro, Portugal

ABSTRACT: The principal aim of this study was to describe some potential risk factors implant loss. A retrospective cohort study design was used. 166 patients received 380 implants of 3 different manufactures. The influence of personal and technical variables was noted. In the full sample on a 10 years study period, we have noticed an overall 92.89% (survival rates of dental implants and 88.6% of success in patient based analysis. Patients were aged from 30 to 75 years old. There were 55 men and 111 women in the full sample... They received an average of 2.29 implants. Clinical parameters involve in implant failures were identified as periodontitis and bruxism. Smoking fewer than ten cigarettes per day is not a risk factor for implant failures. Understanding the effective effect of tobacco, is imperative in order not to exclude some patients from implant placement, or, not recommend this placement due to too high risks failure.

1 INTRODUCTION

Numerous early studies have highlight a direct bone-to-implant contact referred as osseo-integration and obtained encouraging clinical long-term results in treatment of edentulous patients (Adell et al. 1981; Adell et al. 1990; Brånemark et al. 1977; Schroeder et al. 1981; Wedgwood et al. 1992).

Today this treatment modality has become a routine protocol in dentistry and dental implants have been accepted as a viable option for the treatment of edentulous patients supporting the favorable long-term prognosis (Berglundh et al. 2002; Lang et al. 2004; Levin et al. 2005; Levin et al. 2006; Ravald et al. 2012; Romeo et al. 2004).

Correct design of implant surface, a better understanding of the biomechanical properties of the implants and selection of the suitable surgical technique taking in account patient's bone quantity and quality are major parameters affecting the long-term survival and success of dental implants. However, in spite of high success rate, occurrence of implants failure has been reported (Ashley et al. 2003; Bain et al. 2002; Porter et al. 2005).

Potential risk factors attributing to implant failures include local factors (reduced bone volume, reduced bone density, periodontitis), and systemic conditions (diabetes, smoking, osteoporosis, radiation therapy, chemotherapy) (Anner et al. 2010; Baelum et al. 2004; El Assadi et al. 2008; Moy et al. 2005; Roos et al. 2006).

Nevertheless, the scientific literature regarding the risk factors for implant failure is limited (Esposito 1999) concluded that the "treatment of biologic complications and failing implants lacks systemic scientific validation and is based mainly on empirical experience and inference from in vitro findings on a trial-and-error basis." Moreover some studies present a lot of methodological and statistical bias. For exemple, one meta-analysis (Hinode et al. 2006) show an effect of tobacco use but 1) Odds ratio in the analyzed studies were not adjusted 2) there was no report of heterogeneous indice while 9 of 19 studies showed no significant impact of tabacco use. Others studies on tobacco use did not separate smokers in groups (small, moderate or heavy smokers), to our knowledge, just one separate smokers in 3 groups but authors calculated khi-squares while some cells were under 5 so these results are not reliable (Sanchez-Perez et al. 2007). Moreover any studies give the effect-size, while what is important is not also the variance difference between some factors but the load of these differences. We can do the same ascertainments for others risk factors as periodontal diseases or bruxism. Finally, some authors provided recommendations concerning the report of results, as use a patient-basis (Lang et al. 2002), but they did not explained this recommendation and provided no statistical evidence about the value of a patient-basis. However, considering low ratio observed in literature between failure implant and no failure implant groups, according to various risk factors, this recommendation refers to samples-size and statistical puissance issues.

Since periodontal diseases and bruxism are frequently assess as a risk factors in literature, we assume that they are risk factors of failure implants but not tobacco-use for low tobacco dose, that results are based whether on a patient-basis or an implant-basis.

2 METHOD

2.1 *Procedure*

Data were collected from 166 volunteer patients who received dental implant(s) by the same surgeon and prosthetically restored by experienced dentists between 2002 and 2010 in Bordeaux clinic (France).

Patients were selected according to the following inclusion criteria: 1) Presence of any kind of maxillary or mandibular edentulism treated by the mean of implants, 2) A minimal follow up period of 2 years. Patient exclusion criteria were as following: 1) Systemic diseases contra indicating implant treatment, 2) Active periodontal disease, 3) Heavy bruxing or clenching, 4) Heavy smoking (>10/day), 5) Local inflammation and/or and oral mucosal diseases.

All patients had a medical and dental history taken, clinical exams and radiographs were performed. All patients had a periodontal examination and treatment that included oral hygiene instructions. Periodontal treatment, including non-surgical and surgical interventions, was completed if needed. All patients had stable and healthy periodontal conditions at the time of implant placement. The surgical procedures were chosen as a function of the patient characteristics, the anatomic peculiarities of the insertion sites. A 3–6-month healing period was allowed before prosthetic loading. The titanium implants used in this study had a roughened surface.

All patients were seen 10 to 14 days postoperatively, 30 days postoperatively, and at uncovering/testing of the healed implant. If needed, other postoperative visits were scheduled.

If a second-stage surgery was needed to uncover the implant, it was allowed to heal 2 to 4 weeks before initiating prosthetic procedures. Occasionally, soft tissue concerns delayed prosthetic procedures for longer time periods.

After treatment completion, all patients were recalled at least annually. Patients in ongoing periodontal maintenance were seen as frequently as this warranted. All implants were subsequently assessed clinically and radiographically at follow-up examinations.

2.2 *Measures*

We considered three risk-factors: tobacco used with low tobacco use (<10 cigarettes per day), history of treated periodontal diseases, history of bruxism. We also considered covariables such age at implant(s) placement and number of implants and gender.

Implant failure criteria were defined as described previously (Buser et al., 1990). At follow up examinations, the implants were examined for tissue integration according to the strict parameters defined. Specifically, the integration was considered successful if the following parameters were met: 1) absence of recurring peri-implant infection with suppuration; 2) absence of persistent subjective complaints such as pain, foreign body sensation, and/or dysesthesia, 3) absence of a continuous radiolucency around the implant, and 4) absence of any detectable implant mobility.

2.3 *Sample*

Among the 166 volunteers patient, 19 patients had an implant failure, so we extract, with a random solution (bootstrap) 19 patients who had no implant failure. In fact, our study is a case-control study. This new sample is constituted of 12 men (31.6%) and 26 women (68.4%) aged from 30 to 74 years old ($M = 54.63$, $SD = 10.82$). They received 1 to 6 implants ($M = 2.34$, $SD = 1.51$). 5 (13.2%) were smokers (less than 10 cigarettes per day), 8 (21.1%) had an history of bruxism and 11 (28.9%) had an history of periodontal diseases.

2.4 *Statistical analysis*

We transformed the patient-basis ($n = 39$) in implant-basis ($n = 89$) by converting the data-file, so we had two data-file, one implant-basis and one patient basis. For each basis, we performed multivariate Anova (all prerequisites were verified before) in order to calculate effect-sizes of potential variance differences of implant failures number between each risk-factors and for the two data-basis. Then we calculated frequency of risk-factors apparitions in each group (failure/no failure) and Odd-ratio but only for the implant-basis because there were less than 5 observations in some cells for the patient-basis. Finally we compared the results with two indices: internal consistency (Cronbach alpha) and the component of correlation matrix (CCM).

3 RESULTS

On the patient-basis bruxism $D_{bruxims}(1.37) = 4.15$, $p < 0.05$, $\eta^2 = 0.12$, and $D_{pariodontal}(1.37) = 8.72$,

Table 1. Results of multivariate Anovas for numbers of implant failure and risk-factors.

	M	SD	D(ddl)	η^2	Stat. power
Patient-base					
Perio.diseases					
No	0.41	0.64	8.72(1.37)***	0.21	0.82
Yes	1.45	1.13			
Bruxism					
No	0.60	0.89	4.15(1.37)*	0.12	0.51
Yes	1.13	0.99			
Tobacco use					
No	0.61	0.75	0.22(1.37)	0.007	0.07
Yes	1.40	1.67			
Implant-base					
Perio.diseases					
No	0.49	0.71	26.2(1.88)****	0.24	0.99
Yes	1.56	1.22			
Bruxism					
No	0.72	1.04	20.1(1.88)****	0.19	0.99
Yes	1.36	0.95			
Tobacco use					
No	0.72	0.81	1.005(1.88)	0.01	0.42
Yes	1.50	1.58			

****$p < 0.001$, ***$p < 0.01$, *$p < 0.05$

$p < 0.01$, $\eta^2 = 0.21$ were significant but not tobacco use, $D_{tobacco}(1.37) = 0.22$, ns, and, so there was no variance difference of number of implants failure between smokers and no smokers. Statistical power (beta risk) varied from 0.07 (tobacco) to 0.84 (periodontal diseases), which indicates a very low statistical power (Cohen et al.1992) for tobacco or moderate (Bruxism = 0.51). On the implant-basis, we observed the same results, $D_{bruxims}(1.88) = 20.10$, $p < 0.001$, $\eta^2 = 0.19$, and $D_{pariodontal}(1.88) = 26.2$, $p < 0.001$, $\eta^2 = 0.24$ and $D_{tobacco}(1.88) = 1.05$, ns (for means and SD refer to table 1). Statistical power is high for periodontal diseases (0.99) and bruxism (0.99) but moderate for tobacco (0.426).

On the patient-basis, 9(47.4%) of implant-failures occurred in people with no history of periodontal diseases while 10(52.6%) occurred in people with history of periodontal diseases, 13(68.4%) occurred in people with no history of bruxism, and 6(31.6%) in people with history of bruxism, 16 (84.2%) occurred in people who were non smokers, and 3(15.8%) in people who were smokers. On implant-basis, 21(42.9%) implant-failures occurred in people with no history of periodontal diseases and 28 (57.1%) in people with history of periodontal diseases, 31 (63.3%) occurred in people with no history of bruxism and 18 (36.7%) in people with history of bruxism. Finally, 38 (77.6%) occured in people who were non smokers and 11 (61.1%) in people who were smokers. The logistic regression showed that periodontal diseases is a significant risk factor, $\beta = 2.49$, $\chi^2_{wald}(1) = 17.09$, $p < 0.001$, AOR[1] = 12, CI 95% = [3.69, 38.96], $R^2_{Nagelkerke} = 0.309$, as well as bruxism, $\beta = 1.65$, $\chi^2_{wald}(1) = 7.48$, $p < 0.01$, AOR = 5.23, CI95% = [1.59, 17.09], $R^2_{Nagelkerke} = 0.13$ but no low tobacco-use, $\beta = 0.311$, $\chi^2_{wald}(1) = 0.33$, *ns*, AOR = 1.37, CI95% = [0.48, 3.92].

Finally, we observed that the results observed from one base to other are similar, since $\alpha = 0.98$ and CMM = 0.879 for tobacco use, $\alpha = 0.99$, CMM = 0.879 for bruxism and $\alpha = 0.99$ and CMM = 0.867 for periodontal diseases.

4 DISCUSSION

Our findings suggest that smoking fewer than ten cigarettes per day is not a risk factor for implant failures what is congruent with the results of (Sanchez-Perez et al. 2007). They also show that a patient-base decreases too much statistical power increasing beta-risk, which must be over 0.80 (Cohen et al. 1983) while the results of a database to another are similar. This means that if researchers are working on a patient-base, the sample size should be large enough to reduce the beta risk greatly decreased with an implant-basis. Moreover this decrease is observed for periodontal diseases and bruxism which are risk-factors, as already shown in previous researches. However, the effect-size is not very large, which refers to a limitation or our study on sample size. But it also shows another limitation of our study, indeed, the statistical power for tobacco-use remains moderate with implant-base. This means that to determine the real effect of tobacco, it should not only work with different groups of smokers (low, moderate, high) but also with a control group and that the groups should be balanced.

To conclude, understand better the effect of tobacco, including a low consumption, is imperative in order not to exclude some patients from implant placement, or, otherwise, not recommend this placement due to too high risks failure. Future resarches must be control-studies, with an implant-base or with a patient-base, but with a large sample-size.

REFERENCES

Adell, R, Eriksson, B, Lekholm, U, Brånemark, P.-I, & Jemt, T. 1990. Long-term follow-up study of osseointegrated implants in the treatment of totally edentulous jaws. Int J Oral Maxillofac Implants; 5: 347–359.

Adell, R., Lekholm, U., Rockler, B., & Branemark, P.-I. 1981. A 15-year study of osseo-integrated implants in the edentulous jaw. Int J Oral Surg; 10: 387–416.

Alsaadi, G., Quirynen, M., Komarek, A., & van Steenberghe, D. 2008. Impact of local and systemic factors on the incidence of late oral implant loss. Clin Oral Implants Res.; 19: 670–676.

Anner, R., Grossmann, Y., Anner, Y. & Levin, L. 2010. Smoking, diabetes mellitus, periodontitis, 509 and supportive

[1] OR adjusted on age and number of implants

periodontal treatment as factors associated with dental implant 510 survival: a long-term retrospective evaluation of patients followed for up to 511 10 years. Implant Dent; 19: 57–64.

Ashley, E.T., Covington, L.L., Bishop, B.G., & Breault, L.G. 2003. Ailing and failing endosseous dental implants: a literature review. J Contemp Dent Pract.; 4: 35–50.

Baelum, V. & Ellegaard, B. 2004. Implant survival in periodontally compromised patients. Journal of Periodontology 75: 1404–1412.

Bain, C.A., Weng, D., Meltzer, A., Kohles, S.S. & Stach, R.M. 2002. A meta-analysis evaluating the risk for implant failure in patients who smoke. Compendium of Continuing Education in Dentistry 23: 695–69

Berglundh, T., Persson, L. & Klinge, B. 2002. A systematic review of the incidence of biological and technical complications in implant dentistry reported in prospective longitudinal studies of at least 5 years. Journal of Clinical Periodontology 29 (Suppl. 3): 197–212.

Brånemark, P.I., Hannsson, B., Adell, R., Breine, U., Lindström, J., & Öhman, A. 1977. Osseointegrated implants in the treatment of the edentulous jaw. Experience from a 10 year period. Scand J Plast Reconstr Surg; 11: 1–132

Buser, D., Weber, H.P. & Lang, N.P. 1990. Tissue integration of non-submerged implants. 1-year results of a prospective study with 100 ITI hollow-cylinder and hollow-screw implants. Clinical Oral Implants Research 1: 33–40.

Cohen, J. 1992. A power primer. *Psychological Bulletin,* 112(1): 155–159.

Cohen, K.J., Hawawini, G.A., Maier, S.F., Schartz, R.A. & Whitcom, D.K. 1983. Estimating and adjusting for the intervalling-effect bias in beta. Management science, 29(1): 135–148.

Esposito, M. 1999.On biological failures of osseointegrated oral implants. PhD thesis, Institute of Anatomy and Cell Biology, University of Göteborg, Göteborg, Sweden.

Hinode, D., Tanabe, S., Yokoyama, M., Fujisawa, K., Yamauchi, E., & Miyamoto, Y. 2006. Influence of smoking on osseointegrated implant failure: a meta-analysis. Clin Oral Implants Res; 17: 473–478.

Lang, N.P., Pjetursson, B.E., Tan, K., Bragger, U., Egger, M. & Zwahlen, M. 2004. A systematic review of the survival and complication rates of fixed partial dentures (FPDs) after an observation period of at least 5 years. II. Combined tooth-implant-supported FPDs. Clinical Oral Implants Research 15: 643–653.

Lang, N.P., Karring, T., Meredith, N. 2002.Consensus report. Group E summary. Proceedings from the 4th European Workshop on Periodontology. J Clin Periodontol; 29(Suppl. 3): 232–234.

Levin, L., Pathael, S., Dolev, E., Schwartz-Arad, D. 2005. Aesthetic versus surgical success of single dental implants: 1- to 9-year follow-up. Pract Proced Aesthet Dent; 17: 533–8.

Levin, L., Sadet, P., & Grossmann Y. 2006. A retrospective evaluation of 1387 single-tooth implants: A six-year follow up. J Periodontol; 77: 2080–3.

Moy PK, Medina D, Shetty V, Aghaloo TL. 2005.Dental implant failure rates and associated risk factors. Int J Oral Maxillofac Implants; 20: 569–77.

Porter JA, von Fraunhofer JA. 2005.Success or failure of dental implants? A literature review with treatment considerations. Gen Dent.; 53: 423–32.

Ravald N, Dahlgren S, Teiwik A, Gröndahl K. Long-term evaluation of Astra Tech and Brånemark implants in patients treated with full-arch bridges. Results after 12–15 years.Clin Oral Implants Res. 2012 Jul 4.

Romeo, E., Lops, D., Margutti, E., Ghisolfi, M., Chiapasco, M. & Vogel, G. 2004. Long-term survival and success of oral implants in the treatment of full and partial arches: a 7-year prospective study with the ITI dental implant system. International Journal of Oral & Maxillofacial Implants 19: 247–259.

Roos-Jansaker AM, Lindahl C, Renvert H, Renvert S. 2006. Nine- to fourteen-year follow-up of implant treatment. Part I: implant loss and associations to various factors. J Clin Periodontol; 33: 283–289.

Sánchez-Pérez A, Moya-Villaescusa MJ, Caffesse RG. 2007. Tobacco as a risk factor for survival of dental implants. J Periodontol. Feb; 78(2): 351–9.

Schroeder A, van der Zypen E, Stich H, Sutter F. 1981. The reactions of bone, connective tissue, and epithelium to endosteal implants with titanium-sprayed surfaces. J Maxillofac Surg; 9: 15–35.

Wedgwood D, Jennings KJ, Critchlow HA, Watkinson AC, Shepherd JP, Frame JW. Laird WRE, Quatle AA. 1992. Experience with ITI osseointegrated implants at five centers in UK. Br J Oral Maxillofac Surg.; 30: 377–38.

Biodental Engineering II – Natal Jorge et al (Eds)
© 2014 Taylor & Francis Group, London, ISBN 978-1-138-00131-2

Biomodelling partial anodontia case for analysis and surgical implant rehabilitation

Luís Queijo & João Rocha
Departamento de Tecnologia Mecânica – Escola Superior de Tecnologia e Gestão do Instituto Politécnico de Bragança, Bragança, Portugal

André Ramos
Clínica Avenida – Medicina Dentária, Bragança, Portugal

ABSTRACT: Partial Anodontia, also called Hypondontia or Oligodontia is a hereditary disorder occurring as a consequence of disturbances in the ectoderm of the developing embryo and manifests as a lack of development of all or most primary and/or permanent dentition, with or without a cleft lip and palate. In this case, patient is a young adult Caucasian male that suffer from Partial Anodontia and that, after clinical examination, presented the existence of 13th, 16th, 22th, 23th and 27th, with a 26th included tooth in maxilla and the presence of 36th and 46th teeth in mandible. Biomodelling – a technique that join medical imaging with additive manufacturing in order to obtain physical models will be used, and applied to mandible situation, with the manufacturing under 3DP® technique of the needed total or partial models, not only to better understand patient's case and bone condition but also to plan surgical procedures over mandible by defining implants placement and any bone reconfiguration.

1 INTRODUCTION

1.1 *Partial Anodontia disease*

Partial Anodontia, also called Hypondontia or Oligodontia is a sort of manifestation from Ectodermal dysplasia – a hereditary disorder occurring as a consequence of disturbances in the ectoderm of the developing embryo (Nunn et al. 2003; Tarjan et al. 2005).

Oral traits of ectodermal dysplasia (ED) may be expressed as Anodontia or Hypodontia – lack of development of all or most primary and/or permanent dentition, with or without a cleft lip and palate. Anodontia also manifests itself by a lack of alveolar ridge development, once there is an absence of bone production due to physical forces.

The most frequent prosthetic treatment for the dental management of ectodermal dysplasia is removable prosthodontics. Since alveolar bone development is dependent on the presence of teeth, patients with ectodermal dysplasia have little or no bone ridge upon which to construct dentures (Vieira et al. 2007).

1.2 *Biomodelling*

To face difficulty in evaluating bone quality, complementing CT (Computerized Tomography) scan diagnose method it was decided to recur to biomodeling techniques in order to produce both partial and complete physical biomodels from maxilla and mandible, once it has been proved as a valuable auxiliary technique (Queijo et al. 2010).

Biomodelling is a technique that combines image processing and additive manufacturing allowing medical image reconstruction in a 3D digital model and subsequent total or partial physical models construction.

Image processing techniques work with the image data from CT or MRI scanning devices in DICOM format, converting them in a series of sequenced images and are, essentially, based in image segmentation – an image processing technique that using the appropriated algorithms allowing user to define which anatomical structures are to maintain and which can be discarded. Once that operation is performed it is possible to perform a 3D reconstruction, using the processed image sequence, and obtaining a 3D digital model which surfaces can be translated in a triangular mesh and exported under a *.stl* type file.

This file is then transferred to proprietary software from additive manufacturing device that will translate it in a sequence of slices and allow defining additive manufacturing device setup.

Additive manufacturing is a fabrication method that builds physical models, layer by layer, over a wide range of techniques and materials available. These can go from the simplest methods of agglutinating powder composite materials with an aqua based binder, passing by plastic fused deposition or laser sintering and polymerization of resins until the high end of laser metal fusion (Queijo et al. 2009).

2 CASE

2.1 *Case description*

Patient is a young adult Caucasian male that suffer from partial Anodontia and that, after clinical examination, presented the existence of 13th 16th 22th 23th and 27th with a 26th included tooth in maxilla and the presence of 36th and 46th teeth in mandible. There were no variations in facial symmetry and no particular changes in palate or other anatomical structures with exception for light bone atrophy in the areas with dental absence. It was also reported that same situation had occurred in primary dentition and that there were not known similar cases in family.

2.2 *Case objectives*

It was intended the full rehabilitation of the total dentition by recurring to fixed implants. First phase in rehabilitation would be the mandible situation and is the case presented in this study.

3 PROCEDURE

3.1 *Image processing*

Image processing consisted in importing CT scanning images, in DICOM format, to appropriate image processing software, converting them in a sequence of editable images but maintaining CT scanning parameters. First phase of image processing is the segmentation phase. Over these images it is possible to apply a mask by defining a range, in Hounsfield scale (HU), that allow to "paint" each pixel which value lies in that range. The mask creation process is performed using an operation named *threshold*. After this process a first iteration in producing the digital rendered model, also known as 3D reconstruction, can be performed and will allow realizing which corrections in the initial mask need to be done.

Applying *erasing* tools it is possible to retouch the previously applied mask in order to maintain only the wanted anatomical structure – the mandible, without the existence of any noise or adjacent structures.

In figure 1 can be seen the overall look of segmentation process with applied mask visible in the three planes – sagittal, coronal and transverse, plus a view of the obtained 3D digital model.

The obtained 3D model is then exported under a *.stl* file format that translates its surfaces into a triangular mesh and that allow the transfer to proper additive manufacturing device software.

3.2 *Model manufacturing*

Model manufacturing was performed using 3DP® technique in a ZPrinter® 310 from ZCorporation. In print manager – Zprint® are settled up manufacturing parameters like the printing layout, the base material and the binder to be used. This device builds models

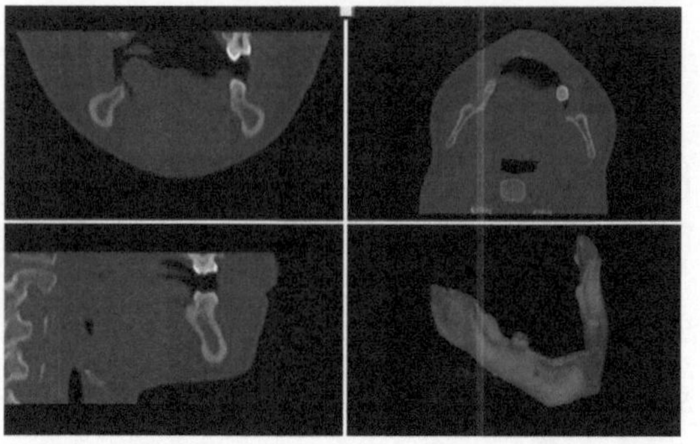

Figure 1. Image segmentation process – three planes view and rendered model.

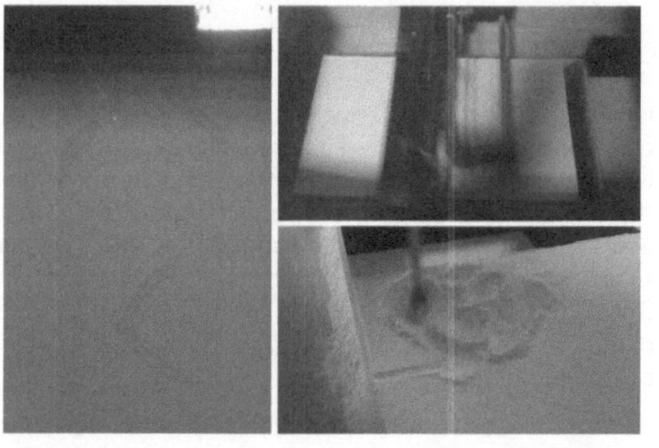

Figure 2. Model manufacturing process: sections printing, printing head working and model removal.

layer by layer by spreading, in a building platform, a thin layer of a composite material similar to plaster. Then, like a common printing head, a section from the wanted model is drawn with the binder in the powder surface. This process repeats spreading successive layers of base material as the building platform moves down and drawing each of the sections until the model is complete.

This model is obtained immersed in a bed of non-bonded material which leads to cleaning and surface stabilizing operations so it can be properly handled.

In figure 2 can be seen some of the manufacturing phase operations.

Cleaning and surface stabilization operations are related with models removal from the manufacturing platform, non-glued powder removal through a compressed air jet and subsequent recycling and, for last, impregnation with cyanoacrylate glue or epoxy resin, so the model gain resistance and could be perfectly handled.

4 SURGERY PLANNING

Surgery planning has been performed recurring to the models analysis, both digital and physical.

Considering complete mandible biomodel (figure 3) it was decided to divide mandible in five different

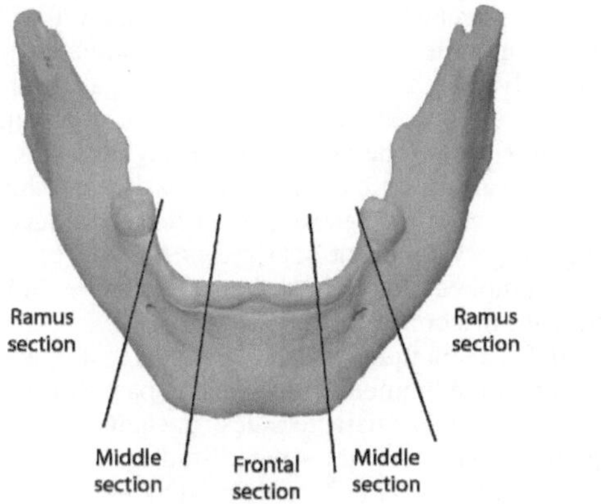

Figure 3. Complete mandible biomodel with sections definition.

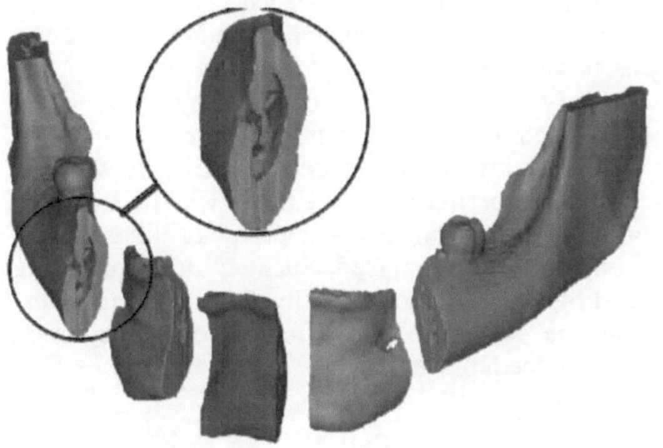

Figure 4. Sections in 3D digital model.

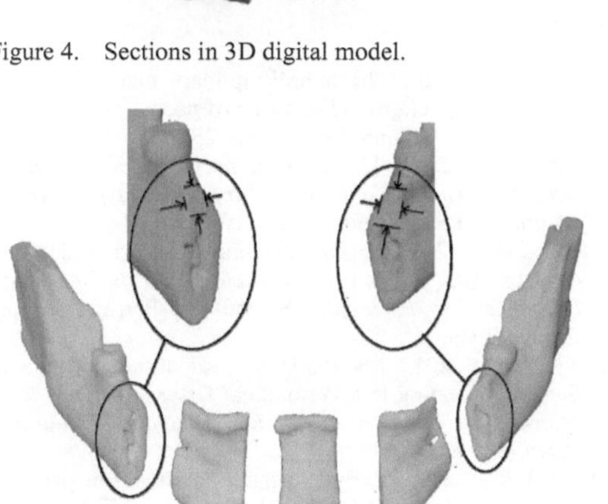

Figure 5. Sections in 3D biomodel with cortical bone evaluation.

sections so the cortical bone thickness in mandible frontal crest could be evaluated.

That way, an individual mask to each section has been created using *Boolean* operations tools in image processing software and individual models have been exported as *.stl* file. Those five individual models have, then, been manufactured following the previously described procedure. In figures 4 and 5 are shown both digital and physical 3D models.

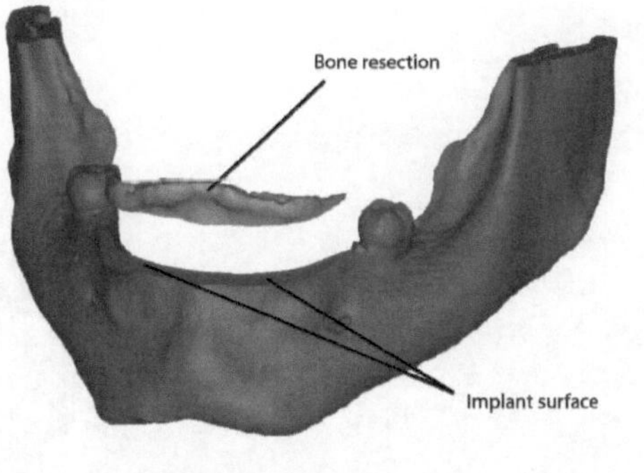

Figure 6. Mandible crest bone resection in 3D digital model.

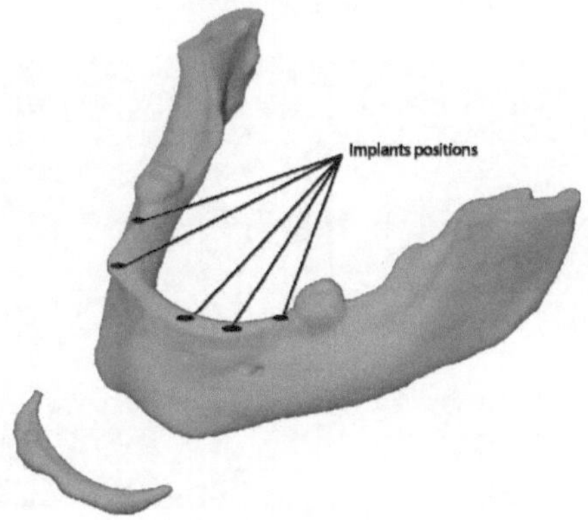

Figure 7. Mandible crest bone resection in 3D biomodel with implant positioning marks.

By measuring biomodels it was found that cortical bone at mandible crest level varied between 3 and 5 mm at a 5 mm depth from the crest top. That resulted in a medium thickness of 4 mm what totally unadvised implant placement.

Once it was considered that the available cortical bone thickness, allied to its irregularity, was unable to allow implants placement, it was decided to lower mandible central crest by performing a bone resection and creating a smother surface with incremented thickness (figures 6 and 7).

That resection should be performed at 7–8 mm from crest top in frontal view, creating a plane that should face the 36th and 46th teeth base, approximately.

The surface should be obtained with a medium thickness of about 6 mm what doesn't fulfill totally the requirements for implant placement.

As said before, after bone resection, the obtained surface still not allowing implant placement due to the bone thickness, so it was planned to perform a bone distraction in implant drilling to gain some more space that could be traduced in 1 to 3 mm what would allow placing the implants without major risks.

5 SURGERY

Surgery procedures start with gingival flap and its detachment with a periosteal elevator that allowed the

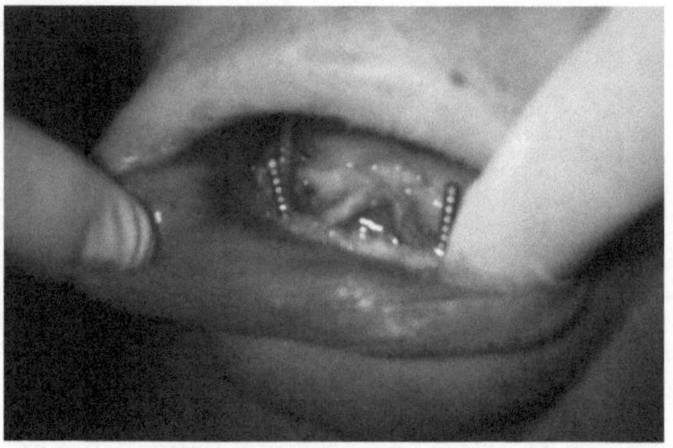

Figure 8. Implant drilling osteotomes.

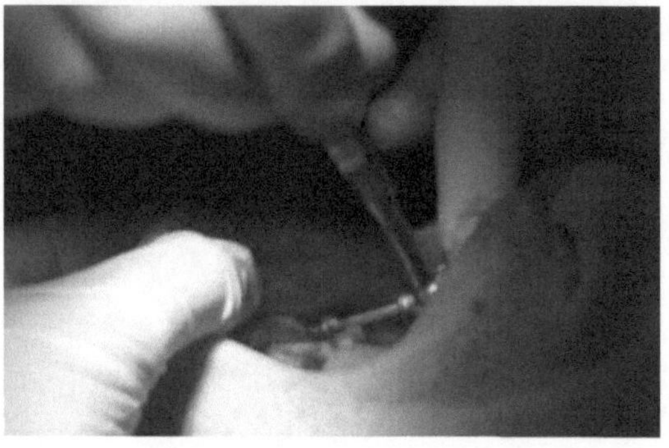

Figure 9. Implant placement.

confirming mandible crest status. Following the previously planned procedures in the physical model, has been made a bone resection of mandible frontal crest, with hand tools and appropriated drills, in order to obtain the needed bone thickness.

In the cut bone surface has been used an initial drill followed by 1.8 mm drill to enlarge the holes. After parallelism confirmation, 1 mm mesial and distal drillings have been performed to turn easier osteotome bone distraction and avoid fractures.

In implants drilling have been used MIS® osteotomes until size 3.5 mm after which have been placed five 3.7 mm diameter TSV (Tapered Screw-Vent®) Zimmer® implants. In figures 8 and 9 can be seen these two last phases.

6 CONCLUSIONS

As conclusion it can be reinterred the suitability of biomodeling techniques as a valuable complementary diagnose tool in bone condition evaluation and surgical planning when applied in dental disease situations (Queijo et al. 2012).

The conventional diagnose means like CT or MRI scanning, allied to biomodelling techniques prove themselves as an outstanding way to gain full perception over a patient bone condition, especially in complex cases. The possibility of having a full scale anatomical structure replica and over it study the procedures that would be executed in surgery reduces not only surgery time but also the possibility of occurring complications due to tissues exposure and also patient's discomfort.

3DP® technique, by having a low cost operation, even that the biomodels don't have, particularly, special mechanical characteristics, presents the needed qualities to perform the wanted studies.

Through the manufactured models was possible to realize patient's bone condition and to preview the type of needed techniques to be used in his rehabilitation, either in surgical procedures as in implant locations and bone reconstruction, if needed.

By combining digital and physical 3D models analysis it was possible to define implant locations and to, clearly, define surgical procedures by realizing that it was not needed to perform bone growth in frontal mandible body, as was expected, and that with the resection to be made at that level would be enough for implant screwing after osteotome drilling.

Implants were placed successfully converting mandible rehabilitation a reality, despite the time that would be needed to allow implant osteointegration and final teeth placement.

REFERENCES

Nunn, J et al. 2003. The interdisciplinary management of hypodontia: background and role of paediatric dentistry. *British dental journal* 194(5): 245–251.

Queijo, L et al. 2010. *Maxilla bone pre-surgical evaluation aided by 3D models obtained by Rapid Prototyping*. Boca Raton, Crc Press-Taylor & Francis Group.

Queijo, L et al. 2009. A prototipagem rápida na modelação de patologias. *3º Congresso Nacional de Biomecânica, Bragança – Portugal*, Sociedade Portuguesa de Biomecânica.

Queijo, L et al. 2012. Maxilla Bone Evaluation and Implant Surgical Planning in a Periodontal Disease Patient. *15th International Conference on Experimental Mechanics, Porto – Portugal.*

Tarjan, I et al. 2005. Early prosthetic treatment of patients with ectodermal dysplasia: a clinical report. *The Journal of prosthetic dentistry* 93(5): 419–424.

Vieira, K A et al. 2007. Prosthodontic treatment of hypohidrotic ectodermal dysplasia with complete anodontia. Case report. *Quintessence international* 38: 75–80.

Biodental Engineering II – Natal Jorge et al (Eds)
© 2014 Taylor & Francis Group, London, ISBN 978-1-138-00131-2

In vitro pilot study on bone heating during surgical implant bed preparation

Sónia Fangaia & Mauro Almeida
Department of Dentistry, Faculty of Medicine, University of Coimbra, Portugal

Lídia Carvalho
Department for Technologies of Diagnosis and Therapeutic, IPSN-CESPU, Porto, Portugal
Centre for Mechanical Technology and Automation, Aveiro, Portugal

Pedro Nicolau
Department of Dentistry, Faculty of Medicine, University of Coimbra, Portugal

ABSTRACT: Introduction: The atraumatic preparation of the implant bed and the presence of healthy bone factors have been considered essential for osseointegration of an implant. Heat generation during bone drilling has been related with the pressure applied by the operator, characteristics of the drill bit, the drilling depth, the type of irrigation, the rotational speed of the drilling time and the density of the bone tissue. Although bone drilling practice has been performed under irrigation, recent studies in the literature propose the use of a clinical protocol without irrigation.

The primary objective of this study was to use an optical fibber Bragg grating sensor to measure thermal variations during implant bed preparation using surgical drills with a new surface coating.

Materials and Methods: A literature review was performed and a pilot study designed using a fresh pig's jaw at room temperature, and three drilling groups were performed:

Group I – Straumann® Drill without irrigation
Group II – Straumann® Drill coated Titanium Nitride and Aluminum (NiTiAl) without irrigation.
Group III (Control) – Straumann®) Drill with irrigation.

The perforations were made sequentially, using drills of 2.2, 2.8 and 3.5 mm, to a depth of 10 mm, at a speed of 800 rpm and 0.2 mm/s under a constant force of 4N. Changes in temperature were recorded using an optical fibber Bragg grating sensor, placed in an intra-osseous location.Results:Implant bed preparation procedure produced a temperature rise of: 0.39°C to 0.53°C, 1.28°C to 2.70°C, and 1.57°C to 4.39°C in group I, II and III respectively. The drills coated with NiTiAl and without irrigation have a lower temperature increase when compared with the uncoated drills, maintaining the procedure without irrigation. Discussion and Conclusions: The optical fibber Bragg gratings sensors have the ability to register changes in temperature that occur during the preparation of the implant bed. The coating of surgical drills with NiTiAl caused a minor increase of temperature in comparison with drills without coating. Perforations without irrigation performed at a speed of 800 rpm with a force of 4 N do not seem to significantly increase the temperature in bone.

1 INTRODUCTION

The atraumatic preparation of the implant bed and the presence of healthy bone factors have been considered essential for osseointegration of an implant (Attard and Zarb 2002). Drilling the implant bed not only causes mechanical damage to the bone but also increases the temperature of the bone directly adjacent to the implant surface (Sener, Dergin et al. 2009). It has been demonstrated that if bone is heated to temperature of 47°C for one minute, bone necrosis, which may impede the osseointegration of an implant, can occur (Eriksson and Albrektsson 1983). Heat generation, during bone drilling, has been related with the pressure applied by the operator, characteristics of the drill bit, the drilling depth, the type of irrigation, the rotational speed of the drilling time and the density of the bone tissue. Although bone drilling practice has been performed under irrigation, recent studies in the literature propose the use of a clinical protocol without irrigation, allowing better visibility and collecting bone for use as graft after placement of the implant.

The literature refers several methods to register the increase or variation of temperature such as optical fibber Bragg (Carvalho, Alberto et al. 2011), thermocouples and infrared Thermography. Thermocouples

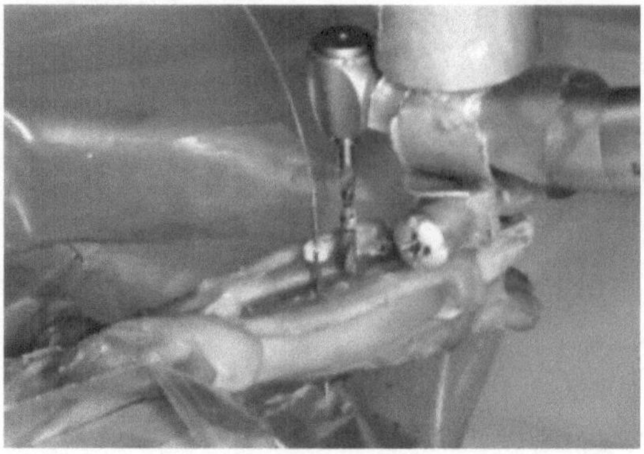

Figure 1. Pig mandible immobilized in a specially designed support and hand piece from the motor drill.

are simple electrical devices, with low cost and very reliable, however its major limitation is the accuracy, since errors of less than 1°C are difficult to obtain (Kerlin 1999). In respect to infrared thermography, despite being a very sensitive method for registering temperature changes, it is only effective for measuring surface temperature changes (Augustin, Davila et al. 2009).

The primary objective of this study was to use an optical fibber Bragg grating sensor to measure thermal variations during implant bed preparation using surgical drills with a new surface coating.

2 MATERIALS AND METHODS

A literature review was performed and a pilot study designed using a fresh pig's mandible at room temperature (25°C), that was immobilized in a specially designed support, with a hand piece from a motor drill (W&H ImplantMED®, Austria), mounted in a Universal testing Machine (Autograph AG-I Shimadzu®, Japan) (fig. 1).

With this apparatus we were able to control the rotational speed of the bur, time and force of perforation. This experimental setup allowed all perforations to be performed in the same conditions. The perforations were made sequentially, using Straumann® drills (Straumann Institute AG, Basel; Switzerland) of 2.2, 2.8 and 3.5 mm diameter to a depth of 10 mm, and at a speed of 800 rpm and 0.2 mm/s under a constant force of 4 N. Thease burs were used as suplied by the manufacturer in group I and III (control) without coating and irrigation, and without coating with irrigation, respectively. In Group II these burs were modified with a Titanium Nitride and Aluminum (NiTiAl) without irrigation. In this work we used a Fibber Bragg Grating sensor to measure the temperature variation.

A perforation was performed to contain the fibber Bragg grating sensor (FBG) that was placed inside in a hollow needle and connected to software to retract and process the data. Data acquisition was made at 1 sample/second, using a sm125 interrogation system from Micron Optics, with 10 pm of wavelength resolution.

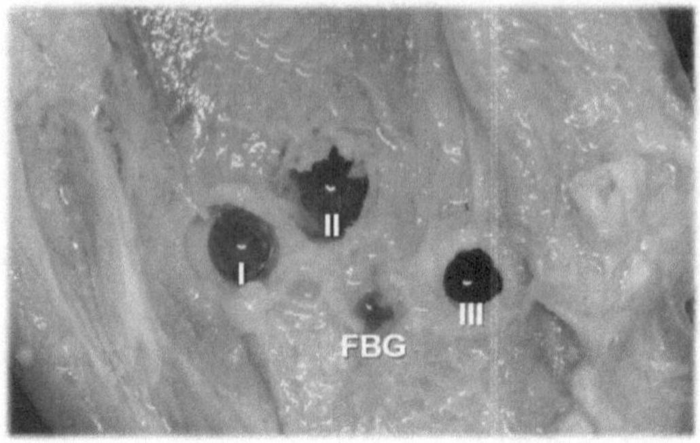

Figure 2. Section of the pig mandible where implant bed preparations were made.

Table 1. Results of the temperature variation.

	temperature variation (°C)		
Drills diameter (mm)	drills without coating and without irrigation	drills with coating and without irrigation	drills without coating and with irrigation
2,2	1,57	1,28	0,39
2,8	4,39	2,70	0,39
3,5	3,25	2,36	0,53

Three drilling groups were performed:

Group I – Straumann® Drill without irrigation.
Group II – Straumann® Drill coated Titanium Nitride and Aluminum (NiTiAl) without irrigation.
Group III – (Control) Straumann® Drill with irrigation (Fig. 2).

3 RESULTS

Implant bed preparation procedure produced a temperature rise of: 0.39°C to 0.53°C, 1.28°C to 2.70°C, and 1.57°C to 4.39°C in group I, II and III respectively (table 1 and graphic 1).

The drills coated with NiTiAl and without irrigation have a lower temperature increase when compared with the uncoated drills, maintaining the procedure without irrigation.

Nevertheless, the test performed with external irrigation with NaCL 0.9% was a temperature variation lower.

Was not registered overheating of the bone tissue with any type of drill, since the temperature variation was between 1.28°C and 4.39°C.

4 DISCUSSION

According to the results obtained in our study, the perforations made without irrigation showed that temperature increase was between 1.28°C and 4.39°C.

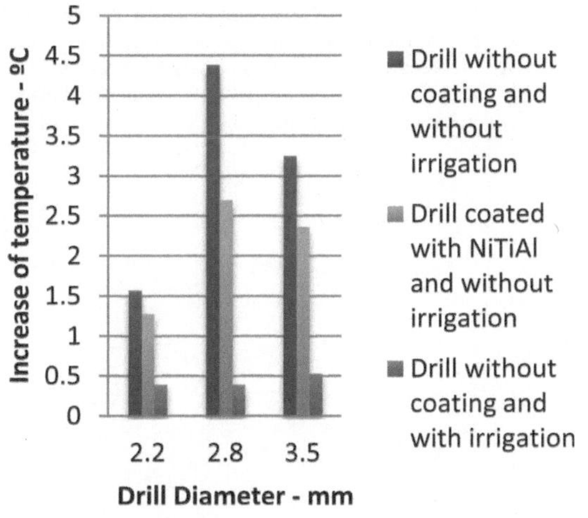

Grafic 1. Results with temperature variation.

The tests carried out with external irrigation had a lower temperature increase, which was between 0.39°C and 0.53°C, which confirms that the temperature variations are lower when using irrigation. However the results obtained in the group II revealed that irrigation may not to be necessary, because under these conditions it is possible to perform the preparation of an implant bed without reaching a temperature of 47°C regarded as the threshold for bone necrosis occurrence (Eriksson and Albrektsson 1983). TiAlN coating, was used because it has shown to have a low coefficient of friction and good resistance to heat and oxidation. Other coatings were used such as Titanium Nitride (TiN) and tungsten carbide/carbon (WC/C) (Ercoli et al. 2004; Golin 2005). However, to our knowledge, up until now these coatings have not been used in burs for implant bed preparation. These coating have also high hardness and an excellent adhesion to the substrate of the burr, chemical stability. As shown in this study the coating improved the performance of the drill bit, allowing a smaller increase of the temperature with respect to uncoated drills. The measurement method that we used was a 1 Hz sensor, capable of registering a temperature measurement per second. The optical fibber Bragg grating had a lower thermal inertia than thermocouples, making this characteristic and the fact that it is measuring inside the bone, close to the implant bed preparation better sensors for temperature measurement than thermocouples or infrared thermography (Reid 1998; Valente et al 2002; Marques 2008; Carvalho, Alberto et al 2011).

This pilot study showed that the optical fibber Bragg grating may be used as temperature sensors in implant bed preparation, measuring accurately changes in temperature during preparation. One aspect however, that needs to be better clarified is its ability to record with irrigation, since in our study, the data obtained in this group leaves us some doubts about this possibility, due to the great variations in temperature rise.

One of the main objectives of our pilot study was to test a protocol on a small sample, thereby minimizing costs and errors that can be avoided in a subsequent study broader and larger. In future work must be taken into account the distance of each drill to the sensor, since the larger diameter drills are closer than the lower ones. Despite these limitations we believe that with some changes to the protocol and an *in vivo* model may be able to contribute more significantly to scientific evidence, that implant bed preparation without irrigation may be recommended for a surgical procedure in implant surgery.

5 CONCLUSIONS

This was a pilot study with some limitations and few repetitions yet it suggest that the optical fibber Bragg gratings sensors, due to this high sensibility, have the ability to register changes in temperature, that occur during the preparation of the implant bed, in real time. The coating of surgical drills with NiTiAl caused a minor increase of temperature in comparison with drills without coating. Perforations without irrigation performed at a speed of 800 rpm with a force of 4N do not seem to significantly increase the temperature in bone, avoiding bone necrosis.

We must have some reservations about the extrapolations to *in vivo.*

REFERENCES

[1] Attard, N., et al. 2002. Implant prosthodontic management of posterior partial edentulism: long-term follow-up of a prospective study *J Can Dent Assoc* 68(2): 118–124.

[2] Sener, B. C., et al. 2009 Effects of irrigation temperature on heat control in vitro at different drilling depths *Clin Oral Implants Res* 20(3): 294–298.

[3] Eriksson R. et al, 1983. Temperature threshold levels for heat-induced bone tissue injury: A vital-microscopic study in the rabbit. *J Prosthet Dent* 50: 101–107.

[4] Carvalho, L., et al. 2011. In the trail of a new bio-sensor for measuring strain in bone: osteoblastic biowithpatibility *Biosens Bioelectron* 26(10): 4046–4052.

[5] Kerlin, T. W. 1999. Practical thermocouple thermometry. Research Triangle Park, NC, Instrument Society of America.

[6] Augustin, G., et al. 2009. Determination of spatial distribution of increase in bone temperature during drilling by infrared thermography: preliminary report. *Arch Orthop Trauma Surg* 129(5): 703–709.

[7] Ercoli, C., et al. 2004. The influence of drill wear on cutting efficiency and heat production during osteotomy preparation for dental implants: a study of drill durability. Int J Oral Maxillofac Implants 19(3): 335–349.

[8] Golin, A. 2005. Análise do comportamento de ferramentas de corte comdiferentes revestimentos e seu efeito sobre a geração de calor no osso. Centro de Ciências Exatas e de Tecnologia. Curitiba, Universidade Católica do Paraná. Tese de Mestrado: 134.

[9] Reid, M. O. M. 1998. Temperature dependence of fiber optic Bragg gratings at low temperatures. *Optical Engineering* 37(1): 4.

[10] Valente, L. et al. 2002. Técnicas de leitura para sensores a fibra óptica baseados em redes de Bragg. *6ª Conferência sobre Tecnologia de Equipamentos. Salvador*: 15.

[11] Marques, L. M. P. 2008. Optimização de Processos de Produção de Sensores de Bragg em Fibra Óptica. Departamento de Engenharia Electrotécnica e de Computadores – Faculdade de Engenharia. Porto, Universidade do Porto: 76.

Biodental Engineering II – Natal Jorge et al (Eds)
© 2014 Taylor & Francis Group, London, ISBN 978-1-138-00131-2

In vivo dental implant micro-movements measuring with 3D digital image correlation method

T. Rodrigues, F. Moreira, F. Guerra & P. Nicolau
Dentistry Area, Faculty of Medicine, University of Coimbra, Portugal

A. Neto
Mechanical Engineering Department, Faculty of Science and Technology, University of Coimbra, Portugal

ABSTRACT: One of the principal factors in the implant's therapy clinical success is implant stability. 3D Digital Image Correlation (3D DIC), is a non-contact optical measurement system that can track an object's surface displacement field in a series of images and it should be capable of direct objective implant micro-movement measuring, despite not being a clinical method. The primary objective of this study was to use 3D DIC technique for implants tridimensional surface micro-movements measurement. Secondarily, to compare the effect of two different prosthetic abutments (Standard (SD) and Platform-Switching (PS)) on implant micro-movement. A total of 18 implants from 13 patients included were measured in the lower posterior jaw (with the two different prosthetic abutments, SD and PS, $n = 9$ for each group), under the application of a bite load of more than 30N (measured with a stainless steel miniature compression load cell). Micro-movements measurements were performed by 3D DIC. The results obtained show no significant statistical differences ($p > 0.05$) between implants with SD and PS abutments for any Direction measured. However, mean micro-movements values were always lower for PS abutments. Micro-movements measured were significantly higher in the W (Bucal-Lingual) Direction. Within the limitations of this study, 3D DIC method is capable to measure dental implants micro-movements.

1 INTRUDUCTION

1.1 *Background*

Implant stability is one of the principal factors in the clinical success of implant therapy. Different methods to measure implant stability have been proposed but, so far, there is no clinical method available to directly measure implants micro-movements. Tridimensional Digital Image Correlation (3D DIC) method is a non-contact optical measurement system that can track an object's surface displacement field in a series of images. This system uses the digital image of two high speed photographic cameras and the principles of optics to stereo-triangulate the tridimensional surface full-field contour of an object. 3D DIC requires a gray value pattern on the object surface. Then an algorithm defines a field of small neighborhoods called subsets which are small N × N pixels boxes with an array of pixel gray-scale values. 3D DIC uses a matching advanced algorithm allows to determine translation, rotation and deformation of these subsets in a series of images with relation to a reference image of fixed subsets. Thereby, the method tracks these subsets on the object surface during deformation which is the principle of digital image correlation. The result is a time history of the objects surface displacements field by video correlation between the initial image (reference image) and the subsequent images. 3D DIC has been used to measure implant micro-movements *In Vitro*, and despite not being a clinical method, it should be capable of direct objective implant micro-movement measuring, useful for clinical studies.

1.2 *Aim*

The primary objective of this study was to use a tridimensional digital image correlation method for full-field tridimensional surface micro-movements measurement. Secondarily, to compare the effect of two different prosthetic abutments (Standard and Platform-Switching) on implant micro-movement [Figure 1].

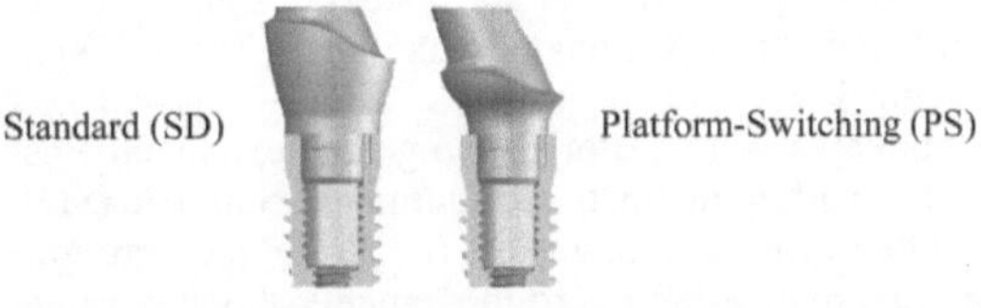

Figure 1. Standard (SD) and Platform-Switching (PS) prosthetic abutments used in this study (Camlog Biotechnologies®, Wimsheim, Germany).

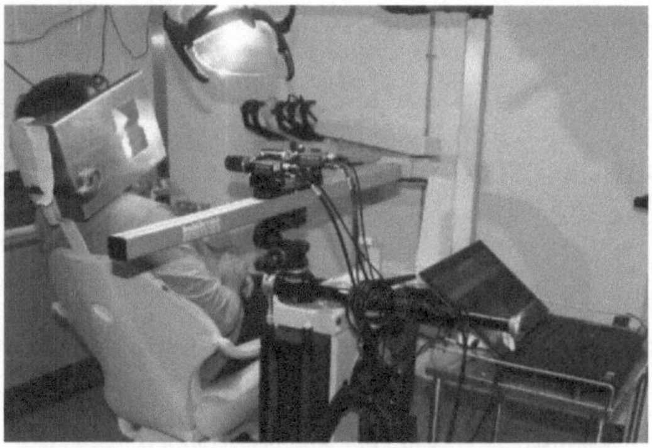

Figure 2. Three-dimensional Digital Image Correlation system *set up* (Correlated Solutions®, Columbia, USA).

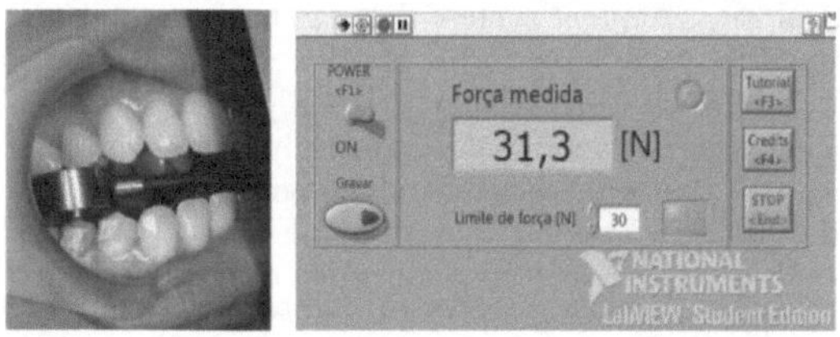

Figure 3. Stainless steel miniature compression load cell in position for images capture (Applied Measurements, Berkshire, UK) in the left image; Interface of the system design software LabVIEW 2010 (National Instruments®, Texas, USA) for measuring and recording the load bite application, in the right image.

2 MATERIAL AND METHODS

13 patients who had placed two or more adjacent dental implants in the lower posterior jaw were included. A total of 18 endosseous implants (Camlog Biotechnologies®, Wimsheim, Germany) were measured (with two different prosthetic abutments, Standard and Platform-switching, n = 9 for each group).

Micro-movements measurements were performed by the optical method of 3D DIC with two high speed photographic cameras (Point Grey GRAS-20S4M-C, 1624 × 1224 pixels) and the video correlation system Vic-3D 2010 (Correlated Solutions®, Columbia, USA) [Figure 2], under the application of a bite load of more than 30N, measured with a stainless steel miniature compression load cell (Applied Measurements Ltd., Berkshire, UK) and the system design software LabVIEW 2010 (National Instruments®, Texas, USA) [Figure 3].

Implants were restored using single unit crowns over two different prosthetic abutments, Standard (SD) and Platform-switching (PS), (n = 9 for each group). In order to measure micro-movements, the gray value heterogeneous pattern on the crown surface over the implant was made with a spray brush over a paper sticker and placed on the buccal side of both the

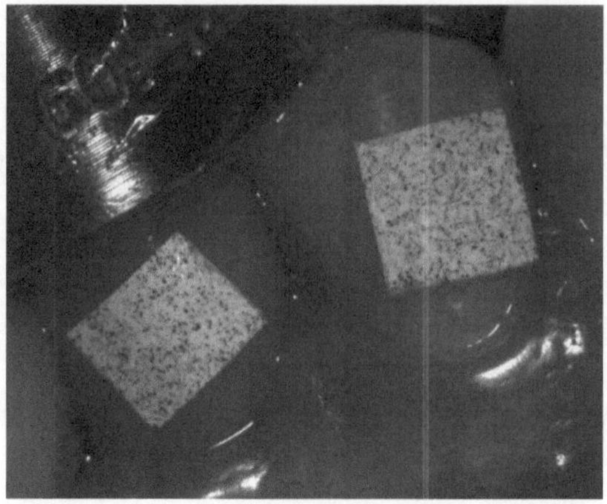

Figure 4. Detail of the speckle pattern on the buccal side of both the crown over the implant and the neighboring natural tooth.

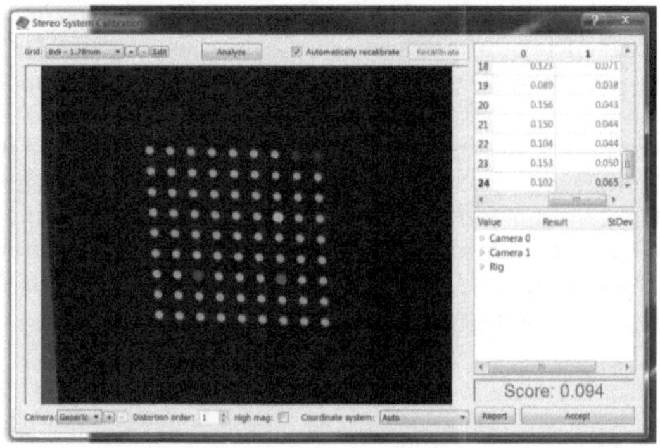

Figure 5. Stereo system calibration procedure performed by Vic-3D 2010 software (Correlated Solutions®, Columbia, USA) with the selected grid target used (example of one clinical case).

crown over implant and the neighboring natural tooth [Figure 4].

For each patient, a *stereo system* calibration was performed using a standardized calibration target sized 14,929 mm, with a pitch of 1,780 mm (9 × 9), before acquiring images [Figure 5].

After images acquisition, micro-movements analysis was done with a post processing application from Vic-3D 2010, in order to remove the rigid body motion. In all these clinical cases, the whole movement of the natural tooth adjacent to the implant was removed, leaving only the absolute implant displacement in the three directions U, V, W which correspond to Mesio-Distal, Oclusal-Apical and Buccal-Lingual Directions, respectively [Figure 6].

In order to verify the existence of significant differences between implants with SD and PS prosthetic abutments ($p \leq 0.05$), the results were statistically analyzed with the paired-samples Mann-Whitney test (PASW Statistics 18 – IBM, USA).

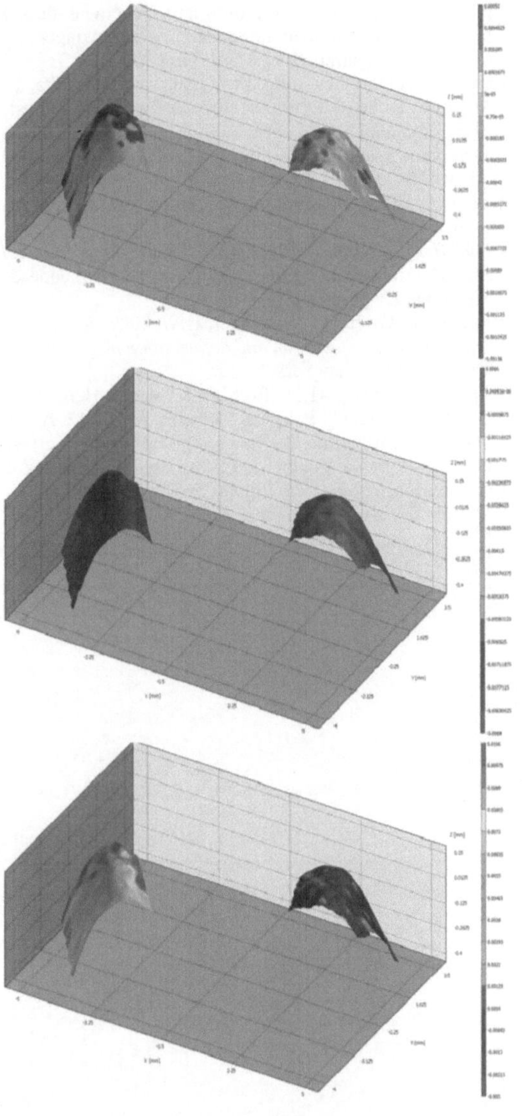

Figure 6. Micro-movements measurements images obtained by digital image correlation with Vic-3D 2010 (Correlated Solutions®, Columbia, USA) after analysis in the three space directions U, V and W (Mesio-Distal, Oclusal-Apical and Buccal-Lingual, respectively) for one clinical case.

3 RESULTS AND DISCUSSION

3.1 *Results*

Results are presented in Table 1.

3.2 *Discussion*

The results obtained show that the values for implants with different prosthetic abutments (SD and PS) do not present significant statistical differences ($p > 0.05$) for any direction measured: U (Mesio-Distal) Direction, $p = 0.171$; V (Oclusal-Apical) Direction, $p = 0.402$; or W (Buccal-Lingual) Direction, $p = 0.085$. This result was possibly due to the small size of the sample, since only 18 implants from the 13 patients included (with two or more implants placed in the lower posterior jaw) were effectively measured, for a total of 9 implants for each group of the two different prosthetic abutments, SD and PS. The reason for not having measured all implants is related to the difficulty of capturing images with both cameras in the posterior dental area, since the angle between the cameras should be superior to 15° and the oral muscles and mucosa have a limit distensibility that do not allow images acquisition backwards.

Table 1. Mean and standard deviation values for implants with the different prosthetic abutments (SD and PS).

	Standard	Platform-Switching
	mean stan. dev.	mean stand. dev.
U (Mesio-Distal) Direction	9.6211 ± 9.5673	4.7806 ± 4.3497
V (Oclusal-Apical) Direction	7.6594 ± 5.7073	4.9761 ± 4.4662
W (Buccal-Lingual) Direction	16.6067 ± 10.8233	10.4767 ± 8.6032

However, mean micro-movements measurements values were always lower for Platform-Switching abutments, for all directions measured, what was according to the results expected. In fact, the current literature seems to show this tendency in the first two years after implant placement, and the results here presented were obtained for osteointegrated implants until 24 months post-loading.

Micro-movements measured in both U (Mesio-Distal) and V (Oclusal-Apical) Directions didn't present significant statistical differences. Although, micro-movements measured in the W (Buccal-Lingual) direction were significantly higher. Once more, this fact is according to what is referred in the existing literature on the subject.

The results obtained seem to indicate 3D DIC as a capable method to measure dental implants micro-movements, although not being a clinical system.

4 CONCLUSIONS

Within the limitations of this study, 3D DIC method is capable to measure dental implants micro-movements, although not being a clinical system. The results do not suggest significant differences between Standard and Platform-Switching prosthetic abutments, however, mean micro-movements measurements values were consistently lower for Platform-Switching abutments, for all directions measured.

ACKNOWLEDGMENTS

Co-financed by the Foundation for Science and Technology via project PTDC/SAU-BEB/108658/2008 and by F.E.D.E.R. via the "Programa Operacional Factores de Competitividade" of QREN with COMPETE reference: FCOMP-01-0124-FEDER-010961.

REFERENCES

Clelland, N.L.; Seidt, J.D.; Daroz, L.G.; McGlumphy, E.A. 2010. Comparison of strains for splinted and nonsplinted implant prostheses using three-dimensional image correlation. *Int J Oral Maxillofac Implants* 25(5): 953–9.

Goellner, M.; Schmitt, J.; Karl, M.; Wichmann, M.; Holst, S. 2010. Photogrammetric measurement of initial tooth displacement under tensile force. *Med Eng Physics* 32: 883–888.

Göllner, M.; Holst, A.; Berthold, C.; Schmitt, J.; Wichmann, M.; Holst, S. 2010. Noncontact intraoral measurement of force-related tooth mobility. *Clin Oral investig* 14(5): 551–7.

Kimura K.; Fukase Y.; Makino M.; Masaki C.; Nakamoto T.; Hosokawa R. 2010 Preoperative assessment of treatment planning on minimization of micro-movement during healing period of immediate-loaded implants using X-ray CT data-based simulation. *J Oral Implantol* 17.

Morita, Y.; Uchino, M.; Todo, M.; Qian, L.; Matsushita, Y.; Arakawa, K. 2010. Dental occlusal deformation analysis of porcine mandibular periodontium using digital image correlation method. *Interface Oral Health Science* 2009 2010: 150–152.

Nicolau, P. 2007. A randomized clinical study between immediate and early loading. In Pedro Nicolau (ed). *Immediate Loading of Endosseous Implants-Clinical and Biomechanical Evaluation*. Coimbra: Faculdade de Medicina, Universidade de Coimbra.

Sutton, M.A.; Orteu, J.J.; Schreider, H.W. 2009. *Image correlation for shape, motion and deformation measurments.* Springer (eds). New York.

Tiossi, R.; Conrad, H.J.; Rodrigues, R.C.; Heo, Y.C.; De Mattos, Mda.G.; Fok, A.S.; Ribeiro, R.F. 2012. A digital image correlation analysis on the influence of crown material in implant-supported prostheses on bone strain distribution. *J Prosthodontic Res* 56: 25–31.

Tiossi, R.; Lin, L.; Rodrigues, R.C.; Heo, Y.C.; Conrad, H.J.; De Mattos, Mda, G.; Ribeiro, R.F.; Fok, A.S. 2011. Digital image correlation analysis of the load transfer by implant-supported restorations. *J Biomech* 44(6): 1008–13.

Biodental Engineering II – Natal Jorge et al (Eds)
© 2014 Taylor & Francis Group, London, ISBN 978-1-138-00131-2

Projection and construction of universal testing machine to simulate fatigue cycles during the insertion/detachment of implant attachments

C. Aroso, S. Silva & J.M. Mendes
Instituto Superior de Ciências da Saúde Norte, Paredes, Portugal

R. Ustrell
Polytechnic University of Catalunya (ETSEIB), Barcelona, Spain

M.C. Manzanares, J.M. Ustrell & T. Escuin
Barcelona University (UB), Barcelona, Spain

ABSTRACT: The authors have projected and built a universal testing machine to simulate fatigue cycles during the insertion/detachment of attachments implants used in oral implantology. This machine may be used for fatigue and rupture tests in cycles of compression and/or traction in several materials used in nowadays odontology. The machine has an automatic data register in excel format and it copies for a digital form with an USB entrance. The machine allows several tests with temperature and ph control. The charge cells are also exchangeable and the engine course may be altered according to the tests to be made. All the machine components obey to international safety rules. Preliminary tests have been made and we have verified that the machine works and fully achieves the intended goals.

1 INTRODUCTION

Mandibular edentulism is as much a public health problem in great economical powers as in less developed nations (Feine, Carlsson et al. 2002). This edentulism has severe consequences as disorders in facial and neck muscular relations and in the temporomandibular joint, where it can cause systemic problems. Due to problems associated to edentulism. It is necessary to rehabilitate these mandibles, being very cautious in what concerns to planning the rehabilitation in a basis of clinical and biomechanical knowledge (Goiato, Garcia et al. 2010). The classical treatments to rehabilitate a mandibular edentulous are the conventional total prosthesis, the implant-retained overdenture and the implant supported denture (Koka and Eckert 2006).

The conventional total prostheses were considered to be the first option to replace the lost structures (Feine, Carlsson et al. 2002). However, a lot of patients that look for the rehabilitation of their mandibular edentulism do not have sufficient existing basal area for a conventional total prosthesis no to move and to assure the needed comfort and safety during chewing and speaking (Duyck, Van Oosterwyck et al. 1999). After Branemark studies (1977) that showed the dental implants success rate in edentulism cases, rehabilitating treatments that combine implants and overdentures have become more and more accessible procedures and with good prognosis (Visser, Raghoebar et al. 2009). According to McGill Consensus Statement on overdentures, in Montreal, Canada, in 2002, evidences show that overdentures retained over two implants will become the standard protocol for the treatment of mandibular edentulous (Feine, Carlsson et al. 2002).

The stability and retention of overdentures are reached through implant/prosthesis connexion systems called attachments. It was in Switzerland, around 1898, that the original concept of attachment emerges (Petropoulos and Smith 2002). Nowadays, there are several types of attachments on the market but the most popular are the bar attachment systems – clip, ball system and internal/external double connexion system like Locator (Evtimovska, Masri et al. 2009; Schmitt, Holst et al. 2009; Gonda, Maeda et al. 2010). Several studies have analysed the biomechanical behaviour of these systems through the retention force needed (Petropoulos and Smith 2002; Porter, Petropoulos et al. 2002; Jemt and Hjalmarsson 2011; Petropoulos and Mante 2011; Rutkunas, Mizutani et al. 2011; Takeshita, Kanazawa et al. 2011; Yang, Maeda et al. 2011; Uçankale, Akoğlu et al. 2012).

The aim of our study was to apply fatigue tests on attachments that we consider to be ideal to be used on implant-retained overdentures. Those tests would be in vitro through the observation and quantification of the insertion and detachment strength of the attachments when subdued to insertion and detachment cycles. We intended to register the strength used along the full cycle duration, that is, if we imagine that a patient puts and removes his overdenture at least 3 times a day we could analyse the strength for periods of 90 cycles,

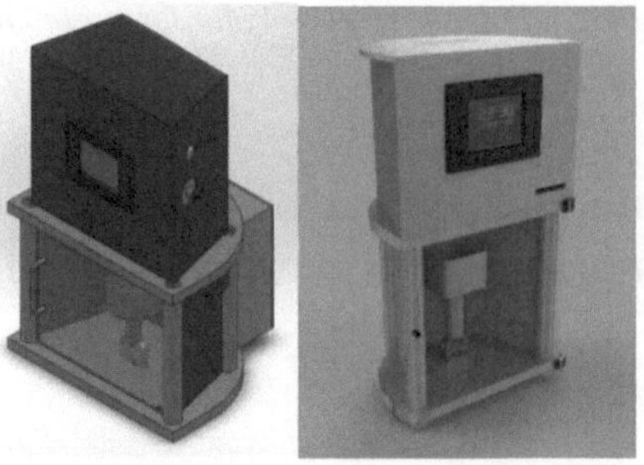

Image 1. Machine structures.

what would represent 1 month, or 5400 cycles that would represent 5 years using the prosthesis. In order to achieve this, we have searched on engineering the possibility of projecting and building a machine that would be useful on evaluating the strength during the insertion and detachment cycles, register and record data in digital form, allowing the change of temperature during the study, allowing the use of continual strength on compression or traction, having an easy use on its initial mechanism, allowing the use of cells with different charges, allowing the register of data with variation of test breaks, allowing the change of the test speed and being safe and reliable.

2 MATERIALS AND METHODS

The machine was developed by the Spanish company Idearum, from Barcelona, and the engineer Raul Ustrell was the one in charge of the project and its design. The machine called "CS – Dental Testing Machine" was assigned to the model ID1-BAD with the serial number 0001. It was finished in the end of 2011 and was put into operation on September 2012 with the electrical connexion of 230 V/50 Hz. This machine is intended for the test of different materials used on Dentistry obeying the Directive 2006/42/EC of the European Parliament and Council on the 17th May 2006 regarding the approach of the member states legislations on machines. This machine does not belong to the Appendix IV of this directive since it is not considered to be a hazardous machine.

The machine comprises two different structures, placed one on top of the other (Image 1).

The first one, placed on the inferior part of the machine, comprises two platforms whose geometry resembles a half-moon form, linked by 4 columns of circular section clamped (Image 2).

On the rear part we have the machine's electrical board whose access is made through the exterior. The front part of this platform comprises a door in transparent polycarbonate. The interior of this platform lodges, at the same time, the charge cell, the vase where the test sample is put, the vase support, the LED lighting and the required ventilator for the extraction of the steam that comes from the liquid's heating (Image 3).

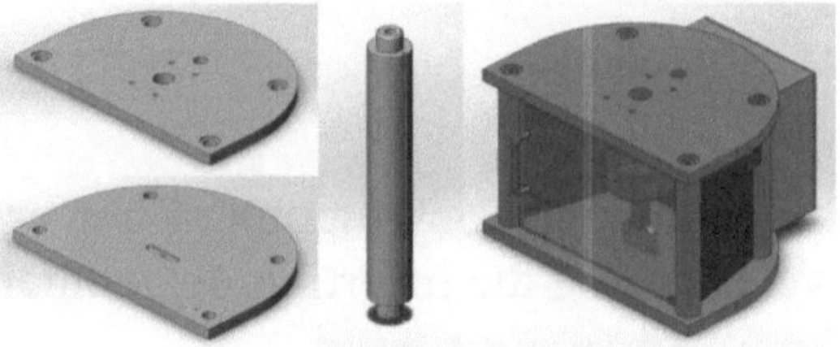

Image 2. Inferior structure of the machine.

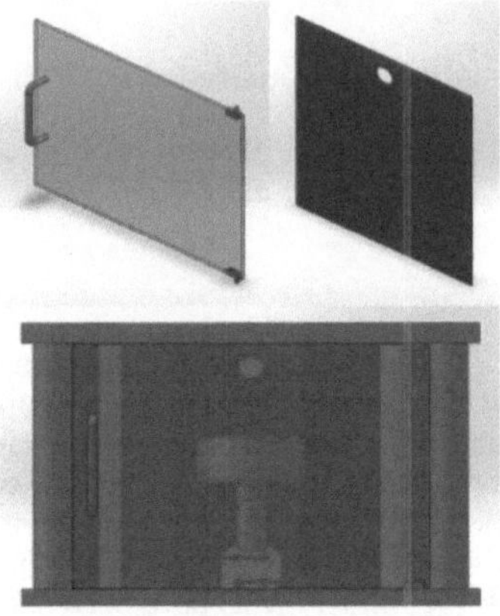

Image 3. Inferior platform's interior.

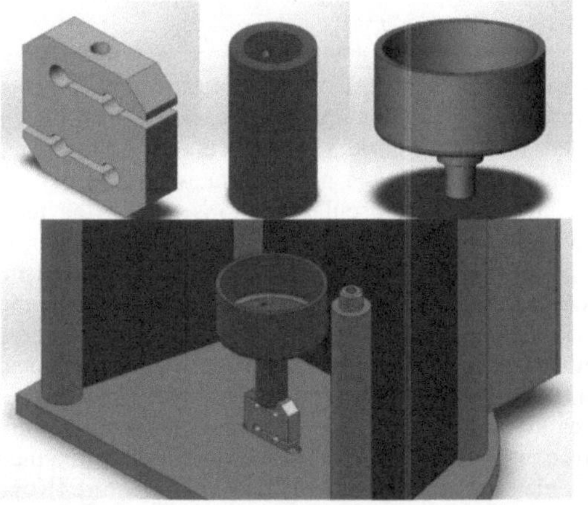

Image 4. Charge cell, vase support, vase.

The vase support placed between both parts conveys these forces from the recipient to the charge cell. The vase is in charge of lodging the liquid (water, artificial saliva, etc.) and the male connector to be tested (Image 4).

In the interior of the vase, along its internal walls, there is a 100 W resistance with a PT100 probe to heat and control the temperature of the liquid that may be used to simulate the test real conditions. This resistance is automatically turned on as soon as the temperature probe detects that the current temperature is less than the one wanted by the operator. On this interior there

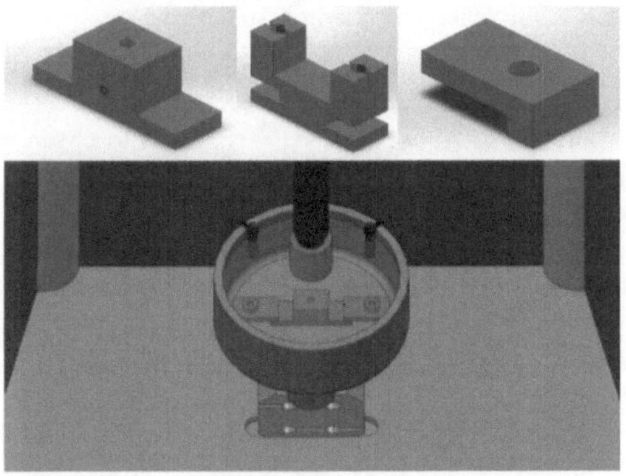

Image 5. Interior of the vase.

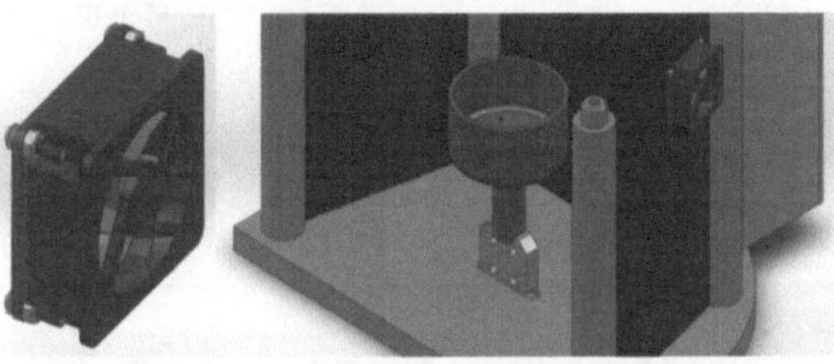

Image 6. Ventilator for steam extraction.

are also placed the supports of the test pieces. These supports vary on their performance according to the pieces tested. On this specific case, we have built two supports to fit the male ball type or Locator and bars. The supports are fixed to the vase by L shaped bonding pads (Image 5).

Ending the interior structure, fixed to one of the lateral walls, there is a ventilator through which it is extracted all the steam that comes from the heating of the liquid that has been put inside the vase. On the interior rear, there has been put a lamp with several LEDs that allows us better lighting during trials. Whenever the resistance is turned on, the ventilator is also on (Image 6).

The second structure of the machine is placed on the upper part, following the superior platform half-moon shaped, as mentioned above. This second structure is formed by a metallic basis of trapezoidal section, whose interior lodges all the electric, mechanic and electronic components of the machine.

Additionally, a second L shaped basis covers the posterior and superior parts of the trapezoidal window already mentioned previously (Image 7).

The first component lodged inside is the actuator/engine. This actuator/engine is in charge of taking a linear movement to a cylinder that is placed inside. Its source of power is electric and we have chosen one form, the Exlar I® Series (Image 8). The second component is the servo motor, which has to pass on the PLC (Programmable Logic Controller) orders to the actuator (Image 9).

The third component is an interfaces module in charge of linking the distinct PLC wires (Image 10).

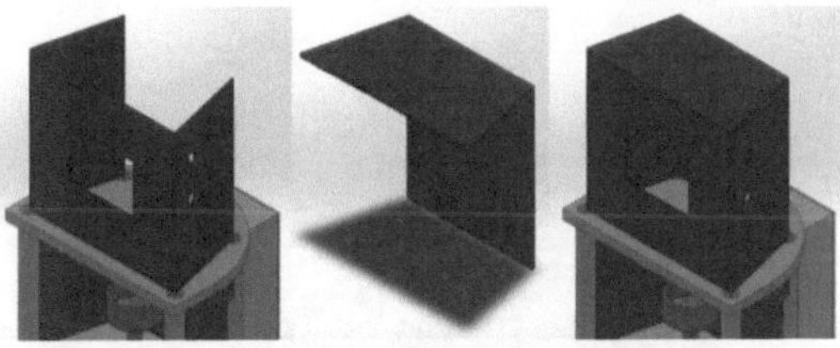

Image 7. Basis of the machine's superior structure.

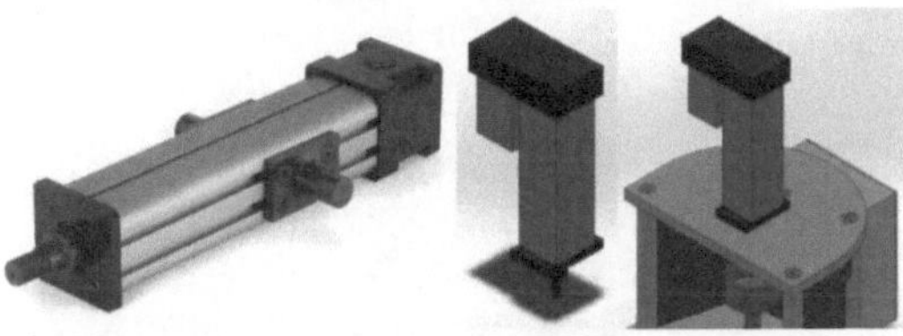

Image 8. Actuator/engine Exlar I® Series.

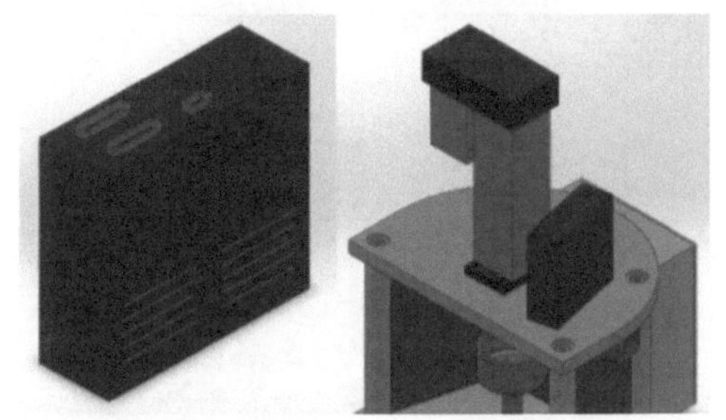

Image 9. Servo motor.

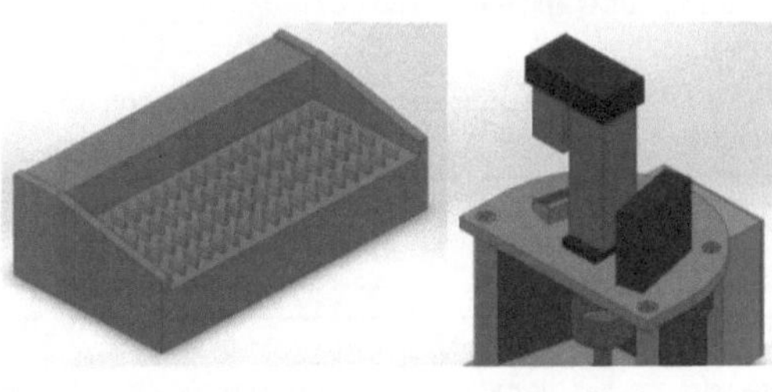

Image 10. Interfaces module.

The fourth component is a touch screen LCD panel that, besides showing the achieved data through the charge cell on the test made, allows the operator to select the intended operations (Image 11).

The fifth component is a USB adapter. It is located on a slot made on the right side of the trapezoidal metallic basis. The sixth component is an emergency stop button placed underneath the USB adapter. The activation of this button immediately stops the machine (Image 12).

At the rear of the machine there is the electric board. Inside we have the PLC, which stores and interprets the machine software, and the power supply. Although it's placed on the inferior structure of the machine, its interaction occurs with the components placed on the superior structure (Image 13).

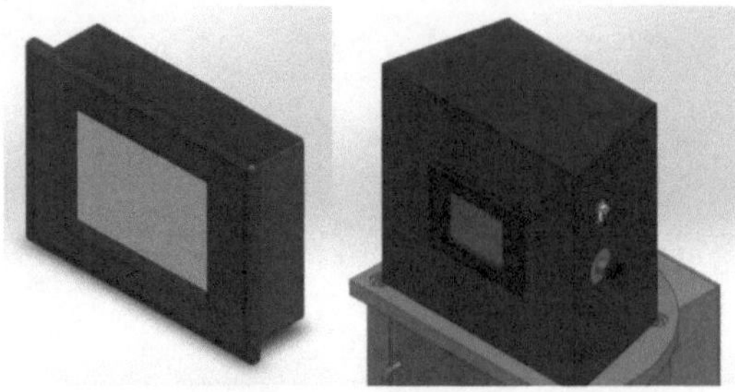

Image 11. LCD screen.

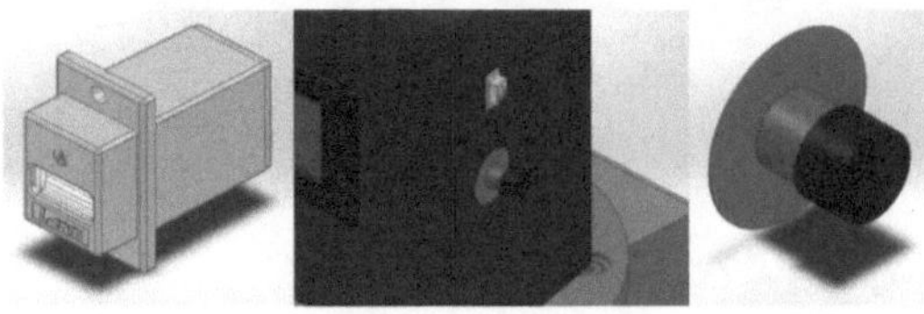

Image 12. USB adapter.

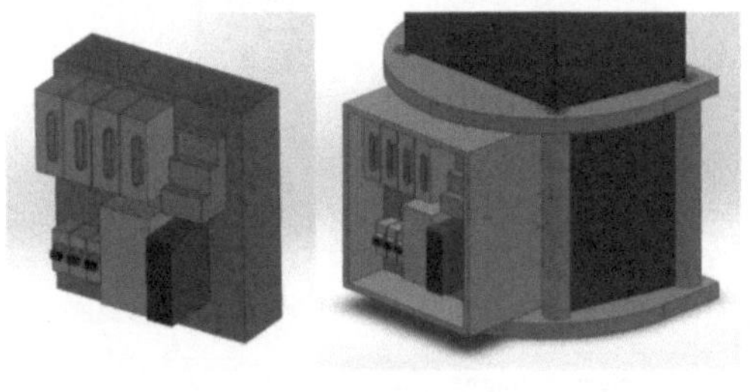

Image 13. PLC and electric board.

Table 1. Stages of preparation and construction of the machine.

Stage 1 Concept	Stage 2 Materialization and design	Stage 3 Conception detail	Stage 4 Construction
• Definition of product specifications • System description • System and mechanism sketches • Identification of critical problems and development of solutions	• Article sizing • Calculation of the functioning systems • Choice of materials • Calculation of strength and fatigue • Assemblage design • 3D presentation	• Global construction plan • Detailed plans of the pieces • Components list • Installation instructions • Documentation on the final project	• Pieces manufacture • Assemblage • Final tests

The electric hazard is kept away with the placing of a separator transformer between the power circuit and the shunting circuit, protecting the user from the 230 V power tension. The preparation and construction of the testing machine comprised 4 stages (Table 1).

The technical characteristics of the machine are summed up on Table 2.

Table 2. Technical characteristics of the machine.

Engine	Charge cell	Generalities
• Course: 150 mm • Maximum force: 1600 Nw • Speed: 210 mm/s	• Precision: 0.01 Nw • Maximum force: 1500 Nw Obs. The maximum force refers to thr charge cell used	• Touch screen control • USB entry for data registration • Electric power Portability

Net weight	49 kg
Actuator maximum power	0.2 kW
Actuator maximum pair	0.64 N.m
Actuator speed	1.06 mm/s
Actuator maximum advance speed	3000 rpm
Dimensions	
Height	740 mm
Width	400 mm
Depth	464 mm
Tension of use	
Power circuit	400 V AC
Shunting circuit	230 V AC
Acoustic pressure level	$L_{eqA} < 70$ dB

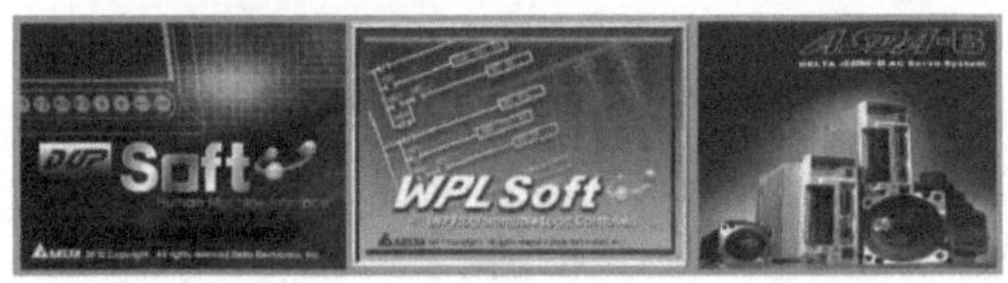

Image 14. Software.

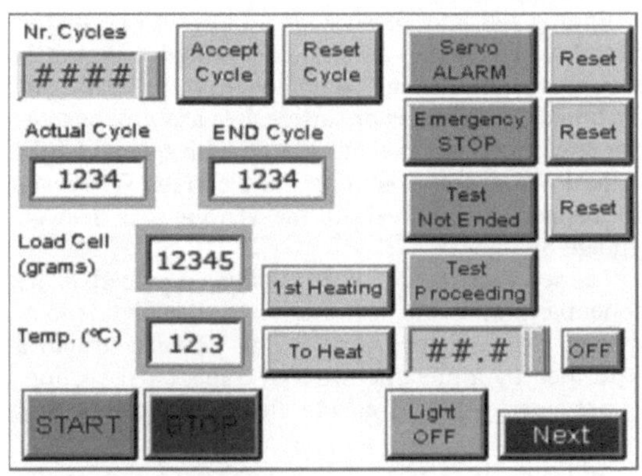

Image 15. 1st control window.

On the case of the LCD, PLC and actuator, we have the required software to reprogram the machine (Image 14).

2.1 *LCD control panel*

The LCD allows the control of the machine and the testing parameters. On the first control window we have several buttons through which we introduce the conditions we want for our test (Image 15).

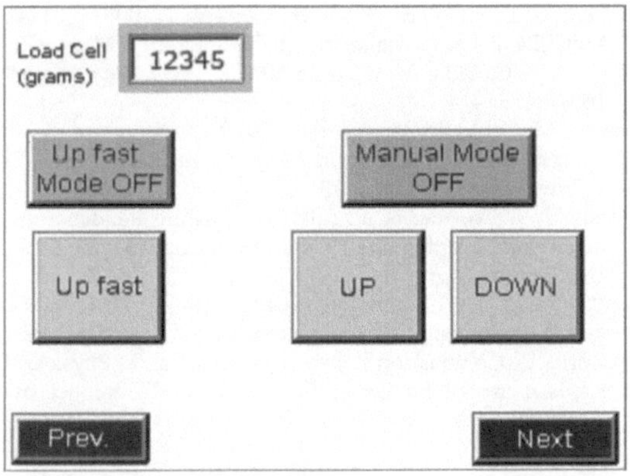

Image 16. 2nd control window.

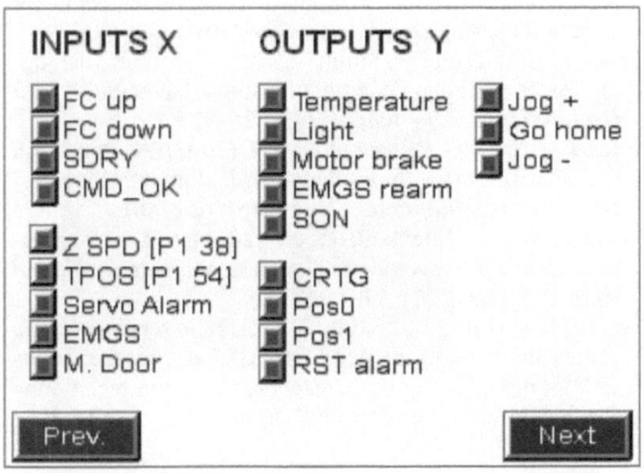

Image 17. 3rd control window.

The second window (Image 16) allows raising or lowering the actuator manually, quickly or slowly, indicating the charge value read by the cell.

The third control window just indicates the state of the system inputs and outputs.

This window is merely indicative and the operator has no need to perform any action on it (Image 17). The fourth control window (Image 18) allows the operator to introduce previous calibration conditions. Here is where the initial stages of the test take place.

The fifth control window shows, in real time, an effort graphic read by the charge cell during testing. The indicators of the charge value, register and removal of the USB memory and data cleaning, for the beginning of a new study, are all present (Image 19).

We end the machine "CS-DENTAL TESTING MACHINE" according to the directive 2006/42/EC on machines security and according to the norm EN 12100-1/2, EN 954-1, EN 1037, EN 61310-1/2, EN 60204-1, EN ISSO 14121-1, EN ISSO 13850 (Image 20).

Preliminary tests on Dalbo – Plus® attachments have been made to test the machine. Attachments samples have been placed on the actuator and, on the vase,

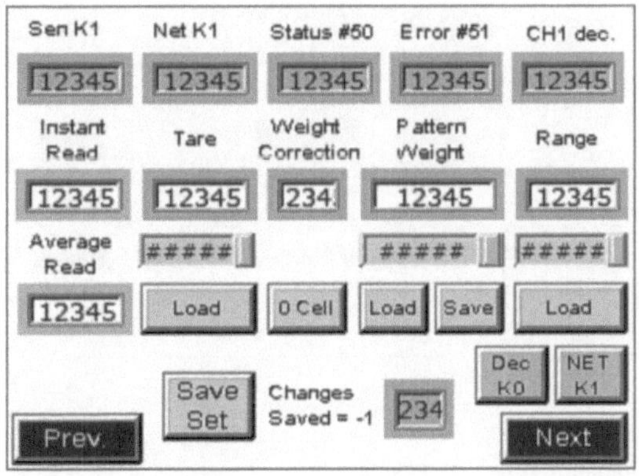

Image 18. 4th control window.

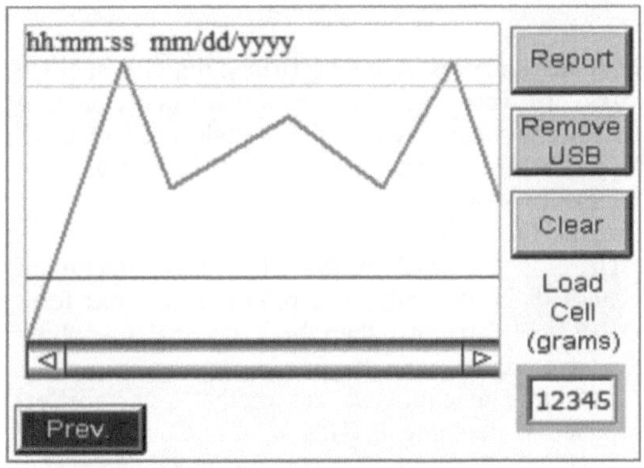

Image 19. 5th control window.

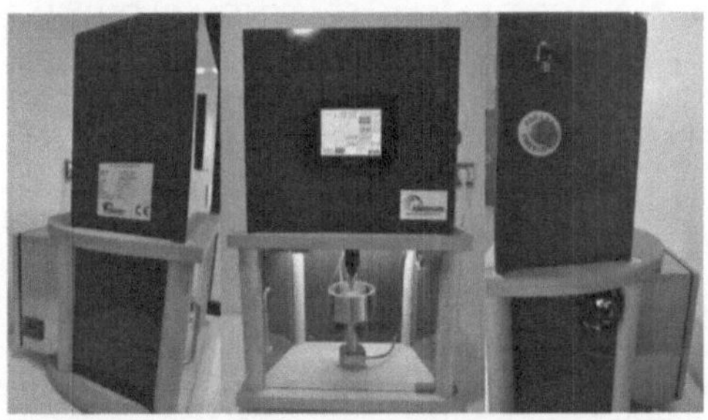

Image 20. CS DENTAL TESTING MACHINE.

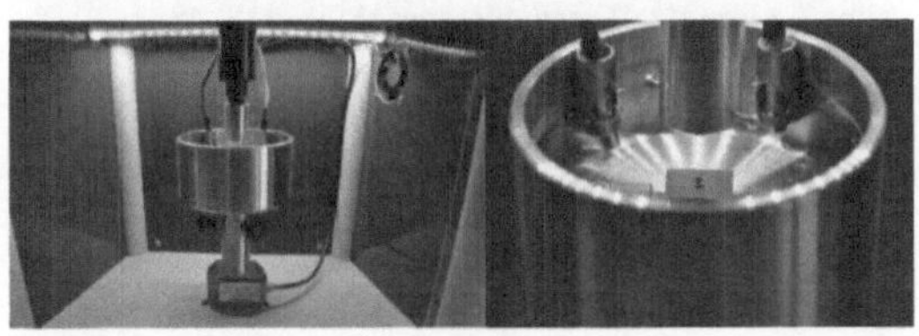

Image 21. Preliminary tests.

there have been put some replicas of implants with ball pillars of the mentioned attachments (Image 21). Cycles of 5400 have been made and results were achieved.

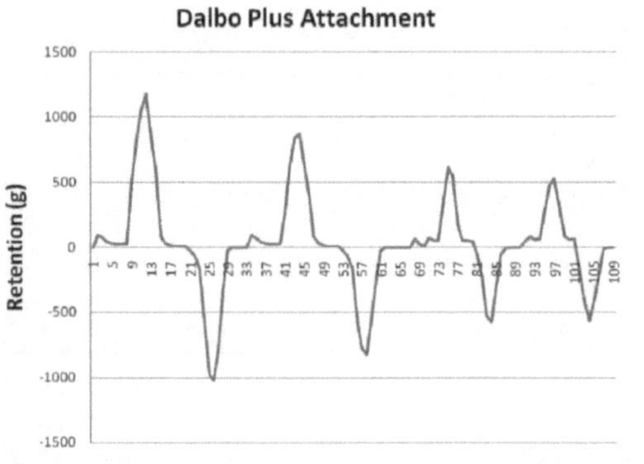

Graphic 1. Test with Dalbo-Plus.

3 DISCUSSION/CONCLUSION

The preliminary tests have confirmed that the machine works, it's very easy to use and allows checking and testing several types of materials used in Dentistry. On these tests we have also verified that Dalbo-Plus attachments have lost its retention capacity (Graphic 1).

There is the need to find the ideal attachment because its components lose retention in short term periods, not fulfilling, therefore, the goal for which they were created.

With this machine we are ready to test different types of attachments (Hader®, Locator®, Dalbo®, Dalbo Plus®, Preci-Clix®, ...) and to check which system is the best, over time, in terms of retention and durability.

And the CS-DENTAL TESTING MACHINE is able to perform several stress/fatigue tests in biological and material sciences, in Prosthodontics, Endodontics, Dentistry, Orthodontics, Periodontics, etc.

REFERENCES

Duyck, J., H. Van Oosterwyck, et al. (1999). "In vivo forces on oral implants supporting a mandibular overdenture: the influence of attachment system." *Clin Oral Investig* **3**(4): 201–207.

Evtimovska, E., R. Masri, et al. (2009). "The change in retentive values of locator attachments and hader clips over time." *Journal of Prosthodontics* **18**(6): 479–483.

Feine, J. S., G. E. Carlsson, et al. (2002). "The McGill Consensus Statement on Overdentures. Montreal, Quebec, Canada. May 24–25, 2002." *Int J Prosthodont* **15**(4): 413–414.

Goiato, M. C., A. R. Garcia, et al. (2010). "Analysis of masticatory cycle efficiency in complete denture wearers." *J Prosthodont* **19**(1): 10–13.

Gonda, T., Y. Maeda, et al. (2010). "Fracture incidence in mandibular overdentures retained by one or two implants." *The Journal of prosthetic dentistry* **103**(3): 178–181.

Jemt, T. and L. Hjalmarsson (2011). "In Vitro Measurements of Precision of Fit of Implant-Supported Frameworks. A Comparison between "Virtual" and "Physical" Assessments of Fit Using Two Different Techniques of Measurements." *Clinical Implant Dentistry and Related Research*.

Koka, S. and S. E. Eckert (2006). "Treatment planning the edentulous mandible." *Compend Contin Educ Dent* **27**(8): 432–434, 436-438.

Petropoulos, V. C. and F. K. Mante (2011). "Comparison of Retention and Strain Energies of Stud Attachments for Implant Overdentures." *Journal of Prosthodontics*.

Petropoulos, V. C. and W. Smith (2002). "Maximum dislodging forces of implant overdenture stud attachments." *Int J Oral Maxillofac Implants* **17**(4): 526–535.

Porter, J. A., Jr., V. C. Petropoulos, et al. (2002). "Comparison of load distribution for implant overdenture attachments." *Int J Oral Maxillofac Implants* **17**(5): 651–662.

Rutkunas, V., H. Mizutani, et al. (2011). "Wear simulation effects on overdenture stud attachments." *Dental materials journal*(0): 1111220201.

Schmitt, J., S. Holst, et al. (2009). "Prosthetic screw detorque values in implants retained as cast bar superstructures or bars modified by the Cresco Ti Precision technique–a comparative in vivo study." *Int J Prosthodont* **22**(2): 193–200.

Takeshita, S., M. Kanazawa, et al. (2011). "Stress analysis of mandibular two-implant overdenture with different attachment systems." *Dental materials journal*(0): 1111220212.

Uçankale, M., B. Akoğlu, et al. (2012). "The effect of different attachment systems with implant-retained overdentures on maximum bite force and EMG." *Gerodontology* **29**(1): 24–29.

Visser, A., G. M. Raghoebar, et al. (2009). "Implant-retained maxillary overdentures on milled bar suprastructures: a 10-year follow-up of surgical and prosthetic care and aftercare." *The International journal of prosthodontics* **22**(2): 181.

Yang, T. C., Y. Maeda, et al. (2011). "Attachment systems for implant overdenture: influence of implant inclination on retentive and lateral forces." *Clinical oral implants research*.

Biodental Engineering II – Natal Jorge et al (Eds)
© 2014 Taylor & Francis Group, London, ISBN 978-1-138-00131-2

3D evaluation of dental impaction using Computed Tomography

S.B. Goncalves & J.H. Correia
Centro Algoritmi, Department of Industrial Electronics, University of Minho, Guimaraes, Portugal

A.C. Costa
Clinica Dentaria Doutor Antonio Carlos Costa, Braga, Portugal

ABSTRACT: Dental impaction is the total or partial lack of eruption of a tooth. Their origins include various local causes, such as supernumerary teeth, which represents excess of teeth in regular dental formula. Treatment of impacted teeth requires a combination of oral surgery and/or orthodontic therapy. Although others radiographic techniques are used to diagnose and assessment dental impaction, Dental Computed Tomography (Dental CT) is the main method for accurately localize and to show orientation and morphology of the supernumerary and impacted teeth. These parameters are essential for allowing surgical and orthodontic successful procedures. This paper presents the role of Dental CT with a clinical case of maxillary central incisor impaction.

1 INTRODUCTION

Computed Tomography (CT) currently has an important role in the aid of diagnostic and the treatment planning in Dentistry. CT examination, complemented by specific dental software (Dental CT), a series of two-dimensional image data sets can be integrated mathematically to generate panoramic and cross-section images of the patients' jaw. These images enable the internal and external viewing and measurement of anatomical structures in slices. Also, provides the ability to perform tridimensional (3D) reconstructions of the entire region.

Impacted teeth are those prevented from erupting by some physical barrier in their path. Common factors in the etiology of impacted teeth include supernumerary teeth, odontogenic tumors such as odotomas or cysts, alteration in the eruption path or formation of scar tissue due to trauma, premature loss of deciduous teeth, abnormal root angulation or tooth dilaceration (Avinash & Aieshya 2011, Reddy et al. 2011, Suri et al. 2004). Although unerupted teeth can occur in both permanent and deciduous dentition, permanent teeth are much more prone for impacting than deciduous teeth, due to the duration of their odontogenesis (Bodner et al. 2001). The most impacted maxillary tooth is the canine, followed by the central incisor with a prevalence of 00.6–0.2% (Avinash & Aieshya 2011).

Supernumerary teeth are those that are in excess of the regular dental formula. The reported prevalence of supernumerary teeth is 0.1–3.8% in Caucasian population (Rajab & Hamdan 2002). Supernumerary teeth can grow in any region of the dental arch, but they are most common in the anterior maxilla, being the main cause of impaction of upper incisors (Rajab & Hamdan 2002, Smailiene et al. 2006, Suri et al. 2004).

The treatment of impacted maxillary permanent incisors is challenging due to these teeth importance to facial aesthetics. The regular approach is to eliminate the cause of the maxillary incisor impaction by surgical remove of the supernumerary tooth (Smailiene et al. 2006). This surgical procedure requires a preoperative knowledge of the position and orientation of supernumerary tooth in dental arch. The position and orientation can be accurately obtained by Dental CT program, which also allows 3D reconstructions of the impaction region.

This paper presents the role of Dental CT in a clinical case related with an unerupted maxillary central incisor associated with supernumerary tooth.

2 CLINICAL CASE

2.1 *Case presentation*

A 9-year-old male patient presented with a complaint of delayed eruption of the left permanent maxillary central incisor. The patient's medical history indicates good health and no previous systemic disease. There was no history of prior trauma to the teeth or jaws.

2.2 *Diagnosis and etiology*

Intraoral examination revealed absence of the left permanent central incisor in anterior maxilla (Fig. 1). Adequate space for the proper alignment of the unerupted central incisor is visible in Figure 1.

The panoramic conventional radiograph showed the patient's mixed dentition and the two impacted maxillary teeth: the permanent left impacted central incisor and a supernumerary tooth (Fig. 2). The etiology of the permanent central incisor's impaction is attributed to the presence of the supernumerary tooth.

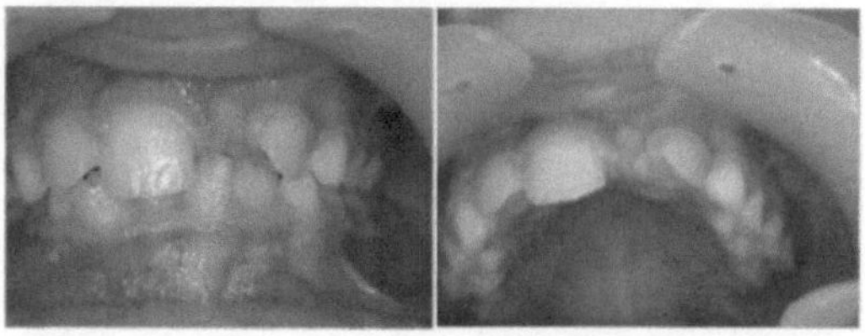

Figure 1. Intraoral views showing the impacted left permanent central incisor in superior dental arch.

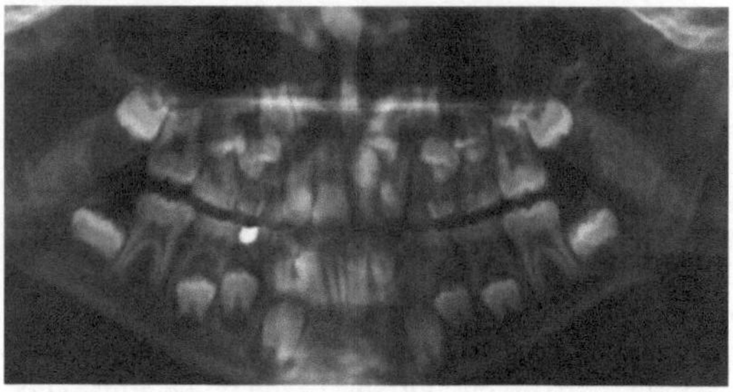

Figure 2. Panoramic conventional radiograph showing a supernumerary tooth associated to the impacted left central incisor.

However, the panoramic image didn't establish the real relation between both impacted teeth and between other dental structures, like adjacent teeth and roots. Thus, CT images were requested to show the localization and orientation of the impacted teeth. All CT images were performed in Siemens SOMATOM Esprit equipment with a slice thickness of 1.5 mm.

3 RESULTS

3.1 *Dental CT examination*

The successful removable of supernumerary tooth is highly dependent on radiographic examination performed to the patient. Thus, a Dental CT exam was made through axial images to acquire at the time of the scanning procedure. During scanning procedure, the patient was instructed to stay motionless in order to avoid motion artifacts. After data acquisition, Dental CT software was used to define the plane and location of the reformatted panoramic and cross-section views. Figure 3 shows topogram and Dental CT evaluation, which was restricted to the patient's maxillary (Figs. 3a, b). The final cross-sectional and panoramic images are defined using transversal (Fig. 3c) and parallel lines (Fig. 3d) overlapped on the arch of the maxilla, respectively. Figures 4 and 5 show the finals cross-sectional (buccolingual) and panoramic images of the patient's premaxilla.

3.2 *3D reconstruction*

In order to assist in accurate localization and orientation of the impacted teeth and for allowing 3D assessment of these teeth and their relationship to others teeth and structures in the dental arch, a 3D Surface

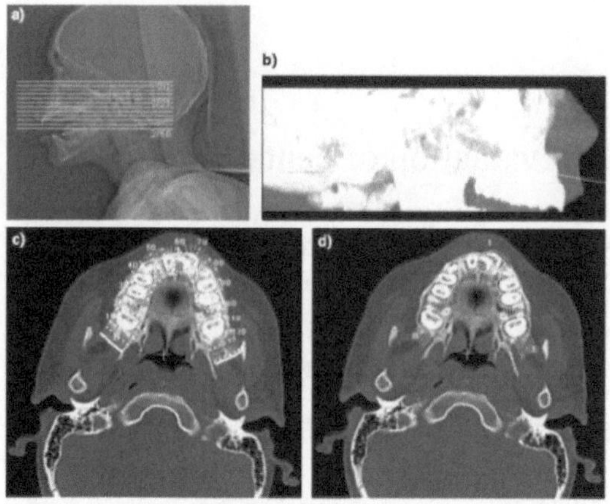

Figure 3. Images obtained in CT exam and Dental CT evaluation. a) Patient's head topogram showing ROI selected (upper jaw); b) Lateral MIP (Maximum Intensity Projection) view of the maxilla. This image has an orientation line in order to choose an image with the best plane (transaxial or oblique) to define reformatted final images; c) Transversal and d) Parallels lines overlapped on the arch of the maxilla in order to generate the cross-sectional and panoramic images, respectively.

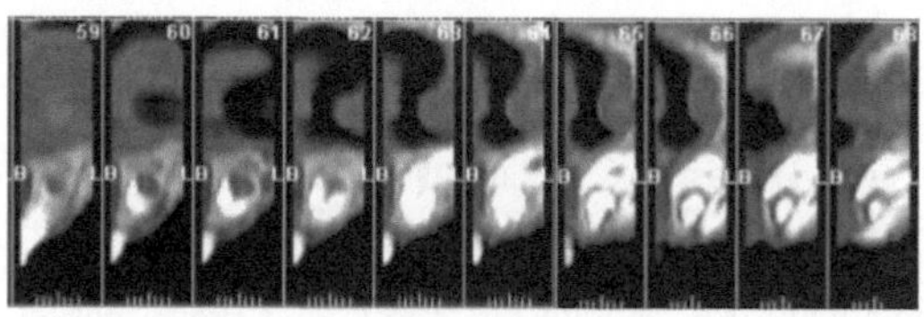

Figure 4. Anterior maxilla cross-sectional images resulting of Dental CT evaluation. These images allow visualization of both impacted teeth and a cyst formation.

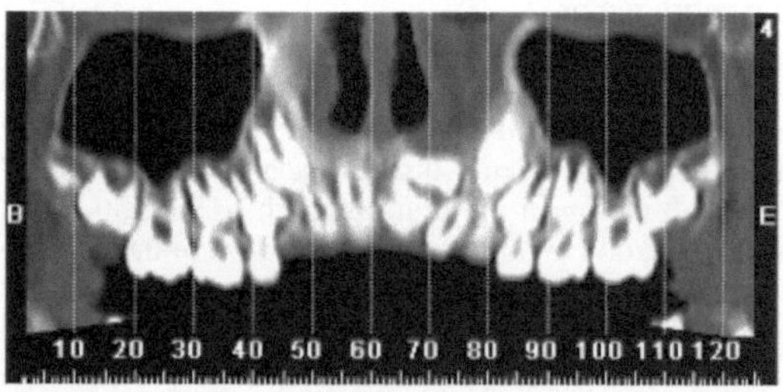

Figure 5. Panoramic image resulting of Dental CT evaluation. The patient's mixed dentition and impacted teeth are clearly shown.

Shade Display (SSD) reconstruction was made. The SSD reconstruction allows reconstruction of the surfaces of volumes. These volumes consist of voxels whose gray-scales are in a range defined by two limit values, an upper and a lower gray-scale limit. This method is especially suitable for displaying bone structures or blood vessels filled with contrast medium. The final 3D SSD reconstruction is shown in Figure 6.

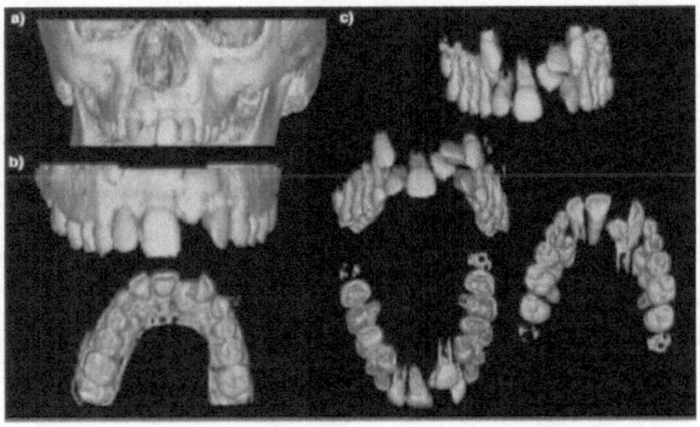

Figure 6. 3D SSD reconstruction of the patient's upper jaw, showing spatial relationship of the impacted central incisor and supernumerary tooth. a) Entire volume reconstruction; b) Upper jaw reconstruction; c) Anterior, superior and inferior view of the teeth reconstruction.

4 DISCUSSION

Impacted teeth are not a rare abnormality in dental arch. These teeth remain embedded in the jawbone due to some obstacle in their eruption path. One of the most causes of impaction is the presence of supernumerary teeth. They are most common in the anterior maxilla, resulting on impaction. Rajab & Hamdan (2002) studied 152 cases of supernumerary teeth: 90% occurred in the premaxilla, of which 92.8% were in the central incisor region. After treatment, 73.5% of the cases were impacted.

In this paper was presented a clinical case diagnosed with an unerupted central incisor in premaxilla due to the presence of a supernumerary tooth in the same region.

The treatment approach of impacted teeth requires cooperation of dental specialties, such oral surgery and/or orthodontics (Avinash & Aieshya 2011). When a supernumerary tooth prevents the eruption of a permanent tooth, the treatment can vary between the removal of the both impacted teeth, the removal of the supernumerary tooth leading to spontaneous eruption of the permanent tooth or the removal of the supernumerary tooth and exposure and traction of the permanent tooth into proper position (Akhare & Daga 2011, Mason et al. 2000). In the permanent dentition, removal of the physical obstruction from the path of eruption is recommended (Suri et al. 2004).

The patient's treatment approach included surgical removal of supernumerary tooth and conservation of the permanent maxillary left central incisor. By extraction of the supernumerary tooth, it is expected that leads to spontaneous eruption of the impacted central incisor.

However, in some instances, eliminating the cause of impaction by removing supernumerary tooth, would not lead to spontaneous eruption of the impacted tooth. Thus, it would be necessary a second surgical exposure of the unerupted tooth in order to perform orthodontic therapy by applying directional traction (Smailiene et al. 2006). Spontaneous eruption of the impacted maxillary tooth has obviously an advantage over orthodontic treatment. Smailiene (2006) found that spontaneous eruption of impacted maxillary incisors occurs in 54% to 76% of cases when supernumerary tooth was removed and there was enough space in the dental arch.

Several factors influence the time needed by an impacted tooth to erupt following removal of the supernumerary tooth, such as initial location and inclination of impacted tooth, the space available in the dental arch and the stage of root development (Avinash & Aieshya 2011, Rajab & Hamdan 2002, Smailiene et al. 2006). The spontaneous eruption of impacted maxillary incisors may take up to 3 years and sometimes orthodontic treatment is necessary to achieve adequate alignment of the erupted tooth in the dental arch (Rajab & Hamdan 2002, Smailiene et al. 2006).

The extraction of supernumerary tooth is not always the treatment's choice. If they are symptomless and do not appear to be affecting the dentition in any way, it is sometimes best left in place and kept under observation (Rajab & Hamdan 2002).

It is important to determine the best surgical approach causing the least harm to adjacent tooth roots while minimizing trauma to surrounding tissues. Thus, to the surgical removal of the supernumerary tooth it is vital the precise location, position and morphology of both impacted and supernumerary teeth and their relationships to the adjacent dental structures.

Dental CT program was used to obtain this information. Figures 4 and 5 shows cross-sectional and panoramic images of the patient's anterior maxilla, respectively. Both images clearly revealed the presence of a supernumerary tooth adjacent to an unerupted left central incisor and the exact location of the impacted teeth in dental arch.

In addition, Figure 4 revealed a cyst formation associated with the supernumerary tooth, which had not been seen on the panoramic radiograph (Fig. 2) because overlapping of the two teeth. Cyst formation is a common complication resulting of permanent teeth impaction (Al-Faleh 2009).

Figure 6 shows a 3D reconstruction of patient's upper jaw. Figures 6a and b allows the visualization of the entire maxilla, however it is difficult to see the whole extent of the impacted tooth root and its relationship to adjacent teeth. Therefore, the threshold level of the 3D reconstructed images was adjusted, in order to remove the surrounding bony structures, allowing evaluation of the entire structure of the teeth (Fig. 6c). Figure 6c presents 3D relationship of the two impacted teeth to the adjacent structures. The supernumerary tooth presents an incomplete root formation, while the root formation of the impacted central incisor has already started.

Mason et al. (2000) in his study assessed the maturity of the unerupted incisors by Cvek's classification (Fig. 7). They concluded that more immature teeth (Cvek groups 1, 2, and 3) erupted spontaneously after removal of the supernumerary than mature teeth (Cvek groups 4 and 5). According to Cvek's classification of

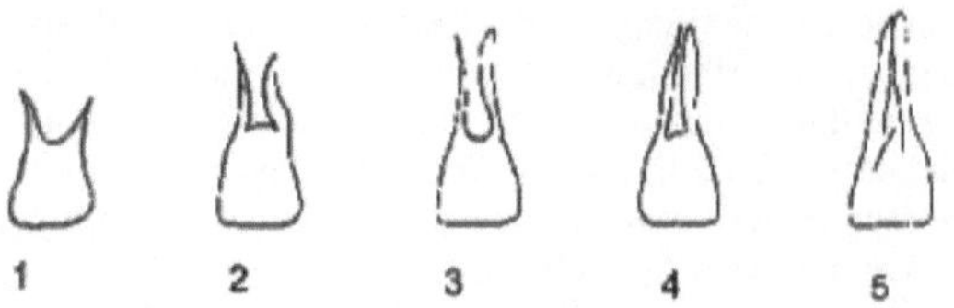

Figure 7. Cvek's classification of maturity of incisors. Group 1 – roots with wide, divergent ends and less than half their final length; Group 2 – roots between one-half and two-thirds their final length; Group 3 – roots two-thirds their final length; Group 4 – teeth with open apical foramina and roots almost full length; Group 5 – teeth with completely formed roots.

the maturity of the unerupted incisors, the patient's impacted teeth can be included on group 3 (see Fig. 6c), and therefore, spontaneous eruption of the left maxillary central incisor is expected.

Radiographic examination is essential to establish the etiology and for accurate diagnosis and planning of treatment, particularly with regard to the surgical approach. Traditionally, conventional periapical, occlusal and panoramic radiographs are used to determined the location and position of impacted teeth (Akhare & Daga 2011, Kim et al. 2003, Rajab & Hamdan 2002). In these images can occur cases of overlapping, magnification or blurred of dental structures. In severe cases of overlapping of impacted teeth, it may be impossible to determine the accurate location of these teeth relative to surrounding structures. Also, these modalities do not provide sufficiently detailed information concerning the 3D relationship between supernumerary or impacted teeth and adjacent structures. The main drawback of conventional radiographic techniques is that the images are two-dimensional.

CT solved these problems, providing accurate information than other imaging methods. This method enables the production of precise 3D images of anatomic structures without overlapping and preserving soft tissue detail. Dental CT software program display multiple axial, cross-sectional, and panoramic images of the jaw, which provides the exact location, inclination and morphology of the impacted teeth in the dental arch and its proximity to the vital structures or to the adjacent teeth (Al-Faleh 2009, Kim et al. 2003, Suri et al. 2004). Thus, surgical access and technique choice are facilitated, also reducing the procedure time.

Based on the images obtained by Dental CT, the supernumerary tooth was easily surgically removed. The patient presents proper space to impacted tooth eruption and, therefore spontaneous eruption of the left maxillary central incisor is expected.

5 CONCLUSION

Dental CT imaging can accurate localize supernumerary or impacted teeth. It can offer useful information for diagnosis and treatment planning that conventional radiograph are unable to provide. Such additional information includes the exact position of the impacted and supernumerary teeth in relation to adjacent roots or anatomic structures, the 3D relationship between dental structures and the absence of overlapping in the final images.

ACKNOWLEDGMENTS

This work is supported by Centro Algoritmi, FEDER funds through the Programa Operacional Fatores de Competitividade – COMPETE and National Funds through FCT – Fundação para a Ciência e Tecnologia with the reference Project: **FCOMP-01-0124-FEDER-022674**.

REFERENCES

Akhare, P. & Daga, A. 2011. Management of impacted teeth in the orthodontic practice. Journal of Clinical and Diagnostic Research. 5(4): 894–898.

Al-Faleh, W. 2009. Completely impacted teeth in dentate and edentulous jaws. Pakistan Oral & Dental Journal. 29(2): 255–260.

Avinash, K. & Aieshya, F. 2011. Impacted maxillary central incisor and over-retained deciduous central incisor: Combined surgical and orthodontical treatment – A case report. *J. Int Oral Health* 3(3): 25–30.

Bodner, L. et al. 2001. Image accuracy of plain film radiography and computed tomography in assessing morphological abnormality of impacted teeth. *Orthod Dentofacial Orthop*. 120: 623–8.

Kim, K. et al. 2003. Personal computer-based three-dimensional computed tomography images of the teeth for evaluating supernumerary or ectopically impacted teeth. Angle Orthod. 73: 614–621.

Mason C. et al. 2000. A retrospective study of unerupted maxillary incisors associated with supernumerary teeth. British Journal of Oral and maxillofacial Surgery. 38: 62–65.

Reddy, V. et al. 2011. Impacted maxillary central incisor with dilacerations. *IJDA* 3(2): 543–545.

Rajab, L. D. & Hamdan, M. A. M. 2002. Supernumerary teeth: review of the literature and a survey of 152 cases. *International Journal of Paediatric Dentistry* 12: 244–254.

Smailiene, D. et al. 2006. Impaction of the central maxillary incisor associated with supernumerary teeth: Initial position and spontaneous eruption time. Stomatologije, Baltic Dental and Maxillofacial Journal. 8: 103–107.

Suri, L. et al. 2004. Delayed tooth eruption: Pathogenesis, diagnosis, and treatment. A literature review. *American Journal of Orthodontics and Dentofacial Orthopedics* 126(4): 432–445.

Biodental Engineering II – Natal Jorge et al (Eds)
© 2014 Taylor & Francis Group, London, ISBN 978-1-138-00131-2

Nasal bone in prenatal ultrasound and genetic changes with orofacial manifestations

P. Vaz
Department of Medical and Orofacial Genetics, The Pregnant and the Baby's Appointment, Faculty of Dental Medicine (FMDUP), University of Porto

M.J. Catita
Dentist, Researcher of the Cooperation Protocol of the Prenatal Diagnosis Unit of the Hospital of Vila Nova de Gaia (CHVNG) and Pregnant and the Baby's Appointment at FMDUP, University of Porto

M.J. Ponces
Department of Orthodontics, The Pregnant and the Baby's Appointment, FMDUP, University of Porto

A.C. Braga
Division of Statistics, Department of Production and Systems Engineering, University of Minho

O. Iskenderva
Geneticist, Researcher of the Cooperation Protocol of the Prenatal Diagnosis Unit, CHVNG

F. Valente
Gynecologist and Obstetrician, Coordinator of the Prenatal Diagnosis Unit of the CHVNG

ABSTRACT: The absence or hypoplasia of nasal bone and the nuchal translucency thickness are of the utmost importance on the detection of birth defects on prenatal ultrasonography. The aim of this study was to determine the prevalence of absence or hypoplasia of nasal bone in a pregnant Caucasian Portuguese population, with a gestational age between 20 weeks and 20+6 days. The sample comprised 79 pregnant women that were divided into two groups: a normal group (A) and a group with fetuses with pathology (B). Measurement of nasal bone was detached through the images and reports obtained in prenatal ultrasonography. It was found a relationship not only between the nasal bone and the existence of pathology but also with the interruption of pregnancy.

1 INTRODUCTION

During pregnancy several congenital anomalies may occur and these result in structural, behaviour, functional, metabolic and neuromuscular defects (Sadler 2010, Lewis 2007, Ferraris & Muñoz 2007).

In the second trimester, ultrasound screening of aneuploidies and fetal malformations is done primarily with fetal morphological study, complemented by biochemical screening (Regateiro 2003, Geipel et al. 2010, Kagun et al. 2009, Benoit & Chaoui 2005). On the ultrasonographic evaluation, the presence or absence of nasal bone and nuchal fold thickness is considered to be an important marker (Geipel et al. 2010, Persico et al. 2008). The presence of hypoplasia of nasal bone happens in 0.4 to 6% of euploid fetuses. However, this is a characteristic often expressed on trisomies 13, 18, and 21 and on Apert, Cri-du-Chat and Lange syndromes. It is also detected in mesomelic dysplasia (Kagun et al. 2009, Benoit & Chaoui 2005, Chung et al. 2010, Persico et al. 2010, Guis et al. 1995, Teoh et al. 2009, Tuxer et al. 2003).

The nasal bone study in prenatal ultrasound may represent a factor of predictability related to the progression of craniofacial development. This is valid not only in aneuploidy cases and genetic syndromes, but also in euploidies situations (Guis et al. 1995, Kouskoura et al. 2011, Sommerlad et al. 2010).

The aim of this study was to determine the prevalence of absence or hypoplasia of nasal bone in a population of pregnant Caucasian Portuguese women.

2 MATERIALS AND METHODS

This investigation was developed in the Unit of Prenatal Diagnosis of CHVNG and in the FMDUP. This retrospective study involved clinical and anamnestic data that were collected from each pregnant woman of a total of 1048 patients, who attended CHVNG from January 2009 to December 2011. The twin pregnancies were excluded. The final sample consisted of 79 pregnant women with gestational age between 20 weeks and 20 + 6 days. The nasal bone length was assessed by transabdominal ultrasound in the mid-sagittal plane.

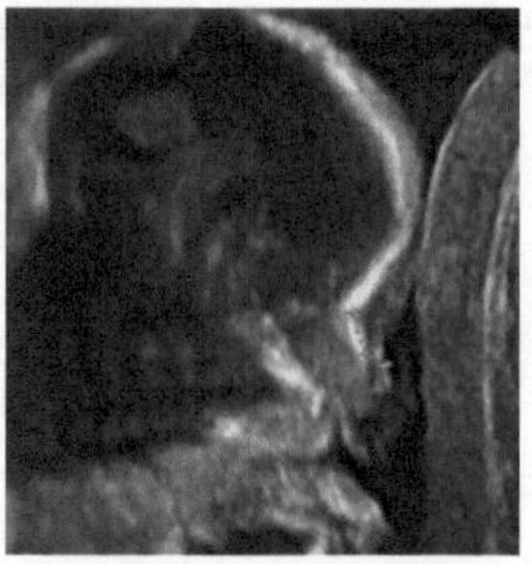

Figure 1. Hypoplastic nasal bone on fetus with 20 weeks + 4days in prenatal ultrasonography.

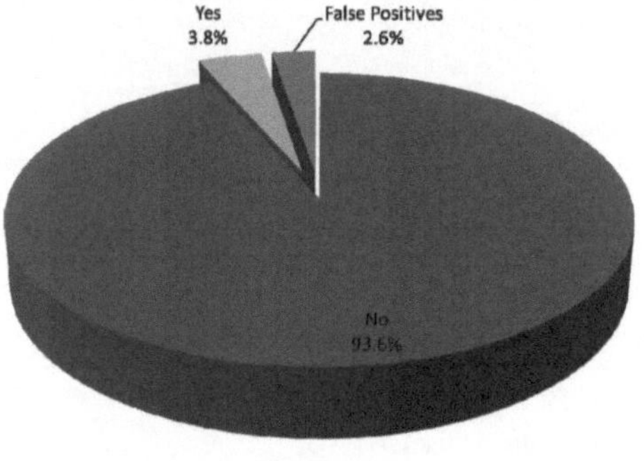

Figure 2. Chromosomal abnormalities.

Measurements of nasal bone were collected from the images and reports obtained in prenatal ultrasonography (Figure 1).

The ultrasound findings were made with the GE Voluson E8 (GE Expert and Toshiba Aplio echographs, USA).

2.1 *Statistical analyses*

The Mann-Whitney U-test for independent samples was used to compare mean nasal bone length between normal fetuses (group A, $n = 71$) and fetuses with pathology (group B, $n = 8$). It was also used to compare the group with and without interrupted pregnancy. Mean nuchal fold thickness and nuchal translucency were also compared between groups A and B.

Collected data were analysed with SPSS Statistics 20.0® (IBM, USA).

3 RESULTS

The final sample involved 79 singleton pregnancies that were divided into two groups (groups A and B). All group B cases presented malformations, which represented 11.5% of the sample. In 6.4% of total cases, there was an increased risk for chromosomal abnormalities, confirmed in 3.8% and with a percentage of 2.6% of false positives (Figure 2).

The mean age of the pregnant women was 31 years old (Figure 3).

The characterization of both groups (A and B) included biometric ultrasound data collection (Table I).

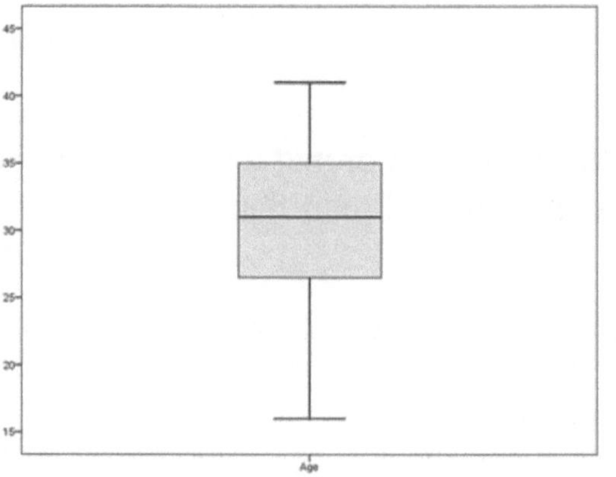

Figure 3. Age distribution of the pregnant women.

It was found that the nasal bone measurement average was lower in the group B (4.3 mm) than in the group A (5.8 mm). Relating to birth weight, higher average was found in fetuses with pathology. However, this discrepancy may be explained by the low number of fetus that survived in group B. Respecting the size of the femur, the cephalic perimeter, the biparietal diameter and cerebellum, these values were lower in the group with pathology (group B). The same was not true in relation to waist circumference, nuchal translucency, nuchal fold, where the values in the group with pathology (group B) were higher.

When comparing the same characteristics between groups with and without interrupted pregnancy, it was clear that most values that were lower in the group B had the same behavior as in the group with interrupted pregnancy (Table II).

The nasal bone tended to be hypoplastic or absent in the group with pathology (B), when compared with the normal group (A) (Figure 4). There were statistically significant differences between the groups with and without interrupted pregnancy (Figure 5).

The nuchal fold thickness showed an increased length in the group B, when compared to group A (Figure 6).

4 DISCUSSION

In this sample there was an increased risk for chromosome disorders, present in 6.3% of the cases, confirmed in 3.8% and with a percentage of 2.5% false positives. These results demonstrate the effectiveness of the screening of aneuploidies and fetal malformations.

There were statistically significant differences between the groups with and without pathology, with higher values in the last for the nasal bone. Benoit et al. (2005) found that in 45% of fetuses with trisomy 21, the nasal bone was absent or hypoplastic. Kagan et al. (2009) showed the same in 59% of fetuses with trisomy 21, in 52% fetuses with trisomy 18 and in 45% fetuses with trisomy 13. The nuchal fold revealed statistically

Table I. Comparison between groups A and B.

		Group	
		A	B
Nasal bone	Valid N	71	8
	Mean	5.779	4.300
	Median	5.900	4.955
	Minimum	2.000	.000
	Maximum	7.600	6.400
	Std. Deviation	.951	2.040
Birth weight	Valid N	63	3
	Mean	2.955	3.348
	Median	3.055	3.515
	Minimum	.680	2.820
	Maximum	4.225	3.710
	Std. Deviation	.679	.468
Length of the femur	Valid N	69	8
	Mean	33.04	31.95
	Median	33.00	32.45
	Minimum	28.80	29.10
	Maximum	37.40	34.30
	Std Deviation	2.00	1.97
Cephalic perimeter	Valid N	71	8
	Mean	176.0	170.3
	Median	176.6	172.7
	Minimum	159.6	146.0
	Maximum	199.3	179.5
	Std. Deviation	8.5	10.4
Waist circumference	Valid N	69	7
	Mean	153.97	154.13
	Median	153.50	154.70
	Minimum	133.40	138.80
	Maximum	175.30	168.60
	Std. Deviation	8.77	9.53
Nuchal translucency	Valid N	53	4
	Mean	1.6	2.1
	Median	1.4	2.1
	Minimum	.8	1.6
	Maximum	2.7	2.5
	Std. Deviation	.5	.5
Nuchal fold	Valid N	38	3
	Mean	4.0	6.2
	Median	4.1	5.9
	Minimum	1.7	4.7
	Maximum	6.0	8.0
	Std. Deviation	1.0	1.7
Cerebellum	Valid N	59	2
	Mean	20.8	20.7
	Median	20.7	20.7
	Minimum	18.8	20.7
	Maximum	23.5	20.7
	Std. Deviation	1.0	.0
Biparietal diameter	Valid N	71	8
	Mean	47.6	45.9
	Median	48.1	46.7
	Minimum	42.0	37.6
	Maximum	53.9	50.8
	Std. Deviation	2.8	4.0

significant differences between groups A and B, the latter presenting higher values. Previous studies have also proved the same (Persico et al 2008, Geipel et al 2010).

Table II. Comparison between groups with and without interrupted pregnancy.

		Pregnancy interrupted	
		No	Yes
Nasal Bone	Valid N	66	5
	Mean	5.842	3.610
	Median	5.900	3.500
	Minimum	3.800	.000
	Maximum	7.600	6.400
	Std. Deviation	.844	2.365
Length of the femur	Valid N	64	5
	Mean	33.08	31.028
	Median	33.01	30.11
	Minimum	28.81	29.11
	Maximum	37.41	33.81
	Std. Deviation	1.91	1.90
Cephalic perimeter	Valid N	66	5
	Mean	175.8	168.9
	Median	176.2	172.8
	Minimum	159.6	146.0
	Maximum	199.3	179.5
	Std. Deviation	8.5	13.1
Waist circumference	Valid N	63	5
	Mean	153.60	152.96
	Median	154.20	154.00
	Minimum	133.40	138.80
	Maximum	175.30	168.60
	Std. Deviation	8.3944	11.2902
Nuchal translucency	Valid N	51	2
	Mean	1.6	2.5
	Median	1.5	2.5
	Minimum	.8	2.5
	Maximum	2.7	2.5
	Std. Deviation	.5	.0
Nuchal fold	Valid N	35	2
	Mean	4.1	6.4
	Median	4.2	6.4
	Minimum	1.7	4.7
	Maximum	6.0	8.0
	Std. Deviation	1.0	2.3
Cerebellum	Valid N	55	1
	Mean	20.8	20.7
	Median	20.7	20.7
	Minimum	18.8	20.7
	Maximum	23.5	20.7
	Standard Deviation	1.0	.
Biparietal diameter	Valid N	66	5
	Mean	47.5	45.1
	Median	47.5	46.1
	Minimum	42.0	37.6
	Maximum	53.9	50.8
	Std. Deviation	2.7	5.0

This study also pointed out statistically significant differences between the nasal bone length and interrupted pregnancies. Many investigations (Benoit et al 2005, Geipel et al 2010, Persico et al 2010) have found a relationship between the absence or hypoplasia of the nasal bone and the existence of aneuploidies.

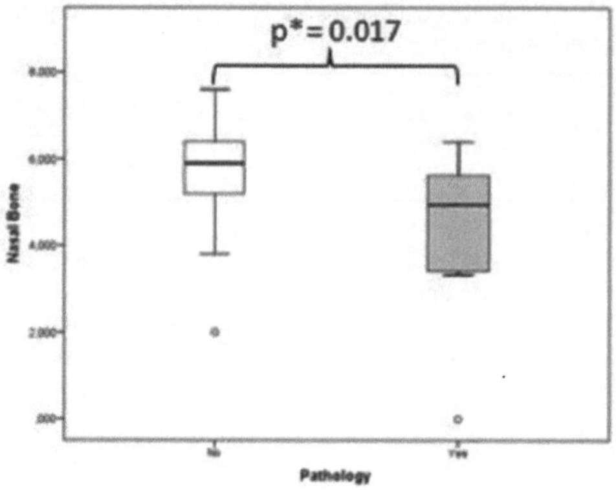

Figure 4. Nasal bone length in groups A and B. *Mann-Whitney test.

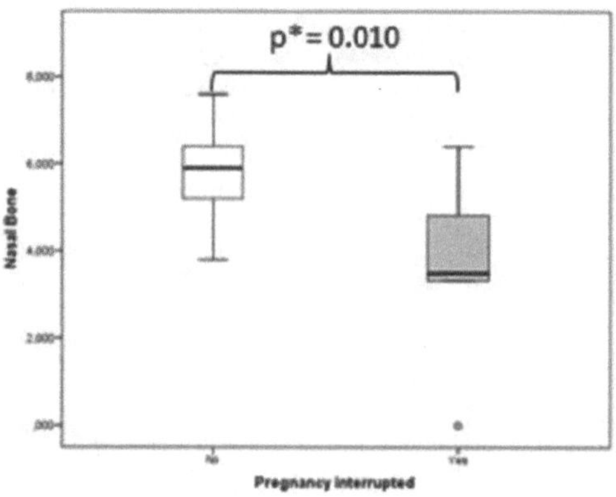

Figure 5. Nasal bone length in groups with and without interrupted pregnancy.

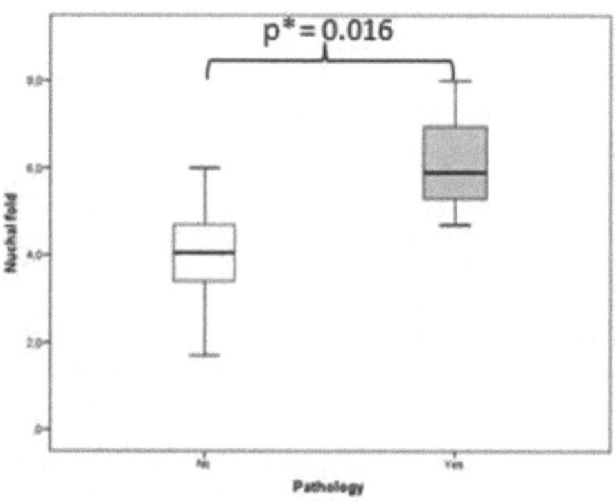

Figure 6. Nuchal fold in groups A and B.

5 CONCLUSION

With a significance level of 5% it can be concluded that there were significant differences in the nasal bone between the groups with and without interrupted pregnancy ($Z = -2.495$, $p < 0.05$).

The nasal bone and the nuchal fold revealed statistically significant differences between normal fetuses and fetuses with pathology ($Z = -2.381$, $p < 0.05$; $Z = -2.304$, $p < 0.05$, respectively). However, the nuchal translucency did not reveal significant differences ($Z = -1.725$, $p > 0.05$).

The results of this study establish a relationship between the extent of the nasal bone and the presence of pathology and between that bone and the medical suspension of pregnancy.

Despite the limitation of the sample, these markers (nasal bone, nuchal fold) demonstrated how important they could be in the detection of aneuploidies and fetal malformations as prognostic pregnancy factors.

REFERENCES

Benoit, B. 2005. Three-dimensional ultrasound with maximal mode rendering: a novel technique for the diagnosis of bilateral or unilateral absence or hypoplasia of nasal bones in second-trimester screening for Down syndrome. *Ultrasound Obstet Gynecol* 25(1): p. 19–24.

Chung, D. 2002. Agenesia do nariz: relato de caso. Rev. *Bras. Otorrinolaringol* 68(4): p. 581–585.

Ferraris, M.; Muñoz, A. 2007. Histología y embriología bucodental. 2ª Ed. Madrid: Editorial *Medica panamericana* 19–43.

Geipel, A. 2010. Nuchal fold thickness, nasal bone absence or hypoplasia, ductus venosus reversed flow and tricuspid valve regurgitation in screening for trisomies 21, 18 and 13 in the early second trimester. *Ultrasound Obstet Gynecol* 35(5): p. 535–539.

Guis, F. 1995. Ultrasound evaluation of the length of the fetal nasal bones throughout gestation. *Ultrasound Obstet Gynecol* 5(5): p. 304–307.

Kagan, K.O. 2009. Fetal nasal bon in screening for trisomies 21, 18 and 13 and Turner syndrome at 11–13 weeks of gestation. *Ultrasound Obstet Gynecol* 33(3): p. 259–264.

Kouskoura, T. 2011. The genetic basis of craniofacial and dental abnormalities. *Schweiz Monatsschr Zahnmed* 121(7–8): p. 636–646.

Lewis, R. 2007. Human Genetics:concepts and applications. 7ª Ed. New York: Mc Graw-Hill *International Edition* 56–62.

Persico, N. 2008. Prenasal thickness in trisomy-21 fetuses at 16–24 weeks of gestation. *Ultrasound Obstet Gynecol* 32(6): p. 751–754.

Persico, N. 2010. Nasal-bone length in euploid fetuses at 16–24 weeks' gestation by three-dimensional ultrasound. *Ultrasound Obstet Gynecol* 36(3): p. 285–290.

Regateiro, F. 2003. Manual de Genética Médica. 1ª Ed; Coimbra: Imprensa da Universidade de Coimbra 307–316.

Sadler, T.; Langman. 2010. Embriologia Médica. 11ª ed. Rio de Janeiro: Guanabara Koogan.

Sommerlad, M. 2010. Detection of lip, alveolar ridge and hard palate abnormalities using two-dimensional ultrasound enhanced with the three-dimensional reverse-face view. *Ultrasound Obstet Gynecol* 36(5): p. 596–600.

Teoh, X. 2009. Prenatal diagnosis of cri-du-chat syndrome: importance of ultrasonographical markers. *Singapore Med J* 50(5): p. 181–184.

Tuxen, A. 2003. A histological and radiological investigation of the nasal bone in fetuses with Down syndrome. Ultrasound *Obstet Gynecol* 22(1): p. 22–26.

Biodental Engineering II – Natal Jorge et al (Eds)
© 2014 Taylor & Francis Group, London, ISBN 978-1-138-00131-2

Guided tissue regeneration and genetics

P. Vaz
Department of Medical and Orofacial Genetics, Faculty of Dental Medicine (FMDUP), University of Porto

B.M. Assunção
Team Member of the Query of Orofacial Genetics of the FMDUP, University of Porto, Portugal

M. Henriques
Department of Biological Engineering, University of Minho, Portugal

C. Pintado
Team Member of the Query of Orofacial Genetics of the FMDUP, University of Porto, Portugal

P. Mesquita
Department of Dental Anatomy and Histology, FMDUP, University of Porto, Portugal

M.H. Figueiral
Department of Removable Prosthesis, FMDUP, University of Porto, Portugal

ABSTRACT: Guided Tissue Regeneration (GTR) is widespread and accepted as an excellent alternative therapy in periodontology and oral implantology. However, there still remain clinical situations for which these procedures do not have predictable results. Several risk factors for developing complications in GTR have been studied. This study had as main objective to present a clinical case of a male patient, with 34 years old and with recurrent failure of GTR surgery on the anterior maxillary sector. A research was carried out on PubMed database, without time limitation, and also in the OMIM database and PUCMINAS, PUCPR. Forty-three articles have been used. According to some researchers, we can assume that, eventually, there may be patients with genotype of increased risk to trigger an exaggerated inflammatory response against bacterial contamination of membranes and various materials of GTR. Therefore, it has been suggested that gene polymorphisms encoding inflammatory cytokines might set the outcome of GTR.

1 INTRODUCTION

The ultimate goal in periodontal therapy is to stop the progression of periodontal disease and regenerate the attachment apparatus lost to periodontal disease. (Christgau *et al.* 2003, Sanctis *et al.* 2000, Hamilton *et al.* 2010).

Guided tissue regeneration (GTR) is widespread and accepted as an excellent alternative therapy in periodontology and oral implantology. However, there still remain clinical situations for which these procedures do not have predictable results (Christgau *et al.* 2003, Vaz *et al.* 2012). The identification and control of significant factors determining clinical outcomes is of paramount importance to improve results of a variety of therapeutic. (Tonetti *et al.* 1996).

Several risk factors for developing complications in GTR have been studied, particularly infection of materials for regeneration. (Christgau *et al.* 2003, Cortellini *et al.* 2000, Kormman *et al.* 2000, Slots *et al.* 2000, Tonetti *et al.* 1995, Tonetti *et al.* 1996; Vaz *et al.* 2012)

The establishment of an infection in guided tissue regeneration in oral surgery has been the subject of several investigations. (Nowzari *et al.* 1995, Nowzari & Slots 1995, Simion *et al.* 1994, Thomas *et al.* 2011) However, it is still urgent an understanding of how the mechanisms can trigger a periodontal destruction and the role of individual susceptibility in establishing biological complications in GTR. (Thomas *et al.* 2011)

According to some researchers, we can assume that, eventually, there may be patients with genotype of increased risk to trigger an exaggerated inflammatory response against bacterial contamination of membranes and several materials of GTR. (Christgau *et al.* 2003, Sanctis *et al.* 2000, Vaz *et al.* 2012, Weiss *et al.* 2004)

Therefore, it has been suggested that gene polymorphisms encoding inflammatory cytokines might set the outcome of GTR therapy. (Vaz *et al.* 2012)

However, this hypothesis is not yet fully clarified – there are still some doubts and it is urgent that further

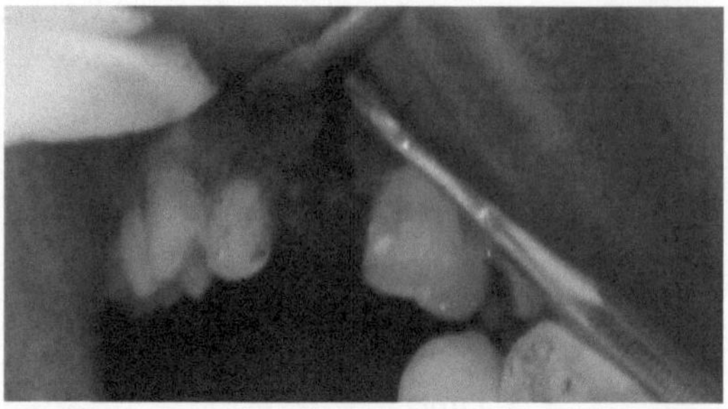

Figure 1. Intrabony defect after the orofacial injury.

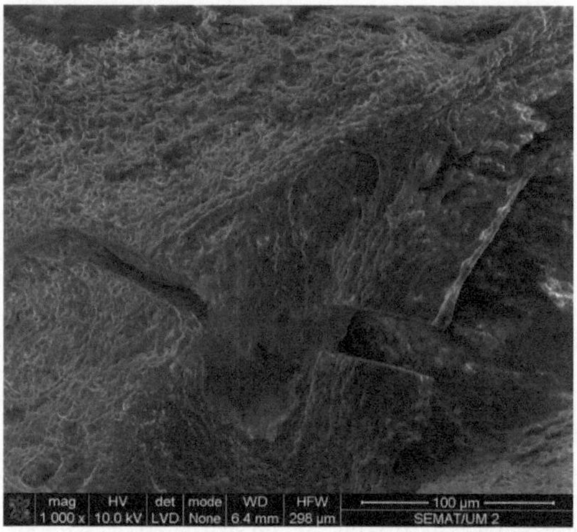

Figure 2. SEM analysis revealed that GTR biomaterial was covered with microorganisms.

studies are developed in order to clarify and assist the dentist in treatment planning in such cases.

This study had as main objective to present a clinical case of a male patient, who suffered an orofacial injury (that led to the loss of the tooth 11), with 34 years old and had recurrent failure of GTR procedure on the anterior maxillary sector (Fig. 1).

2 MATERIALS AND METHODS

The treatment performed on the patient comprised 3 GTR therapies (all of them with resorbable collagen membrane 3I® and lyophilized bovine bone Bio-Oss®), removable and fixed prosthetic rehabilitation on dental implant.

Awaiting the usual healing period of GTR, it was placed an acrylic removable partial denture (RPD). In the second GTR, after 8 months, a sample was removed from the regeneration material and a surface analysis was performed with scanning electron microscopy (SEM). It was also performed a genotyping study of interleukin-1 (IL-1) gene polymorphisms.

Clinical controls were made quarterly, after the first GTR and monthly after the second and third GTR,

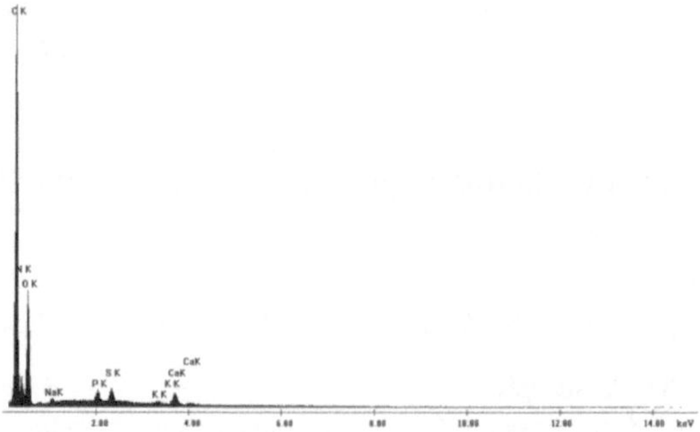

Figure 3. EDS of the sample showed high amount of Carbon and Oxygen and confirmed its organic origin.

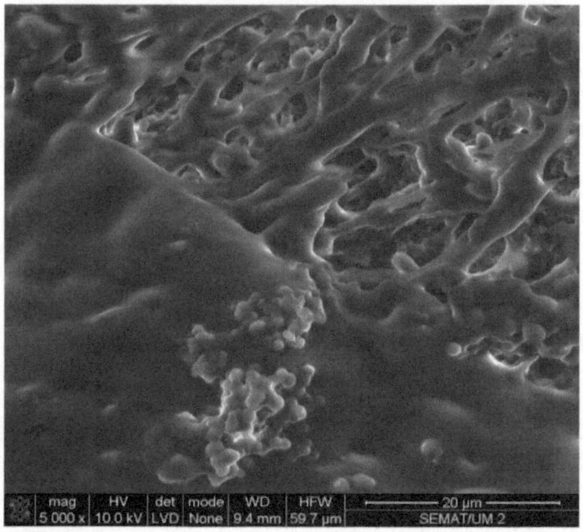

Figure 4. SEM analysis showed the presence on the sample of a complex structure of microorganisms (bacteria and yeast) and a viscous layer.

which did not indicate any evidence of infection on GTR material. The sample, removed after the second GTR surgery (biomaterial used in the procedure), was dehydrated and after coated with gold it was observed under SEM (Fig. 2 and 4).

Some EDS analysis were also performed in some points to confirm the origin of the material present in the sample (Fig. 3).

The identification of the IL-1 gene polymorphisms (positions −889 of *IL1A* gene and +3953 of *IL1B* gene) was performed through a CGC Genetics Kit (CGC Genetics, Portugal) and included the DNA extraction, amplification and reverse hybridization. These positive results were identified in a DNA strip.

The results of SEM analysis revealed that the biomaterial had microbial colonization in several areas (Fig. 4) and the study of the gene polymorphisms identified a positive-genotype (presence of the allele 2 – Thymine in the two positions of the studied genes).

Aware of the risks, but because of the patient's age, the authors chose to perform the elimination of all material from GTR, waited for a healing period of

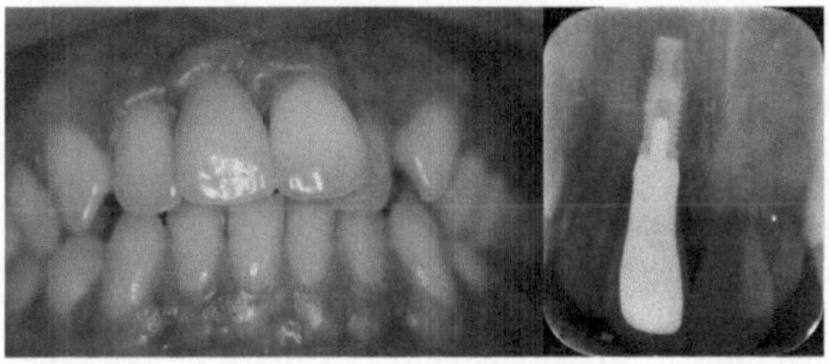

Figure 5. Final result of the dental rehabilitation after GTR procedures and dental implant placement – a metal-ceramic crown screwed into the implant and its x-ray.

3 months, repeated GTR-therapy and, after 6 months, placed a dental implant and crown on implant (Fig. 5).

A research was carried out on PubMed database (File digital biomedical literature and life sciences at the National Institute of Health of the United States) and OMIM detabase (Online Mendelian Inheritance in Man), without time limitation. We used, as search terms, in PubMed: "Biofilm guided oral regeneration" and "Guided bone regeneration Il-1gene polymorphims." We used the keyword "Interleukin-1" in research directed to OMIM. It was also performed a search in the database of PUCMINAS (Catholic University of Minas Gerais) and PUCPR (Catholic University of Paraná) using the terms "polymorphism Il-1." We excluded articles whose first language was not English, Spanish or Portuguese. For articles obtained from PubMed, we excluded items with incomplete abstract or with full text unavailable. After analysis according to the inclusion and exclusion criteria, 43 articles were selected, with interest for the study of the subject.

3 GTR-THERAPY

The biological principle of guided tissue regeneration has been discovered by Karring and Nyman in the early 80's, as a result of the desire to regenerate lost periodontal tissues. (Nyman *et al.* 1982) Almost immediately, the guided tissue regeneration was applied in other tissue, particularly in bone tissue regeneration. (Hämmerle *et al.* 2002)

Thus, could be re-establishing the lost supporting tissue with the gain of a new clinical attachment (Sanctis *et al.* 2000) and alveolar bone growth, so that the form, function and original architecture were restored. (Hamilton *et al.* 2010)

Indeed, the use of membranes for periodontal regeneration is well established. (Ricci *et al.* 1996) In the early 90's, and beyond, case reports or case series were presented describing the use of resorbable membranes for GTR on exposed surfaces of implants. Later there were published randomized clinical trials and in all of them were a low rate of complications, including inflammation of the flap that covered the local regeneration and the exposure of the membranes. (Hämmerle *et al.* 2002)

However, there is also a general consensus that guided bone regeneration is difficult to achieve and requires skills and experience of the professional. (Hämmerle *et al.* 2002) The guided tissue regeneration is a periodontal regenerative technique which promotes selective repopulation of a periodontal defect by those cells most likely to result in tissue regeneration. (Nyman *et al.* 1982, Needleman *et al.* 2006, Thomas *et al.* 2011) This is achieved through the use of barrier materials (e.g., membranes) that are used to exclude gingival epithelium from the root surface and provide physical space for the in growth of the desired tissue. (Thomas *et al.* 2011) Thus, it is allowed that the space maintained by barrier membranes is filled by new bone. (Hämmerle *et al.* 2002). Through selecting the type of cells that will repopulate the wound we aim to allow periodontal ligament cells to regenerate the lost tissue, inhibiting the early migration of epithelial cells. (Lindhe *et al.* 2005, Thomas *et al.* 2011)

Although, bone regeneration using the membrane barrier is normally achieved successfully in clinical practice, many problems remain and must be studied and solved to increase the success rate. (Hämmerle *et al.* 2002)

These treatments may fail because of shortcomings in surgical techniques, restriction in the size and shape of the defect, anatomical features that may interfere with surgery or infectious complications. (Nowzari *et al.* 1995) Problems encountered more frequently include partial or total collapse of the membrane, soft tissue dehiscence with concomitant exposure of the membrane, resulting in infection of the site and incomplete regeneration. (Hämmerle *et al.* 2002)

In order to overcome these difficulties, which usually result in unsatisfactory clinical results, several attempts were made to improve the materials and surgical techniques. It is evident that it is fundamental to improve the knowledge of the biological mechanisms and temporal dynamics of new bone formation under the conditions of the guided regeneration. Researchers and clinicians consider this knowledge as a requirement to better understand the steps of wound healing, leading to a mature and fully regenerated bone and to be able to positively influence the healing process and thus increasing the predictability of clinical outcomes. (Hämmerle *et al.* 2002)

Undoubtedly, premature membrane exposure is common in GTR procedures and results in microbial colonization of the membrane, in a way that leads to the establishment of periodontal infections. These membrane barriers may serve as substrates for the formation of biofilms. The non-resorbable membranes are rapidly colonized with periodontal microorganisms after surgical placement. Many investigators have reported that such exposure is the main factor for the failure in the healing process of GTR (Sanctis *et al.* 2000, Ricci *et al.* 1996, Thomas *et al.* 2011).

In recent years the role of several risk factors has been analyzed with respect to their influence on the final result of the treatment of bone defects. High plaque and bleeding on probing (HPS) scores, cigarette smoking and lack of compliance, are often associated with clinical attachment loss. (Sanctis *et al.* 2000) Numerous studies have shown the importance of an adequate pre- and postoperative infection control to obtain periodontal regeneration. (Christgau *et al.* 2003, Nowzari & Slots 1995; Slots *et al.* 2000) It is known, that the control of periodontal pathogens in the oral cavity prior to placing of barrier membrane around implants might improve the prognosis of bone regeneration. (Slots & Nowzari 1995) Control of the patient's oral hygiene and residual periodontal infection of the oral cavity are strongly associated with clinical outcomes of regenerative techniques and conventional surgical procedures and should receive proper attention. (Tonitti *et al.* 1996)

Although it is desirable to regenerate lost tissue, the oral cavity is a challenging environment that is colonized by an impressive variety of microorganisms, many of which can colonize the materials often used in regenerative procedures. (Thomas *et al.* 2011)

The subgingival insertion of the barrier membrane in a potentially highly infected environment as well as the relatively open periodontal wound healing situation facilitate the bacterial contamination of these foreign bodies. (Christgau *et al.* 2003, Sanctis *et al.*, 1996a, Ricci *et al.* 1996) An important role in this process is performed by *Porphyromonas gingivalis*. (Ricci *et al.* 1996)

One of the disadvantages associated with the use of membranes is their premature clinically exposure with consequent bacterial contamination through plaque colonization. (Simion *et al.* 1994, Sanctis *et al.* 1996a) In fact, there is an inverse proportional relationship between the extent barrier membrane bacterial contamination and the gain in clinic attachment. (Christgau *et al.* 2003, Sanctis *et al.* 2000, Nowzari & Slots 1995) Studies have shown that bacterial colonization in the mid part of the membrane reduces by 50% the potential gain in probing attachment following GTR-therapy. (De Sanctis *et al.* 1996b)

4 GENE POLYMORPHIMS OF IL-1

It is known that the course and extent of the host response are influenced by genetic factors. (Christgau *et al.* 2003) However, relatively little is known about the impact of genetic factors on the wound healing process. (Christgau *et al.* 2003) Most genetic research in oral disease has focused on gene polymorphisms that play a role in immune responses, specifically in tissue destructive process or its metabolic mechanism. (Vaz *et al.* 2012)

With the discovery of a specific genetic marker for susceptibility to periodontitis and the availability of a laboratory test for diagnosis and prognosis of periodontal or peri-implant tissue destruction now becomes possible to assess the patient's genetic risk. (Sanctis *et al.* 2000, Vaz *et al.* 2012) While, there is a growing body of evidence demonstrating that family history has an impact on disease susceptibility, only recently has a specific genetic marker for identifying an individual's predisposition to develop periodontitis been reported. (Sanctis *et al.* 2000) In this context, knowledge of the human genome associated with numerous studies of genetic polymorphisms combined with many diseases has demonstrated the existence of a genetic basis for most of them. (Kinane *et al.* 2003) In some situations, genetic polymorphisms cause an alteration in the protein or its expression, causing effects on the phenotype of the individual conferring thus susceptibility to developing certain diseases. (Vaz *et al.* 2012, Greenstein *et al.* 2002) Moreover, genetic polymorphisms may also act like a protector or a destructive factor for a disease. (Vaz *et al.* 2012) Precisely, many forms of genes and allelic variations can produce variations in tissue structure, the adaptive immune response and expression of inflammatory mediators. (Vaz *et al.* 2012, Kinane *et al.* 2003) While the effect of allelic variation may have some clinical significance, the other is probably less or no significance. (Kinane *et al.* 2003)

There are currently three known regulatory genes productions of IL-1. *IL1A* and *IL1B* genes produce IL-1α and IL-1β, respectively. The third gene, *IL1RN*, encodes a protein called receiver antagonist of IL-1 (IL-1ra). These genes (*IL1A*, *IL1B* and *IL1RN*) are close together and located on the long arm of chromosome 2 (2q13-q21). (Sanctis *et al.* 2000, Vaz *et al.* 2012, Nicklin *et al.* 1994, Montes et al. 2009, Cafesse *et al.* 2002, Armitage *et al.* 2000) *IL1A, IL1B* and *IL1RN* genes are potential candidates as genetic markers for inflammatory conditions, including periodontitis and peri-implantitis. (Moreira *et al.* 2005, Laine *et al.* 2006, Montes *et al.* 2009)

Effectively, there are polymorphisms in the set of genes that regulate the production of IL-1 (Kornman *et al.* 1998, Montes *et al.* 2009). The polymorphisms are alterations in the gene sequence which generate variants, designated by alleles, the frequency of which the most common is less than 99%. At position −889 of the promoter of the *IL1A* gene was described a polymorphism characterized by the switch of a cytosine base (C) by a thymine (T), yielding two possible alleles: the C allele (allele 1) and T allele (allele 2). (McDowell *et al.* 1995; Montes CC *et al.* 2009).

Studies have shown that patients with the T allele at position −889 of the *IL1A* gene could produce higher levels of IL-1α protein. (Shirodoria *et al.* 2000, Montes *et al.* 2009). At position −511 of the promoter and at position +3954 of *IL1B* exon 5 of the gene were also described bi-allelic polymorphisms, characterized by substitution of a C for a base T. The T alleles of the two polymorphisms were associated with an increased production of IL-1β protein. (Pociot *et al.* 1992, Montes *et al.* 2009) Therefore, it was noted that two of these polymorphisms (the T allele of the gene-889 *IL1A* and *IL1B* gene T allele +3954), when together, are associated with the presence of severe periodontitis in non-smoking adults (Kornman *et al.* 1998, Montes *et al.* 2009). Subsequently, it was demonstrated linkage disequilibrium between these polymorphic loci. (Asano *et al.* 1976, Gore *et al.* 1998, Montes *et al.* 2009) Patients with this haplotype – allelic composition with both T polymorphisms – were called positive genotype. (Kornman *et al.* 1998, Montes *et al.* 2009)

The both polymorphisms, in the gene of IL-1α (at position – 889) and in the gene of IL-1β (at position +3953) [corresponding to the same reference the position +3954, due solely to a change in nomenclature] appears to be associated with a almost 7 times higher risk for developing chronic adult periodontitis in non-smoking patients of Caucasian origin. (Kornman *et al.* 1998; Kornman *et al.* 2000)

In vitro studies, monocytes from patients with polymorphism in the IL-1 gene, secrete 2 to 4 fold more IL-1β in response to bacterial lipopolysaccharide (LPS) than patients without this polymorphism. (Christgau *et al.* 2003, Sanctis *et al.* 2000, Montes *et al.* 2009, Kornman *et al.* 1998)

The presence polymorphism in the gene IL1B (C +3954 T-presence of Thymine at position 3953) has been implicated in the risk and severity of many immune-inflammatory disease (Takamatsu *et al.* 2000, Karjalainem *et al.* 2002, Montes *et al.* 2009), including periodontitis. (Rogers *et al.* 2002)

Specific IL-1 gene polymorphisms seems to be associated with increased susceptibility to severe periodontitis, increased inflammation and increased likelihood of tooth loss during the maintenance phase after conventional periodontal treatment. (Sanctis *et al.* 2000) Such a situation occurred because periodontitis is a disease caused by bacterial biofilms (dental plaque), which progressively destroys the periodontal tissue supporting the teeth. (Murakami *et al.* 2007)

According to existing knowledge, a limited result of regeneration would be expected on IL-1 genotype positive patients, due to an increased secretion of IL-1 in response to bacterial challenge. (Christgau *et al.* 2003) IL-1 also has significant effects on bone tissue. (Masada *et al.* 1990, Tatakis *et al.* 1993, Montes *et al.* 2009) In vitro and in vivo studies demonstrated the inhibition of bone formation by IL-1 and the important role of IL-1 in periodontal bone destruction. (Meikle *et al.* 1990, Montes *et al.* 2009, Christgau *et al.* 2003) Osteoblasts have surface receptors for IL-1 that, when activated, stimulate the production of prostaglandins and their own IL-1, and modulate gene expression of several other cytokines. Thus, it was suggested that IL-1 participate in the pathogenesis of diseases involving bone tissue. (Masada *et al.* 1990, Tatakis *et al.* 1993, Montes *et al.* 2009)

Elevated levels of IL-1 in gingival fluid of periodontitis patients, suggests that local production of interleukin contribute to the destruction of periodontal tissues. (Masada *et al.* 1990, Montes *et al.* 2009, Vaz *et al.* 2012)

5 DISCUSSION

According to existing knowledge, it can be hypothetically assumed that IL-1 genotype positive patients respond with an increased proinflammatory reaction to bacterial contamination of GTR membranes. (Christgau et al. 2003)

In fact, in the presented case the bacteria contamination, associated with the positive genotype of Il-1 polymorphisms, seemed to be the basis of the recurrent failure of the GTR procedures. The SEM images showed that the biomaterial of the GTR was covered with a very complex structure of microorganisms, which could include both bacteria and yeast (frequent colonizers of the oral cavity). Moreover surrounding those microbial cells it was very clear a viscous layer, which might be an exopolymeric matrix that is often produced be microorganism within biofilms (heterogeneous communities of microbial cells embedded in a polymeric matrix, that confers them high resistance) (Fig. 2 and 4). EDS analysis confirmed (by the high amount of Carbon and Oxygen) that the material present in the sample was organic matter (Fig. 3).

Since IL-1 is an important component of periodontal tissue homeostasis, it is logical to consider that individuals with a predisposition to excessive production of IL-1, due to this genotype, would respond differently to regenerative periodontal therapy. (Weiss *et al.* 2004) In the study of Weiss *et al.* 2004, there was no evidence that IL-1 polymorphism influenced the treatment outcome of GTR therapy with bone replacement grafts, as evaluated by probing depth and the level of clinical adhesion (CAL). However, it should be well-known that the study sample (44 patients) was too small to test for significant differences between positive and negative genotype. (Weiss *et al.* 2004)

The only study that found such an influence was the Sanctis & Zucchelli 2000 study, in which patients were evaluated 4 years after GTR therapy. (Weiss *et al.* 2004) This study demonstrated that the expression of positive genotype had no influence on the clinical and radiographic regeneration results following GTR therapy in the first year (Christgau *et al.* 2003, Sanctis *et al.* 2000, Weiss *et al.* 2004), but had a great impact on long-term stability (four years). (Sanctis *et al.* 2000) In a 3-year period, patients with positive genotype IL-1 lost about 50% of the clinical adhesion level acquired in the first year when compared to patients with negative genotype. (Sanctis *et al.* 2000) This high-risk group (IL-1 genotype-positive) showed a 10-time more probability of losing $\geq$2 mm CAL between the first year and the fourth year after GTR-therapy. (Sanctis *et al.* 2000) The prevalence of this polymorphism is about 30% on the north Europe population. Few studies have investigated the possible influence of this IL-1 gene polymorphism on the outcome of different methods of periodontal therapy. (Christgau *et al.* 2003, Sanctis *et al.* 2000, Vaz *et al.* 2012) In the Portuguese Caucasian population with dental implants, the estimated prevalence of polymorphisms in the −889 position of *IL1A* gene and +3953 position of *IL1B* gene was 33.5%, with an estimated error of about 7%. (Vaz *et al.* 2012)

In Spain, a study of these polymorphisms revealed a prevalence value of 43% in a population control of patients consulting a private clinic of periodontics. (Arregui *et al.* 2000, Vaz *et al.* 2012) Another similar study, in a Hispanic population (Mexicans) of a private clinic patients, with unknown periodontal status at the recruitment, presented values of 26% prevalence of IL-1positive genotype. (Caffesse *et al.* 2002, Vaz *et al.* 2012) The variability in the results of different studies on the same genetic polymorphisms analysis does not necessarily represent a controversy. Genetic associations can have a different strength based on distinct populations and in different settings. (Vaz *et al.* 2012)

6 CONCLUSIONS

Surgical techniques based on the principles of GTR are an effective treatment to solve intrabony defects. The host response seems to be determinant in tissue destruction and may affect tissue regeneration and promote undesirable bone loss. In this context, pro-inflammatory mediators play a crucial role. Polymorphisms in genes encoding inflammatory cytokines may change its expression rate, increasing its share. The increase of proinflammatory cytokines may indicate a susceptibility to complications in GTR surgery. The analysis of levels of interleukins through genetic markers allows us to detect individuals who produce more inflammatory cytokines. Therefore, as clinicians, we should concentrate our efforts on controlling these variables that influence the response to GTR treatment, as well as the maintenance of the results. However, this hypothesis is not yet fully clarified and there are some doubts, so it is urgent that further clinical studies are developed in order to clarify and assist the dentist in treatment planning such cases.

REFERENCES

Armitage, G.C. 2000. Low prevalence of a periodontitis-associated interleukin-1 composite genotype in individuals of Chinese heritage. J Periodontol 71: 164–171.

Arregui, I. 2000. IL-1 genotype distribution in a periodontally diseased population in Spain. J Clin Periodontol 27 (Suppl. 1): 86.

Asano, S. & Magari, S. 1976. Electron microscopic studies on the development of the post-capillary venules in the rabbit lymph nodes. Kaibogaku Zasshi 51: 426–439.

Caffesse, R.G. 2002. Prevalence of interleukin1 periodontal genotype in a Hispanic dental population. Quintessence Int 33:190–194.

Christgau, M. 2003. Influence of interleukin-1 gene polymorphism on periodontal regeneration in intrabony defects. J Periodontal Res 38:20–27.

Cortellini, P. 2000. Focus on intrabony defects: guided tissue regeneration. Periodontol 2000 22:104–132.

Gore, E.A. 1998. Interleukin1beta+3953 allele 2: association with disease status in adult periodontitis. J Clin Periodontol 25:781–785.

Greendtein, G. 2002. A critical assessment of interleukin-1 (IL-1) genotyping when used in a genetic susceptibility test for severe chronic periodontitis. J. Periodontol 73:231–47.

Hamilton, D.W. 2010. Migration of periodontal ligament fibroblasts on nanometric topographical patterns: influence of filopodia and focal adhesions on contact guidance. PLoS One 1;5(12):e15129.

Hämmerle, C.G. 2002. A systematic review of the survival of implants in bone sites augmented with barrier membranes (guided bone regeneration) in partially edentulous patients. J Clin Periodontol 29:226–231.

Karjalainen, J. 2002. The IL-1beta genotype carries asthma susceptibility only in men. J Allergy Clin Immunol 109: 514–516.

Kinane, D.F. 2003. Genes and gene polymorphisms associated with periodontal disease. Crit Rev Oral Biol Med 14(6):430–49.

Kornman, K.S.1998. F.S. Genetic variations in cytokine expression: a risk factor for severity of adult periodontitis. Ann Periodontol 3:327–338.

Kornman, K.S. 2000. Fundamental principles affecting the outcomes of therapy for osseous lesions. Periodontol 2000 22:22–43.

Laine, M.L. 2006. IL-1RN gene polymorphism is associated with peri-implantitis. Clin Oral Implants Res 17:380–385.

Lindhe, J. 2005. Tratado de periodontia clínica e implantologia oral. 4ª ed. Rio de Janeiro: Guanabara Koogan.

Masada, M.P. 1990. Measurement of interleukin-1 alpha and -1 beta in gingival crevicular fluid: implications for the pathogenesis of periodontal disease. J Periodontal Res 25:156–163.

McDowell, T.L. 1995. A genetic association between juvenile rheumatoid arthritis and a novel interleukin-1 alpha polymorphism. Arthritis Rheum 38: 221–228.

Meikle, M.C. 1990. Interleukins and their relevance to the pathogenesis of periodontal disease. J Parodontol 9: 103–115.

Montes, C.C. 2009. Analysis of the association of IL1B (C+3954T) and IL1RN (Intron 2) polymorphisms with os-seointegrated implant loss in a Brazilian population. Clin Oral Implants Res 20(2):208–17.

Moreira, P.R. 2005. A functional interleukin-1 beta gene polymorphism is associated with chronic periodontitis in a sample of Brazilian individuals. J Periodontal Res 40:306–311.

Murakami, S. 2007. Periodontal regeneration by FGF2, Clin Calcium 17(2):249–255.

Needleman, I.G. 2006. Guided tissue regeneration for periodontal infrabony defects. Cochrane Database Syst Ver 2:CD001724.

Nicklin, M.J. 1994. A physical map of the region encompassing the human interleukin-1 alpha, interleukin-1 beta, and interleukin-1 receptor antagonist genes. Genomics 19: 382–384.

Nowzari, H. 1995. The importance of periodontal pathogens in guided periodontal tissue regeneration and guided bone regeneration. Compend Contin Educ Dent 16(10): 1042–1058.

Nowzari, H.1995. Microbiologic and clinical study of polytetrafluoroethylene membranes for guided bone regeneration around implants. Int J Oral Maxillofac Implants 10(1):67–73.

Nyman, S. 1982. New attachment following surgical treatment of human periodontal disease. J Clin Periodontol 9:290–296.

Pociot, F. 1992. A TaqI polymorphism in the human interleukin-1 beta (IL-1 beta) gene correlates with IL-1 beta secretion in vitro. Eur J Clin Invest 22: 396–402.

Ricci, G. 1996. In vitro permeability evaluation and colonization of membranes for periodontal regeneration by Porphy-romonas gingivalis. J Periodontol 67(5):490–496.

Rogers, M.A. 2002. Do interleukin-1 polymorphisms predict the development of periodontitis or the success of dental implants?. J Periodontal Res 37: 37–41.
Sanctis, M. 1996a. Bacterial colonization of barrier material and periodontal regeneration. J Clin Periodontol 23(11):1039–46.
Sanctis M. 1996b. Bacterial colonization of bioabsorbable barrier material and periodontal regeneration. J Periodontol 67(11):1193–200.
Sanctis M. 2000. Interleukin-1 Gene Polymorphisms and Long-Term Stability Following Guided Tissue Regeneration Therapy. J Periodontol 71(4): 606–613.
Shirodaria, S. 2000. Polymorphisms in the IL-1A gene are correlated with levels of interleukin-1alpha protein in gingival crevicular fluid of teeth with severe periodontal disease. J Dent Res 79: 1864–1869.
Simion, M. 1994. A preliminary report on a method for studying the permeability of expanded polytetrafluoroethylene membrane to bacteria in vitro: a scanning electron microscopic and histological study. J Periodontol 65(8):755–61.
Slots, J. 1999. Infectious aspects of periodontal regeneration. Periodontol 200019:164–172.
Takamatsu, M. 2000. Genetic polymorphisms of interleukin-1beta in association with the development of alcoholic liver disease in Japanese patients. Am J Gastroenterol 95:1305–1311.
Tatakis, D.N. 1993. Interleukin-1 and bone metabolism: a review. J Periodontol 64: 416–431.
Thomas, M.V. 2011. Infection, inflammation, and bone regeneration: a paradoxical relationship. J Dent Res 90(9):1052–61. Epub 2011 Jan 19.
Tonetti, M. 1995. Effect of cigarette smoking on periodontal healing following GTR in infrabony defects. A preliminary retrospective study. J Clin Periodontol 22: 229–234.
Tonetti, M. 1996. Factors affecting the healing response of intrabony defects following guided tissue regeneration and access flap surgery. J Clin Periodontol 23:548–556.
Vaz, P. 2012. IL1 gene polymorphisms and unsuccessful dental implants. Clin Oral Implants Res. 23(12):1404–1413.
Weiss, O.I. 2004. Effect of the interleukin-1 genotype on outcomes of regenerative periodontal therapy with bone replacement grafts. J Periodontology 75:1335–1342.

Biodental Engineering II – Natal Jorge et al (Eds)
© 2014 Taylor & Francis Group, London, ISBN 978-1-138-00131-2

Different methods for composite removal after bracket debonding

F.M. Lourenço
Dentist, Graduated from Faculty of Dental Medicine, University of Oporto

S. Castro, M.J. Ponces & J.D. Lopes
Department of Orthodontics, Faculty of Dental Medicine, University of Oporto

P. Vaz
Department of Medical and Orofacial Genetics, Faculty of Dental Medicine, University of Oporto

L. Rocha
Department of Mechanical Engineering, University of Minho

ABSTRACT: In contemporary orthodontics, simplification of the methodology has been one of the primary objectives, in order to decrease the treatment time, without neglecting the conditions of functional balance and aesthetic. This paper presents methods for removal of the composite remaining after debonding of orthodontic *brackets*, with the aim of obtaining a smooth surface and as close as possible to the conditions presented pre-treatment. The sample comprised 30 human premolars in which we used three different methods for composite removal. The results were analyzed using the SPSS® program. Evaluating the differences between the 1st and 2nd moment of the evaluation of the three methods we found that no statistically significant differences between them ($P > 0.05$).

1 INTRODUCTION

There has been a simplification of contemporary orthodontics methodology in order to decrease treatment time without neglecting functional balance and aesthetics (Buonocore 1995, Newman 1965).

Direct bonding of brackets to the enamel surface became possible after Buonocore (1955) studies. This researcher showed that enamel conditioning with phosphoric acid solution, as a mechanical union method, promoted a significantly stronger bond between enamel and restorative material surfaces (Buonocore 1995). Afterwards, Newman (1965) introduced this adhesive technique in orthodontics. Therefore, enamel conditioning promotes a more efficient mechanical bonding of brackets, contributing not only to an improvement in the settlement of orthodontic appliances but also adding numerous advantages as superior aesthetics, less discomfort, technical simplicity, greater precision in positioning brackets, better hygiene, less risk of caries and minor periodontal problems (Newman 1965).

With the development of materials and the improvement of techniques, collages were no longer a technical barrier. However, the possibility of damages on the enamel surface caused by resin waste removal is still a problem, as it can affect the outer layer of enamel which, in normal conditions, has a high resistance to the establishment of dental caries lesions (Bishara 2007, Brosh 2005, Campbell 1995, Katona 1997).

There are still some doubts concerning the best method for braces and composite removal (Brosh 2005, Campbell 1995, Katona 1997). There are several factors that can affect the process of bracket removal, being the most important the type of tools and methodology used to eliminate the remaining composite (Dagriff 1979, Rouleau 1982). When a bracket is removed, the rupture may occur at different levels: at the interface bracket/adhesive (adhesive), at the interface adhesive/enamel (adhesive), at the adhesive layer (cohesive) or it may be mixed (adhesive, cohesive) (Bishara 2007). When the interface between adhesive and enamel is broken, there is a greater risk of enamel fragments being removed along with the base of the brackets (Stratmann 1996, Naini 2008, van Waes 1997, Schuler 2006). Therefore, the orthodontist should consider the use of techniques that render the detachment interface bracket/adhesive easier and simultaneously prevent enamel structure damage.

The search for a safe and effective method for composite remnants removal resulted in the introduction of a wide range of instruments and procedures (Boyer 1995, Eliades 2004, Ulusoy 2009, Miksic 2003, Albuquerque 2010, Chen 2008, Hong 1995, Roush 1997, Watanabea 2003). Some clinicians prefer the conventional diamond drills. It is important to note that, despite the careful cutting removal, the sharp and powerful drill tips can scratch the enamel (Retiel 1979, Zarrinnia 1995). Eliades (2004) reported that conventional finishing diamond burs should not be used for composite removal, because they cause deep grooves on the enamel surface (Eliades 2004).

Other methods, which have proved to be more effective, include manual removal using pliers or a wire band, different forms of tungsten carbide burs, low or high rotation handpiece and Sof-Lex® (3M Brasil) (Campbell 1995, Eminkahyagil 2006). New approaches involving the application of carbon dioxide laser seem to represent a promising alternative, while Nd: YAG laser® (DMT Italy) has demonstrated a high potential for structural resin composite degradation (Obata 1999). Therefore, it has been suggested the use of laser technology as a complement for residual composite removal (Hayakawa 2005, Thomas 19996). Along with the introduction of new methods, conventional instruments have been improved leading to new bur designs. These were specially conceived for composite removal after previous debonding, which result in a less aggressive effect to the enamel (Karan 2010). All the reported techniques produce various degrees of enamel surface roughness. Some of them are so abrasive that produce a significant loss of enamel tissue. The methods for composite removal can also have harmful effects on pulp, if the cooling is not appropriate (Watanabea 2003).

Hence, bracket debonding and improper finishing and polishing at the end of treatment can potentially cause iatrogenic damage to enamel (Eliades 2004), such as excessive accumulation of plaque, gingival irritation and stained enamel (Joo 2011).

The primary goal of this study was to assess the in vitro changes on enamel surface roughness after using different techniques for composite removal post bracket debonding. Another purpose of the study was the finding of the method that produces minor changes on the enamel surface and that it allows it to keep pre-treatment conditions.

The assessed composite removal methods were the pliers, the carbamide drill (8 blades) with inactive tip and the latest method – the Nd: YAG laser (LaserMaq®).

2 MATERIALS AND METHODS

The sample of this study comprised 30 recently extracted human premolars. The teeth were collected and stored till further use in distilled water at room temperature. Before being used, the teeth were cleaned and polished with prophylactic paste.

After this preparation the next step was the settlement of brackets on the teeth labial surface. The protocol included etching with ortophosphoric acid gem 37% (Ormco®, France) during 30 seconds, washing with water, drying and an applying of composite. The adhesive Enlight® (Ormco®, France) and the composite Orthosolo (Ormco®, France) were selected and used according to the manufacturer's recommendations.

After fixing the brackets, the teeth were stored in water at 37°C for a 24 hour period. After the storage period, we removed the brackets with pliers.

Then, the teeth were randomly divided into 3 groups ($n = 10$), each group relating to a different method for composite removal.

In group 1, the plier was the method used for composite removal (Ormco®, France). One tip of the plier was supported on the occlusal surface, while the other edge scraped the remaining resin, detaching it from enamel.

In group 2, a tungsten carbide drill with 8 blades (H22ALGK, Komet, Germany) was used for the composite removal. Its action was based on the application of light pressure with mesiodistal movements during 10 seconds. The drills were replaced every 5 uses.

In group 3, it was used a drill plus the Nd: YAG laser DM200® PLUS (DMT, dental Medical Technologies, Italy) application in the resin removal. Firstly, the exceeding resin was removed with the same type of drill used in group 2, leaving only a thin resin layer on the enamel surface. Then, this layer was removed by laser, using 100 Hz for 3 periods of 3 seconds. The neodymium YAG laser (Nd: YAG) offers predefined programs with specificities for different areas in dentistry. The power and frequency are adjustable directly in the equipment: the average power of the pulse varies from 0.5 to 10 watts and frequency of 5 Hz to 200 Hz (with steps of 1 Hz). The optical fibers may be 320–200 microns with a wavelength of 1064 nm. The operation is performed in pulsed mode, with pulse duration variable 50/500 microseconds.

After the removal of composite by different procedures, a new polishing was carried out with prophylactic paste and rubber cup (changed every five procedures).

The surface roughness was analyzed with a rugosimeter (Mahr Perthen, USA) in two stages – before the bracket bonding and after polishing.

3 RESULTS AND DISCUSSION

Since there was a small sample that did not follow a normal distribution, as evidenced by the histograms and box-plots, the differences between initial and final roughness of the various groups were evaluated by the Wilcoxon test.

The hypotheses equated for search in this study were:

- Null hypothesis: there are no statistically significant differences between the two measurements;
- Alternative hypothesis: there are statistically significant differences between the two measurements.

Table 1. Wilcoxon test with 95% confidence[b].

	Pliers_final – Pliers_initial	Drill_final – Drill_initial	Laser_final – Laser_initial
Z	−0,357[a]	−1,682[a]	−1,304[a]
Asymp. Sig. (2-tailed)	0,721	0,093	0,192

a. Based on positive ranks.
b. Wilcoxon signed rank test.
Asymp Sig (2-tailed) – 2 tailed significance

Table 2. Kruskal Wallis test[a,b].

	Diference
Chi-square	0,502
df	2
Asymp. Sig.	0,778

a. Kruskal Wallis test
b. Agroupment variable: Method
df – Degree of freedom
Asymp Sig – Significance

In table 1 it can be seen that there are no statistically significant differences between the 1st and the 2nd moment of evaluation of the procedures, since p-value > 0.05 for all methods.

Concerning the comparison of differences between initial and final roughness on the different procedures the following hypotheses were developed:

- Null hypothesis: there are no statistically significant differences among the three procedures;
- Alternative hypothesis: there are statistically significant differences among the three procedures.

Through observation of Table 2 it can be seen that there are no statistically significant differences among the three procedures, since p-value > 0.05.

However, the differences in roughness produced by the drill and laser were lower than with the use of pliers. The drill and the laser became, thus, more effective procedures than the pliers.

The development of biomaterials for dental use, particularly composite resin and adhesive systems, led to a more effective adhesion between enamel and resin, reducing the rate of interface bracket enamel link fracture during orthodontic treatment. Yet, due to the higher adhesion to enamel, the removal of remnant resin after the bracket debonding became more difficult. Researchers agree that there is a loss of tooth structure after composite removal; however, it is not clinically significant (Campbell, 1995, Hong 1995, van Waes 1997). The thickness of enamel was quantified from 2000 μm to 2500 μm. With bonding, debonding and removal of composite resin, approximately 40 μm and 80 μm in tooth enamel is lost (van Waes 1997, Schuler 2003). Several researchers analyzed a wide variety of tools and techniques for composite removal and, even so, there is still no consensus on the best method to measure the damage caused on tooth enamel (Boyer 1995, Eliades 2004, Ulusoy 2009, Miksic 2003, Albuquerque 2010, Chen 2008, Hong 1995, Roush 1997, Watanabea 2003).

A method used in several studies to analyze the enamel surface after composite removal is the surface rugosimetry (Ra) and electron microscopy (Eliades 2004, Albuquerque 2010, Chen 2008, Hong 1995, Roush 1997, Karan 2010).

The tungsten drill used in this study is also considered, according to various studies, the best method for composite removal (Campbell 1995, Eliades 2004, Ulusoy 2009, Miksic 2003, Albuquerque 2010, Retief 1979, Zarrinnia 1995, Karan 2010). The use of the drill, at a high or low speed, is controversial, since the results of the study diverge. It should be noted that the larger the number of the drill blades, the smaller the cutting power and the larger the smoothing/polishing ability. Other important features are the space between the blades and the blade shape. The H22ALGK drill (Komet®, France) used in this study has 8 rounded blades (no bevel) and presents a bigger distance between them, providing thus a greater resistance and polishing ability without damaging the enamel (Ulusoy 2009, Karan 2010).

Another important aspect that should also be considered is that air and water spray were concomitantly used with the high speed rotary instrument. The use of water spray results in a decrease of contrast between the composite and enamel structure, thus affecting the visual perception of the operator during the finishing procedures.

In accordance to literature data, the results of this study suggest that the roughness of the enamel after cleaning with the tungsten drill at high speed was lower than with the other methods, although not statistically significant (p > 0.05).

Hong & Lew did not indicate the use of pliers as a method of removal because they said it did not remove efficiently the remaining composite, causing scratches and depressions in the enamel (Hong 1995). The results obtained are coincident, being the pliers the least effective method, with greater differences between final and initial roughness.

As to the neodymium laser there are few studies related to the composite removal and there are no studies yet that relate the laser with other methods (Hayakawa 2005, Thomas 1996). Thus, there are no comparative methods on this type of procedure. In our study, the laser presented interim results on the surface roughness showing, however, the disadvantage of being more time consuming, once it implied the use of the drill for removing the outermost surface of the remaining resin, leaving only a thin layer in contact with the enamel. Furthermore, the laser presented also a higher overheating and a higher incidence on the discolorations of the enamel surface.

4 CONCLUSIONS

According to the methodology and based on the analysis and discussion of the results it was concluded that:

- Drill and laser presented less final roughness after residual resin removal.
- Pliers showed the worst results, with a higher final enamel surface roughness.

Nevertheless, no statistically significant differences were found among these three methods.

Further studies are needed to clarify the remaining doubts.

REFERENCES

Albuquerque, G., et al. 2010. Evaluation of enamel roughness after ceramic bracket debonding and clean-up with different methods. *Braz J Oral Sci*. 9(Orthodontics): 4.

Bishara, S.E., et al. 2007. Shear bond strength comparison of two adhesive systems following thermocycling. A new self-etch primer and a resin-modified glass ionomer. *Angle Orthod*, 77(2): 337–41.

Boyer, D.B., et al. 1995. Debonding orthodontic ceramic brackets by ultrasonic instrumentation. *Am J Orthod Dentofacial Orthop*, 108(3): 262–6.

Brosh, T., et al. 2005. In vivo debonding strength and enamel damage in two orthodontic debonding methods. *J Biomech*, 38(5): 1107–13.

Buonocore, M.G. 1955. A simple method of increasing the adhesion of acrylic filling materials to enamel surfaces. *J Dent Res*, 34(6): 849–53.

Campbell, P.M. 1995. Enamel surfaces after orthodontic bracket debonding. *Angle Orthod*, 65(2): 103–10.

Chen, C.S., et al. 2008. Failure analysis: enamel fracture after debonding orthodontic brackets. *Angle Orthod*, 78(6): 1071–7.

Dragiff, D. A. 1979. A new debonding procedure. *J. Clin. Ortho*, 13(2): 107–11.

Eliades, T., et al. 2004. Enamel surface roughness following debonding using two resin grinding methods. *Eur J Orthod*, 26(3): 333–8.

Eminkahyagil, N., et al. 2006 Effect of resin-removal methods on enamel and shear bond strength of rebonded brackets. *Angle Orthod*, 76(2): 314–21.

Hayakawa, K. 2005. Nd: YAG laser for debonding ceramic orthodontic brackets. *Am J Orthod Dentofacial Orthop*, 128(5): 638–47.

Hong, Y.H. & Lew, K.K. 1995. Quantitative and qualitative assessment of enamel surface following five composite removal methods after bracket debonding. *Eur J Orthod*, 17(2): 121–8.

Joo, H.J., et al. 2011. Influence of orthodontic adhesives and clean-up procedures on the stain susceptibility of enamel after debonding. *Angle Orthod*, 81(2): 334–40.

Karan, S., et al. 2010. Enamel surface roughness after debonding. *Angle Orthod*. 80(6): 1081–8.

Katona, T.R. 1997. Stresses developed during clinical debonding of stainless steel orthodontic brackets. *Angle Orthod*, 67(1): 39–46.

Miksic, M. 2003 Stereomicroscope analysis of enamel surface after orthodontic bracket debonding. *Coll Antropol*. 27 Suppl 2: 83–9.

Naini, F.B. & Gill D.S. 2008. Tooth fracture associated with debonding a metal orthodontic bracket: A case report. *World J Orthod*, 9(3): e78–82.

Newman, G.V. 1965. Epoxy adhesives for orthodontic attachments: progress report. *Am J Orthod*, 51(12): 901–12.

Obata, A., et al. 1999. Super pulse CO2 laser for bracket bonding and debonding. *Eur J Orthod*. 21(2): 193–8.

Retief, D.H. & Denys F.R. 1979. Finishing of enamel surfaces after debonding of orthodontic attachments. *Angle Orthod*. 49(1): 1–10.

Rouleau Jr., B.D., et al. 1982. Enamel surface evaluations after clinical treatment and removal of orthodontics brackets. *Am. J. Orthod*., 81: 423–26.

Roush, E.L., et al. 1997. In vitro study assessing enamel surface roughness subsequent to various final finishing procedures after debonding. *Northwest Dent Res*, 7(2): 2–6.

Schuler, F.S., et al. 2003. SEM-evaluation of enamel surfaces after removal of fixed orthodontic appliances. *Am J Dent*, 16(6): 390–4.

Stratmann, U., et al.1996. The extent of enamel surface fractures. A quantitative comparison of thermally debonded ceramic and mechanically debonded metal brackets by energy dispersive micro- and image-analysis. *Eur J Orthod*, 18(6): 655–62.

Thomas, B.W., et al. 1996. Laser-aided degradation of composite resin. *Angle Orthod*, 66(4): 281-6.

Ulusoy, C. 2009. Comparison of finishing and polishing systems for residual resin removal after debonding. *J Appl Oral Sci*, 17(3): 209–15.

van Waes, H., et al. 1997. Three-dimensional measurement of enamel loss caused by bonding and debonding of orthodontic brackets. *Am J Orthod Dentofacial Orthop*. 112(6): 666–9.

Watanabea H., et al. 2003. In vitro and in vivo studies on application of erbium: YAG laser for dentine hypersensitivity. *International Congress Series*, 1248(Periodontology): 3.

Zarrinnia, K., et al. 1995. The effect of different debonding techniques on the enamel surface: an in vitro qualitative study. *Am J Orthod Dentofacial Orthop*, 108(3): 284–93.

Biodental Engineering II – Natal Jorge et al (Eds)
© 2014 Taylor & Francis Group, London, ISBN 978-1-138-00131-2

Modified core design in an all-ceramic CAD-CAM crown – a numerical stress analysis

I. Lopes
Dental Medicine PhD Course, Faculty of Dental Medicine of the University of Porto (FMDUP)

A. Correia
Faculty of Dental Medicine of the University of Porto (FMDUP); Institute of Mechanical Engineering and Industrial Management (INEGI)

J.C. Sampaio
Faculty of Dental Medicine of the University of Porto, Fixed Prosthodontics Department

Z. Kovacs
DentalMaia Dental Lab

N.V. Ramos & M. Vaz
Laboratory of Optics and Experimental Mechanics – Faculty of Engineering of the University of Porto, Portugal; Institute of Mechanical Engineering and Industrial Management (INEGI)

ABSTRACT: The aim of this research was to perform a numerical stress analysis in zirconia framework crown designs virtually inserted in a dental implant. The framework designs were obtained using a CAD-CAM dental system. A 3D geometry .stl file was exported and processed into a numerical model to perform finite elements (FE) simulations. A qualitative stress analysis of the interproximal areas was performed using unitary loads in a vertical and oblique direction. Results of the stress analysis with FEM showed that the highest stresses were obtained in the conventional framework design, decreasing in the other designs, especially in the last one with the rounded cervical-middle projection. Therefore, it seems that the new designs shows improvement in stress distribution in the interproximal areas showing an overall improvement in the final strength of the framework.

1 INTRODUCTION

The use of ceramic materials for frameworks of fixed dental prosthesis has increased considerably in the last decade (Manicone 2007). Although the success in function and aesthetic has been described in the literature, it has also been reported the occurrence of chipping in the ceramic veneer (Bonfante 2009, De Backer 2006 & Tsumita 2008).

In the posterior regions of the oral cavity, the masticatory loads are very high (98-714N with 448N average in men and 357N in women). Due to this load, chipping is relatively frequent, with values of 18% of occurrence, mostly in interproximal areas (Coelho 2009, De Backer 2006 & Tsumita 2008).

These complications in dental prosthetic rehabilitations may be studied through stress analysis techniques (experimental and numerical), commonly used in engineering, that are increasinlgy being used in Dentistry for the past two decades (Correia 2009, Correia 2010, Correia 2012, Imanishi 2003 & Piloto 2009).

The aim of this preliminary research is to analyse the stress distribution in a single dental crown with a different core design.

2 MATERIAL AND METHODS

The CAD-CAM dental system Zirconzahn (Brunneck®, Italy) was used to design three different framework configurations of a single dental crown supported by a dental implant (Figure 1–2).

The idealized designs were created to increase the support area of the veneer ceramic in the interproximal

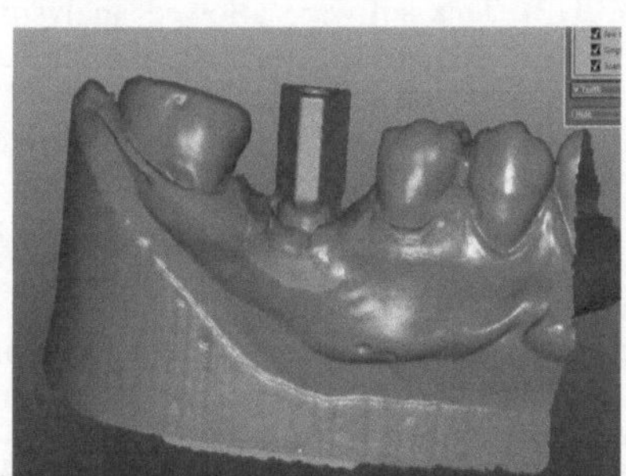

Figure 1. CAD image of the scanned dental model with a scan body element inserted in the dental implant.

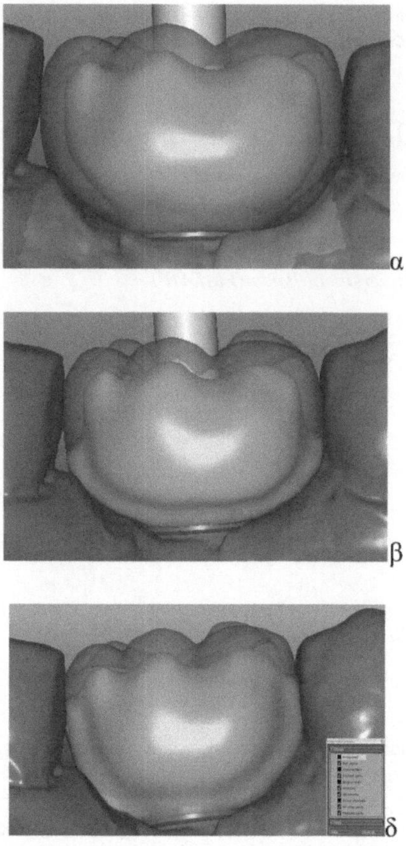

Figure 2. Designs obtained with Zirconzahn® dental system (α) – no interproximal projection; (β) – 1/3 height interproximal projection; (δ) – 2/3 height interproximal projection.

area. This area has been divided in thirds (cervical, middle and occlusal) and three designs were studied: conventional (alfa), 1/3 height projection (beta), and 2/3 height projection of the framework (delta) [5].

The .STL files generated by this system were then exported to Solidworks® (Dassault Systemes S.A, France), a CAD software available in the Laboratory of Optics and Experimental Mechanics (LOME) of the Faculty of Engineering of the University of Porto (FEUP). This software allowed analysing the computer-aided design and correcting some surface geometries as necessary (Figure 3).

Then, this file was exported to Abaqus® (Dassault Systemes S.A, France) to generate a FE mesh in the referred designs. To analyse the stress distribution under different load conditions, the finite element analysis (FEA) was used.

Later on, was decided to create two improved designs based on the three first ones, were identified by $\beta 1$ and $\delta 1$ and differed from the first one by having smoother edges in the interproximal projections. (Figure 4).

This methodology of importing the 3D design file of the CAD-CAM dental system to Solidworks® and

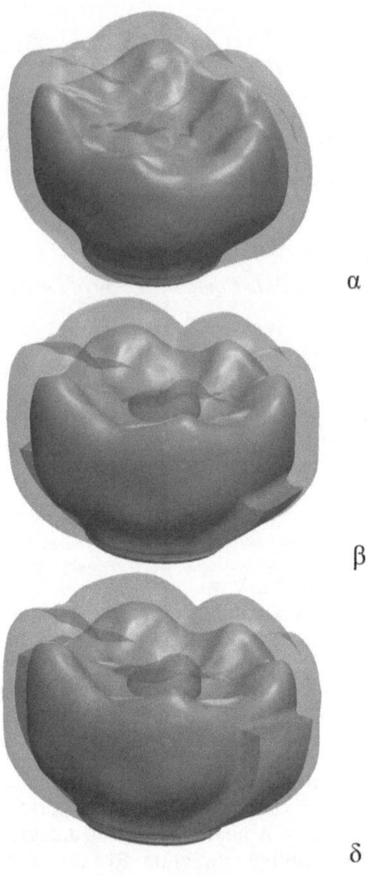

Figure 3. (α) – CAD of a single dental crown with a translucent outer layer of ceramic and an opaque inner layer of zirconia; (β) – CAD 1/3 height interproximal projection; (δ) – CAD 2/3 height interproximal projection.

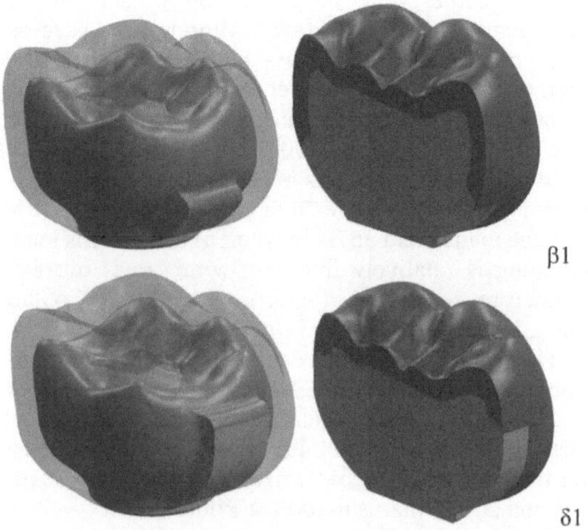

Figure 4. ($\beta 1$) – CAD 1/3 height interproximal projection; ($\delta 1$) – CAD 2/3 height interproximal projection.

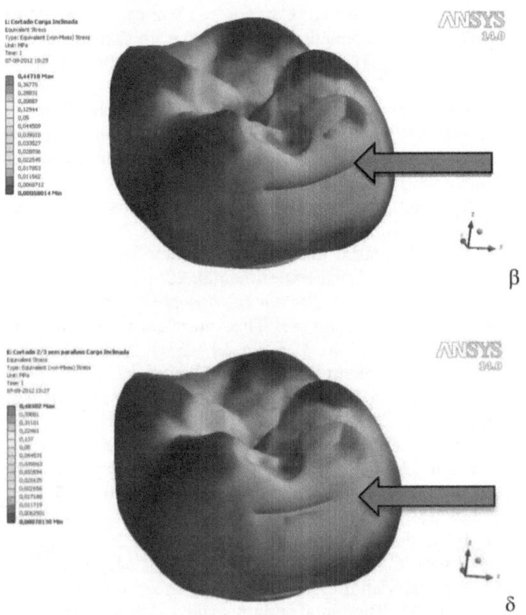

Figure 5. FEA analysis in β and δ design. Higher stresses obtained in the interface ceramic veneer – framework.

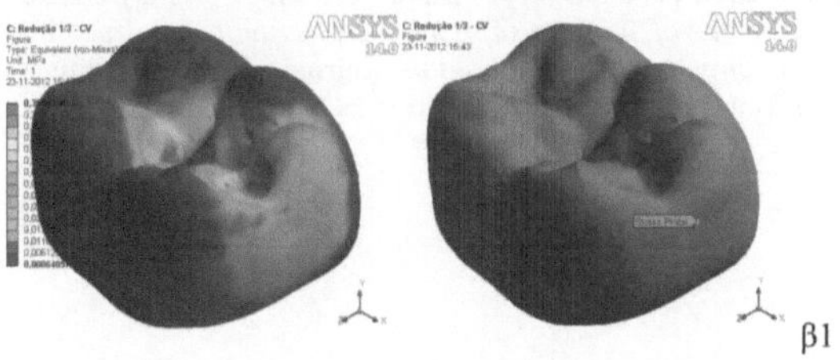

Figure 6. $\beta 1$ FEA analysis. Decreased stresses in the interface ceramic veneer – framework, with vertical loads.

finally to Abaqus®, was adopted from the articles of Correia (2009, 2010 & 2012). Also, the smoother edges were also derived from the researches of this author that introduced fillets (roundings) in the gingival embrasure of fixed partial dentures.

3 RESULTS AND DISCUSSION

Increased stress distribution in the interproximal contact point area was obtained, in the interface between the framework projection and the veneering ceramics, by applying single vertical an oblique loads in the crowns occlusal table.

Although the aim of this research was to optimize the interproximal design to better support occlusal loads, this results proved exactly the opposite.

In the optimized designs (Figure 6–9) decreased stress values were obtained, both in vertical and oblique loads. Stress probe values showed that the smoother round edges create a transition interface between the two ceramic materials. Therefore, the

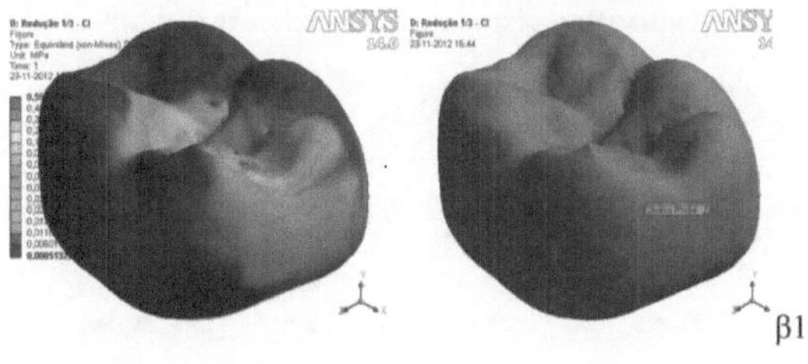

Figure 7. $\beta 1$ FEA analysis. Decreased stresses in the interface ceramic veneer – framework, with oblique loads.

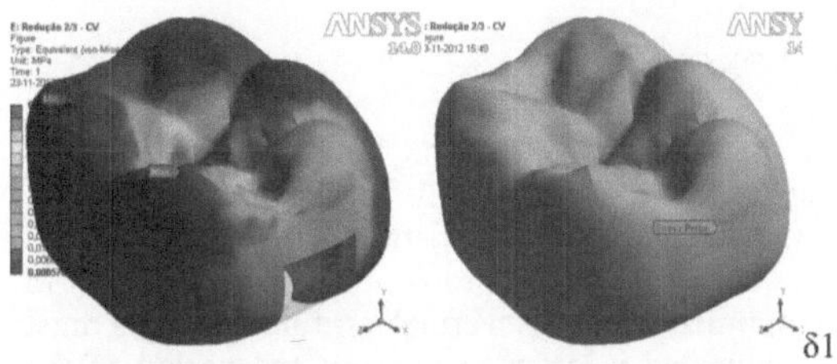

Figure 8. $\delta 1$ FEA analysis. Decreased stresses in the interface ceramic veneer – framework, with vertical loads.

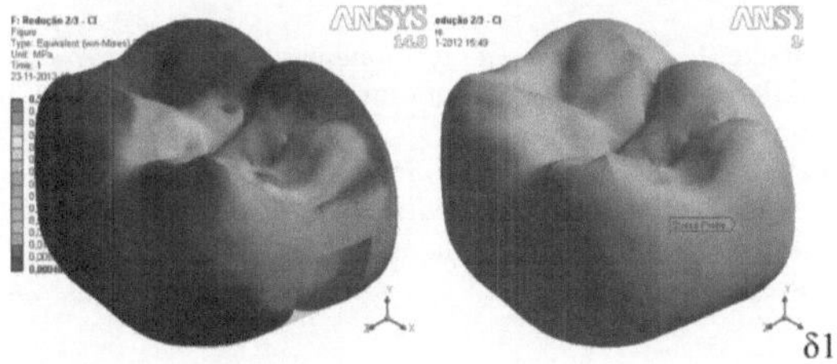

Figure 9. $\delta 1$ FEA. Decreased stresses in the interface ceramic veneer – framework, with oblique loads.

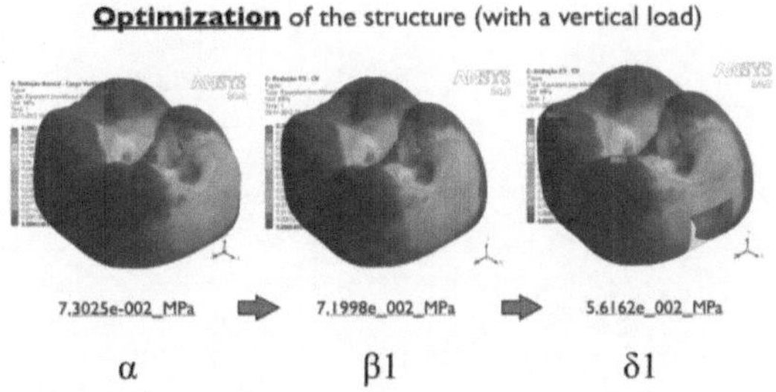

Figure 10. Decreased stresses in the interface ceramic veneer – framework, with vertical loads.

stress distribution in the interproximal contact point have lower values than the previous ones showing that this is the right path way to follow, as can be seen in the images below (Figure 6–9).

The stress distribution decreases from the $\beta 1$ to the $\delta 1$ design suggesting that the best design so far might be last (Figure 10–11).

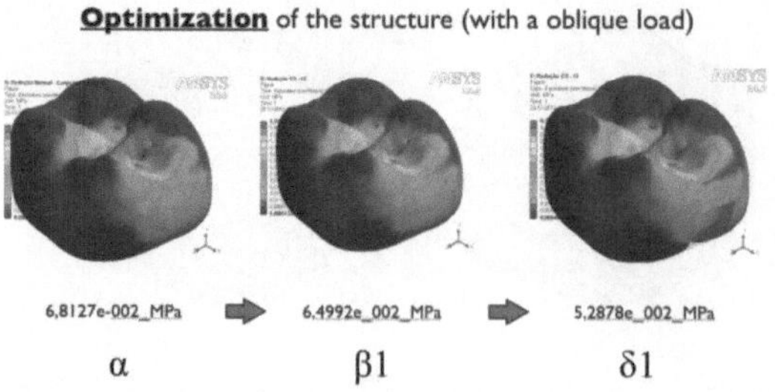

Figure 11. Decreased stresses in the interface ceramic veneer – framework, with oblique loads.

4 CONCLUSIONS

For the present work it can be concluded that the designs tested in this study reveal an optimization of the stress distribution between the two materials that compose a dental crown, from the first ones to the optimized ones. Nevertheless, future studies must be conducted in order to improve the design of the frameworks to better support the veneering ceramic.

REFERENCES

Bonfante, E.A., et al., *Effect of framework design on crown failure.* European journal of oral sciences, 2009. 117(2): p. 194–9.

Coelho, P.G., et al., *Effect of proximal wall height on all-ceramic crown core stress distribution: a finite element analysis study.* The International journal of prosthodontics, 2009. 22(1): p. 78–86.

Correia A., Fernandes JC, Campos JC, Vaz M & Silva JM. 2009. Effect of connector design on the stress distribution of a cantilever fixed partial denture. J Indian Prosthodont Soc, 9: p. 13–7.

Correia A, Sampaio Fernandes JC, Reis Campos JC, Vaz M, Ramos NV & Silva JM. Stress distribution on cantilever dental prostheses. Biodental Engineering. Taylor & Francis; 2010. p. 205–208.

Correia A., Sampaio Fernandes JC, Reis Campos JC, Vaz M, Piloto P & Ramos NV. 2012. Sistemas CAD-CAM em Medicina Dentária: integração com métodos de análises de tensões. Mecânica Experimental, 20: p. 131–34.

De Backer, H., et al., *A 20-year retrospective survival study of fixed partial dentures.* The International journal of prosthodontics, 2006. 19(2): p. 143–53.

Imanishi, A., T. Nakamura, and T. Ohyama, *3-D Finite element analysis of all-ceramic posterior crowns.* Journal of oral rehabilitation, 2003. 30(8): p. 818–22.

Manicone, P.F., P. Rossi Iommetti, and L. Raffaelli, *An overview of zirconia ceramics: basic properties and clinical applications.* Journal of dentistry, 2007. 35(11): p. 819–26.

Piloto P, Alves A, Correia A, Reis Campos JC, Sampaio Fernandes JC, Vaz MAP & Viriato N. 2010. Metal ceramic fixed partial denture – fracture resistance. In Natal Jorge et al. (eds), Biodental Engineering – Proceedings of the I International Conference on Biodental Engineering, Porto, Portugal, 26–27 June 2009: 125–28. Taylor & Francis Group, London, UK.

Tsumita, M., et al., *Effect of framework shape on the fracture strength of implant-supported all-ceramic fixed partial dentures in the molar region.* Journal of prosthodontics: official journal of the American College of Prosthodontists, 2008. 17(4): p. 274–85.

Biodental Engineering II – Natal Jorge et al (Eds)
© 2014 Taylor & Francis Group, London, ISBN 978-1-138-00131-2

New method and software prototype for automatized measurement of crestal bone levels around implants

A. Messias, R. Reis, S. Rocha & P. Nicolau
Department of Dentistry, Faculty of Medicine, University of Coimbra, Portugal

P. Cunha & M. Lopez
Institute of Mechanical Engineering and Industrial Management, Faculty of Engineering, University of Oporto, Portugal

ABSTRACT: Digital radiographic images are currently the most popular method for evaluation of the proximal bone level around implants. **Aim:** This study aimed at both the elaboration of a new automatized method for detecting implant edges and crestal bone line on digital x-ray images based on the suitable combination of pre-processing and image segmentation techniques and the development of a software system prototype named DISIAT (Dental Image System for Implants Analysis and Tracking). **Methods:** two independent examiners using the DISIAT application analyzed sixty standardized digital radiographs of CAMLOG Screw-line implants. The method uses pre-processing tools such as noise suppression filters, histogram thresholding and mathematical morphology for bone line and implant contour determination and subsequent extraction of mesial and distal bone levels measurements. These results were compared with the matching readings from a group of experts (PASW® Statistics 20 – IBM, USA). **Results:** No significant differences were found between the 94 manual measurements and the 94 measurements obtained by either of the two examiners using the DISIAT prototype ($p = 0.802$ for examiner 1 and $p = 0.806$ for examiner 2). The intraclass correlation coefficient (ICC) found for the measurements obtained by the three examiners was 0.839 [0.783–0.884, 95% CI]. The two examiners using DISIAT presented an ICC of 0.880 [0.824–0.918, 95% CI]. **Conclusions:** Automatized image segmentation with determination of implant boundaries and crestal bone line is a promising technique for simple bone level measurement around dental implants. The new proposed method has proven to be a robust tool, as no significant differences were found between the manual measurements and those produced with the DISIAT application. The reliability analysis showed a very good agreement between examiners using the prototype and between the DISIAT measurements and those obtained manually.

1 BACKGROUND

The radiographic analysis is the best non-invasive method for bone level determination proximal to osseointegrated dental implants and is mandatory to ascertain the outcome of both routine practice and clinical trials. (Hermann et al. 2001, De Smet et al. 2002, Hanggi et al. 2005) In 1986, Albretksson et al. proposed criteria for the assessment of the long-term efficacy of implant therapy and established as radiologically acceptable a marginal bone level change inferior to 1.5 mm in the first year, and less than 0.2 mm of continuing annual vertical bone loss. However, the diagnosis of progressive bone loss or the identification of bone gain from one radiographic examination to the next may be difficult to interpret due to confounding issues such as projection errors in the alignment of successive images or the lack of examiner training and measurement calibration on the evaluation of radiographs that generates intra and inter-examiner variability. (Benn 1992, Mol & Dunn 2003, Huh et al. 2005, Lanning et al. 2006, Wakoh et al. 2006, Cochran et al. 2009)

Recently, dedicated imaging software such as ImageJ (http://rsbweb.nih.gov/ij/) or VixWin (Gendex Dental Systems, Hatfield, USA) have been introduced to carry out diverse measurements in radiographs. (Grandi et al. 2012) However, these programs only make use of a simple pixel-counter ruler to measure linear distances between two points identified by the operator, which can arise intra and inter-examiner errors. This is particularly true in conventional periapical radiographs of dental implants where projection errors lead to superimposition of structures and image distortion. The operator can be misguided in the correct identification of the first bone-to-implant contact and other landmarks that correspond to the edge points of the distance to be determined, as the implant shoulder. Image distortion can also induce miscalculations in the calibration procedure, thereby inflating inaccuracies in the measurements obtained.

This paper aims at the description of a graphics user interface developed for simple bone level determination in standardized radiographs of dental implants that includes a new automatized image segmentation method to detect implant edges and crestal bone line, based on thresholding algorithms and on trained active shape models. The paper also intents to determine the reproducibility, reliability and accuracy of the segmentation method and measurements extraction by intra and inter-rater agreement analysis of bone levels around Camlog® Screw-line implants (Basel, Switzerland) using both platform-switching and standard abutments.

2 MATERIALS AND METHODS

2.1 *DISIAT (Dental Image System for Implants Analysis and Tracking)*

A user interface named DISIAT was designed for importing the image files, exploring the segmentation method (image preprocessing plus deformable models application phase) and for automatized extraction of the calculated bone levels into a spreadsheet, from both single or DICOM files.

2.2 *Definition and training of the Active Shape Models (ASM)*

In this case, the ASM models of the left and right implant profiles were built over a representative image of CAMLOG® SCREW-LINE Promote® plus implants, considering specific landmarks for each side. The bone line profile was trained simply by the selection of 5 landmarks.

2.3 *Implant shoulder detection*

The first step required by the user interface DISIAT is the implant shoulder detection, according to the type of platform.

2.4 *Measurement extraction tool*

The bone line segmentation combines the application of noise suppression filters to enhance the intended structures (Guevara et al. 2003) with histogram thresholding and mathematical morphology operations (Cunha et al. 2012), that generate the bone segmentation. Afterwards the user interface recovers the ASM for the bone line and requests the operator to place it close to the respective site. The good fit of the model is achieved through 125 iterations searching for the correct positioning and adaptation in the image. The final result is suitable for operator-driven changes. Implant detection begins with binary thresholding (Glasbey 1993), and a pop-up menu recovers the ASM for the left and right sides of the implant and requests the operator to place them close to the respective site in the segmented image of the implant

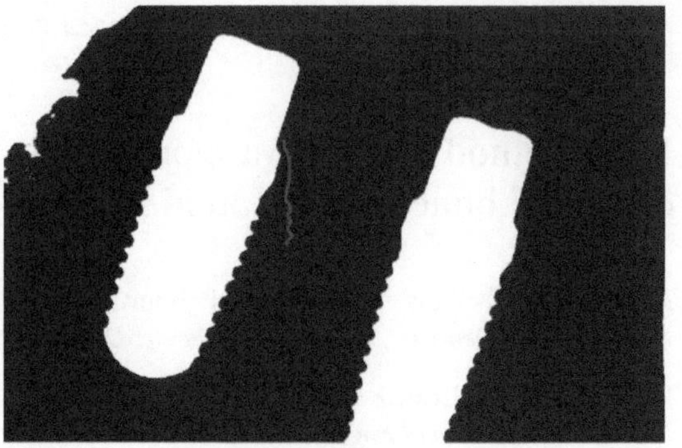

Figure 1. Binary thresholding of the image in order to achieve implant segmentation and right ASM application (blue).

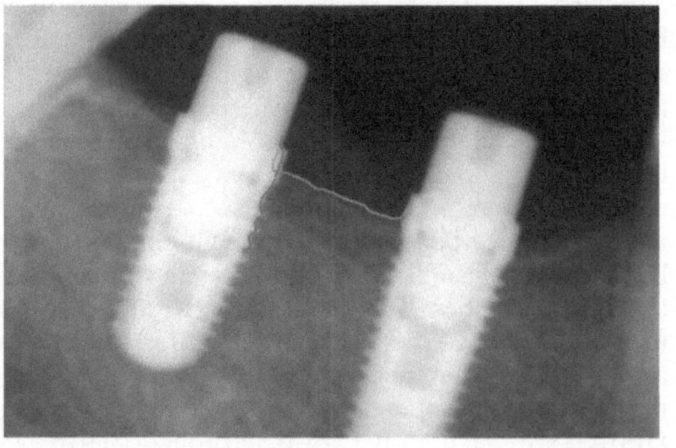

Figure 2. Final segmentation of both the right side of the implant (red) and the bone level (green).

(fig. 1). The following processes run by iteration, as described for the bone line, without the manual adjustment possibility (fig. 2).

2.5 *Bone level extraction*

The bone level is set by the calculation of the distance between the implant shoulder and the first point of implant-to-bone contact, which takes into consideration the implant dimensions. After the intersection point determination, the DISIAT makes the optimization and then the operator selects the export tool in order to send the values determined into a spread sheet where type of appointment, implant positions and side are specified for each radiograph or set of radiographs. Two experts from the Faculty of Medicine of the University of Coimbra trained on implant radiograph analysis executed the bone level extraction process in 60 radiographs of patients enrolled for a RCT to access bone level changes and success rates of CAMLOG® SCREW-LINE Promote® plus implants. Each expert, blinded to the RCT, imported the images, performed the segmentation, applied the ASM and extracted bone level measurements to identified spreadsheets as detailed previously. Procedures were replicated by the examiners to all images.

Data were analysed with PASW® Statistics 20.0 (SPSS Inc., 233 South Wacker Drive, 11th Floor Chicago, IL 60606-6412). Bias of 0.15 mm was determined as the maximum clinically acceptable difference between two radiographic measurements (Cochran et al. 2009). Significance level was set to $\alpha = 0.05$.

3 RESULTS

Ninety-four measurements were obtained by the two examiners using the DISIAT application and considered for comparison with those provided by the professionals involved in the RCT. The results obtained by the first examiner using the DISIAT software are referred as DISIAT 1, the results obtained by the second examiner are referred as DISIAT 2 and the manual measurements obtained by the experts are referred as manual.

Descriptive statistics for the manual, DISIAT 1 and DISIAT 2 measurements are shown in table 1. Presented results are in mm.

The measurements obtained manually and by the two examiners, were considered repeated measures performed on the same subject. Thus, repeated measures ANOVA was conducted testing for null mean differences ($\alpha = 0.05$). The three measurements obtained for each subject were introduced as the within-subject variables and the implant platform as the between-subject variable, since the method used for determination of the implant shoulder differed from platform-switching abutments and standard abutment implants. No differences were found between the three groups as $F(2, 186) = 0.16$, $p = 0.852$. Pairwise comparisons, obtained with the paired samples T-test, are summarized in table 2 ($\alpha = 0.05$).

Reliability analysis of the measurements obtained by the three raters revealed an intraclass correlation coefficient of 0.839 [0.783–0.884, 95% CI] calculated for single measures of the three groups using the absolute agreement definition ($p < 0.01$). The correlation of the measurements obtained by the two examiners using DISIAT was 0.880 [0.824–0.918, 95% CI] ($p < 0.01$). Approximately 60% of the measurements obtained with the DISIAT prototype by either examiner had less than 0.15 mm difference from the manual measurements and were considered perfect hits.

Table 1. Descriptive statistics for the measurements performed manually, with DISIAT 1 and with DISIAT 2.

Group	Mean (mm)	SD (mm)	95% CI (mm)
Manual	0.605	0.491	[0.505–0.706]
DISIAT 1	0.614	0.601	[0.490–0.737]
DISIAT 2	0.596	0.665	[0.459–0.732]

4 DISCUSSION

Peri-implant bone levels are a key factor for the determination of success of implant therapy (Albrektsson et al. 1986, Al-Nsour et al. 2012). However, up to this moment few studies focus on rater agreement, arising the problem of the correctness of the peri-implant bone levels reported (Tonetti & Palmer 2012). Cochran et al. (Cochran et al. 2009) report the marginal bone level error between raters to be 0.193 mm in average. In our study, the mean marginal bone level error of 0.018 mm between examiners using the DISIAT prototype was minute when compared to those values. More, Cochran et al refer small result variability within consecutive readings by presenting 77.5% of values with less than 0.5 mm difference, whereas the overall chance of agreement for the measurements obtained by either examiner using DISIAT for the same limit is superior to 90%. However, when considering 0.15 mm difference for the correct value, the DISIAT chance of agreement decreases to approximately 60%, which is still close to the value reported by Lanning et al for accurate rating of bone loss by trained clinical instructors (Lanning et al. 2006, Cochran et al. 2009).

The measurements discrepant from those obtained manually could be related to the manual identification of the first bone-to-implant contact, which could be underestimated (Eickholz & Hausmann 2000, Hermann et al. 2001, Scaf et al. 2006).

Due to projection errors (Benn 1992, Eickholz & Hausmann 2000) the bone line could have been distorted and consequently the first bone-to-implant contact miscalculated (Schulze & d'Hoedt 2002). Crestal bone line delineation could also be influenced by the densitometry calibration of the image. Brighter images have low contrast and present unbalanced histograms that have an impact on the thresholding and algorithm segmentation method, influencing the bone line positioning and consequently biasing the first bone-to-implant-contact.

Table 2. t-test results for the pairwise comparisons of the three groups. Significance level $\alpha = 0.05$.

Pair	Mean difference	SD	95% CI	Max	*t*	*p*
Manual – DISIAT 1	−0.008	0.32	[−0.07–0.06]	1.30	−0.25	0.80
Manual – DISIAT 2	0.009	0.37	[−0.07–0.09]	1.15	0.25	0.80
DISIAT 1 – DISIAT 2	0.018	0.31	[−0.05–0.08]	1.17	0.56	0.58

5 CONCLUSIONS

Automatized image segmentation with determination of implant boundaries and crestal bone line is a promising technique for simple bone level measurement around dental implants. The new proposed method/prototype has proven to be a robust tool, as no significant differences were found between the manual measurements and those produced with the DISIAT application. The reliability analysis showed a very good agreement between the measurements of different examiners using the prototype and between the DISIAT measurements and those obtained manually.

ACKNOWLEDGMENTS

This study was co-financed by the Foundation for Science and Technology via project PTDC/SAUBEB/108658/2008 and by FEDER via the "Programa Operacional Factores de Competitividade" of QREN with COMPETE reference: FCOMP-01-0124-FEDER-010961.

REFERENCES

Al-Nsour MM, Chan HL and Wang HL (2012). "Effect of the platform-switching technique on preservation of peri-implant marginal bone: a systematic review." *Int J Oral Maxillofac Implants* **27**(1): 138–145.

Albrektsson T, Zarb G, Worthington P and Eriksson AR (1986). "The long-term efficacy of currently used dental implants: a review and proposed criteria of success." *Int J Oral Maxillofac Implants* **1**(1): 11–25.

Benn DK (1992). "Estimating the validity of radiographic measurements of marginal bone height changes around osseointegrated implants." *Implant Dent* **1**(1): 79–83.

Cochran DL, Nummikoski PV, Schoolfield JD, Jones AA and Oates TW (2009). "A prospective multicenter 5-year radiographic evaluation of crestal bone levels over time in 596 dental implants placed in 192 patients." *J Periodontol* **80**(5): 725–733.

Cunha P, Guevara M, Messias A, Rocha S, Reis R and Nicolau PG (2012). "A method for segmentation of dental implants and crestal bone." *International Journal of Computer Assisted Radiology and Surgery*: 1–11.

De Smet E, Jacobs R, Gijbels F and Naert I (2002). "The accuracy and reliability of radiographic methods for the assessment of marginal bone level around oral implants." *Dentomaxillofac Radiol* **31**(3): 176–181.

Eickholz P and Hausmann E (2000). "Accuracy of radiographic assessment of interproximal bone loss in intrabony defects using linear measurements." *Eur J Oral Sci* **108**(1): 70–73.

Glasbey CA (1993). "An analysis of histogram-based thresholding algorithms." *CVGIP: Graphical Models and Image Processing* **55**(6): 532–537.

Grandi T, Garuti G, Guazzi P, Tarabini L and Forabosco A (2012). "Survival and success rates of immediately and early loaded implants: 12-month results from a multicentric randomized clinical study." *J Oral Implantol* **38**(3): 239–249.

Guevara M, Silva A, Oliveira H, de Lourdes Pereira M and Morgado F (2003). "Segmentation and morphometry of histological sections using deformable models: A new tool for evaluating testicular histopathology." *Progress in Pattern Recognition, Speech and Image Analysis*: 282–290.

Hanggi MP, Hanggi DC, Schoolfield JD, Meyer J, Cochran DL and Hermann JS (2005). "Crestal bone changes around titanium implants. Part I: A retrospective radiographic evaluation in humans comparing two non-submerged implant designs with different machined collar lengths." *J Periodontol* **76**(5): 791–802.

Hermann JS, Schoolfield JD, Nummikoski PV, Buser D, Schenk RK and Cochran DL (2001). "Crestal bone changes around titanium implants: a methodologic study comparing linear radiographic with histometric measurements." *Int J Oral Maxillofac Implants* **16**(4): 475–485.

Huh KH, Lee SS, Jeon IS, Yi WJ, Heo MS and Choi SC (2005). "Quantitative analysis of errors in alveolar crest level caused by discrepant projection geometry in digital subtraction radiography: an in vivo study." *Oral Surg Oral Med Oral Pathol Oral Radiol Endod* **100**(6): 750–755.

Lanning SK, Best AM, Temple HJ, Richards PS, Carey A and McCauley LK (2006). "Accuracy and consistency of radiographic interpretation among clinical instructors using two viewing systems." *J Dent Educ* **70**(2): 149–159.

Mol A and Dunn SM (2003). "The performance of projective standardization for digital subtraction radiography." *Oral Surg Oral Med Oral Pathol Oral Radiol Endod* **96**(3): 373–382.

Scaf G, Sakakura CE, Kalil PF, Dearo de Morais JA, Loffredo LC and Wenzel A (2006). "Comparison of simulated periodontal bone defect depth measured in digital radiographs in dedicated and non-dedicated software systems." *Dentomaxillofac Radiol* **35**(6): 422–425.

Schulze RK and d'Hoedt B (2002). "A method to calculate angular disparities between object and receptor in "paralleling technique"." *Dentomaxillofac Radiol* **31**(1): 32–38.

Tonetti M and Palmer R (2012). "Clinical research in implant dentistry: study design, reporting and outcome measurements: consensus report of Working Group 2 of the VIII European Workshop on Periodontology." *J Clin Periodontol* **39 Suppl 12**: 73–80.

Wakoh M, Harada T, Otonari T, Otonari-Yamamoto M, Ohkubo M, Kousuge Y, Kobayashi N, Mizuta S, Kitagawa H and Sano T (2006). "Reliability of linear distance measurement for dental implant length with standardized periapical radiographs." *Bull Tokyo Dent Coll* **47**(3): 105–115.

Biodental Engineering II – Natal Jorge et al (Eds)
© 2014 Taylor & Francis Group, London, ISBN 978-1-138-00131-2

X-ray fluorescence technique to evaluate in vitro the de/remineralization in bovine enamel

F.S. Calazans, R.F. Moreira & M.S. Miranda*
*Universidade do Estado do Rio de Janeiro, Faculdade de Odontologia, Departamento de Dentística, Rio de Janeiro, RJ. Brazil *Coordenador do Doutorado em Odontologia-Dentística*

R.S. Santos & M.J. Anjos
Universidade do Estado do Rio de Janeiro, Instituto de Física, Laboratório de Física Aplicada e Termodinâmica, Rio de Janeiro, RJ. Brazil

J.T. Assis
Universidade do Estado do Rio de Janeiro, Instituto Politécnico, Nova Friburgo, RJ. Brazil

ABSTRACT: The aim of this in vitro study was to evaluate the efficacy of X-Ray fluorescence technique on the measurements of de-remineralization in bovine enamel subject to erosion and treated with three products. We obtained 15 specimens (CP) who were randomly divided into 3 groups. All teeth were initially evaluated to obtain the count of elements phosphorus (P) and calcium (Ca) interpreted from a range of X-Ray Fluorescence obtained by Artax 800. After one week of the initial measurement, each group of samples was immersed in a solution of 10 ml of 2% citric acid (pH 2.6) for 90 minutes. Immediately after obtaining the spectra of teeth subjected to the erosive challenge, each group received their treatment accordingly. Group 1 (Saliva) – saliva, Group 2 (Fluor) – Fluoride and Group 3 (Nano P) – Desensibilize Nano P. Reading and treatments were carried out every seven days and repeated for 3 weeks. It was first used the Bonferroni test for comparison of parametric average loss of P and Cain each stage of treatment in the groups, with a significance level of 0.05 ($p = 0.05$). We used thet Student test for comparison between means of different treatment groups with a significance level of 5% ($p = 0.05$). The Nano P was more effective than all the groups and Saliva less effectiveness than Fluor after three weeks of treatment. It can be concluded that this methodology was effective on the measurement of de-remineralization in bovine enamel subject to erosion and their treatments in correspondence.

1 INTRODUCTION

The quantitative analysis of chemical elements plays an important role in the Biomedical, since these elements may be essential to the physiology of the biological tissue. Several diseases are associated with a deficiency or excess of these elements, interfering with the metabolism of human beings. Elements such as phosphorus (P), sulfur (S), potassium (K), chlorine (Cl), iron (Fe), zinc (Zn), copper (Cu), bromine (Br), manganese (Mn), nickel (Ni), and chromium (Cr) are responsible for biochemical and physiological processes. Furthermore, non-essential elements such as lead (Pb), cadmium (Cd), silver (Ag), etc., even in small concentrations produce toxic effects, which may lead the individual to death (Santos & Anjos, 2009). The X-ray fluorescence (XRF) is a physical phenomenon that occurs in the process of transition electron orbitals. The analysis by X-ray Fluorescence is a non-destructive analytical technique based on the measurement of the intensities (the number of X-rays detected by unit time) of the characteristic X-rays emitted by elements that constitute one sample (Klockenkamper & Bohlen, 1996). The X-ray beam on the sample and focuses on the process of interaction of X-rays with the sample occurs release of electrons bound to the atom, and consequently less bound electrons in the outermost orbitals migrate to these orbitals with "holes" left by electrons that have been released. The result of this process is the release of energy as electromagnetic radiation called characteristic X-rays. The energy of the emitted radiation is represented by the difference of the energies of electrons in the outermost orbital and orbital energy of the electrons in the innermost. This energy difference is characteristic of each element (This can be used as an elemental XRF signature). Thus, by detecting the radiation that is emitted in the process of interaction we have the signatures of the elements in the sample represented in the XRF spectrum (Lachance & Claisse, 1995).

The aim of this in vitro study was to evaluate the efficacy of X-Ray fluorescence technique on the measurements of de-remineralization in bovine enamel subject to erosion and treated with three products.

2 MATERIALS AND METHODS

2.1 *Sample preparation*

We used 15 bovine incisors. The samples were stored in 0.05% thymol for up to one week before the tests. The teeth were sectioned at the cementum-enamel line, discarding the root portion and were stored in ultrapure water at a temperature of 4°C. Then the teeth were fixed epoxy resin with the aid of a delineator so that the buccal stay parallel to the horizontal plane of the bench and were contained in PVC tubes (nominal diameter 22 mm) for 24 hours to wait for the polymerization the resin. The set tooth/base was taken to a metallographic polishing (Arotec® model-APL-4), employing silicon carbide abrasives (abrasives water) abrasive 600 and copious irrigation, thus, made by standardizing planning area.

After inclusion and planning, the specimens were immersed for 5 minutes in an ultrasonic bath (ultrapure water – Water Distiller® and Megapurity ultrasonic tank – Ultra Cleaner 700, Unique® – Indaiatuba, SP, Brazil) and then insulated with tape and white enamel so that only six nozzles were exposed to the external environment. We obtained 15 specimens (CP) who were randomly divided into 3 groups, each with 5 CP. Each group was designated as their treatment to be used. Group 1 (G1) Saliva: artificial saliva; Group 2 (G2) Fluor: Fluoride gel neutral; Group 3 (G3) Nano P: Dessensibilize Nano P (nanoparticles of calcium hydroxyapatite and Fluoride).

2.2 *Instrumentation*

All teeth of the three groups were initially evaluated to obtain the count of elements P and Ca obtained from the X-ray fluorescence spectra by the X-ray equipment micro X-ray Fluorescence Artax™ 800. This equipment is installed in the Laboratory for Electronic Instrumentation and Analytical Techniques (Lieta – Block F – 3005) of the Institute of Physics Armando Dias Tavares (Centre of Technology and Science – UERJ). The experimental conditions were such as: X-ray tube high voltage of 30 kV, X-ray tubeanode current of 400 μA, molybdenum target and X-ray spectra acquisition time of 100 s. The figure 1 shows geometric set-upof the X-ray beam on the sample.

In each CP was performed XRF measurement at predefined 6 points and the X-ray beam is positioned in the central region of the points. The measurement system has a laser for positioning the X-ray beam at the measurement point (Figure 2).

XRF spectra were analyzed using the equipment's software ARTAX. The values generated by the program represent areas on the photon peak of each element. Figure 3 shows an XRF spectrum with the peaks of the elements P and Ca discriminated.

After XRF measurements of all the teeth, they were stored for 7 days in distilled water at a temperature of 4°C.

After a week of the initial steps of the XRF samples of bovine teeth without any treatment, the specimens

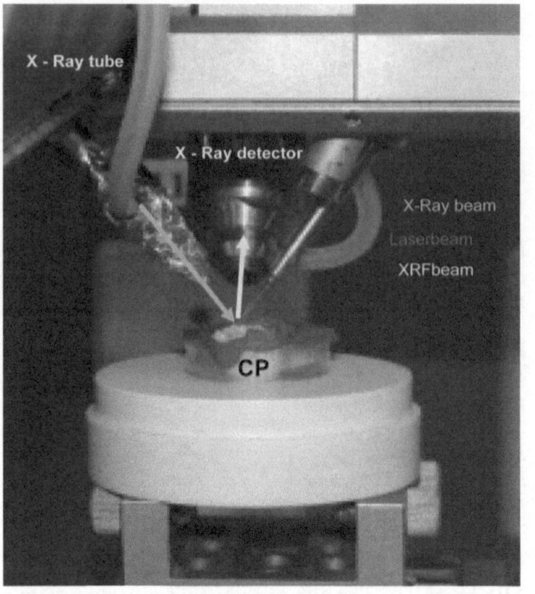

Figure 1. Geometric set-up of the X-ray beam on the sample.

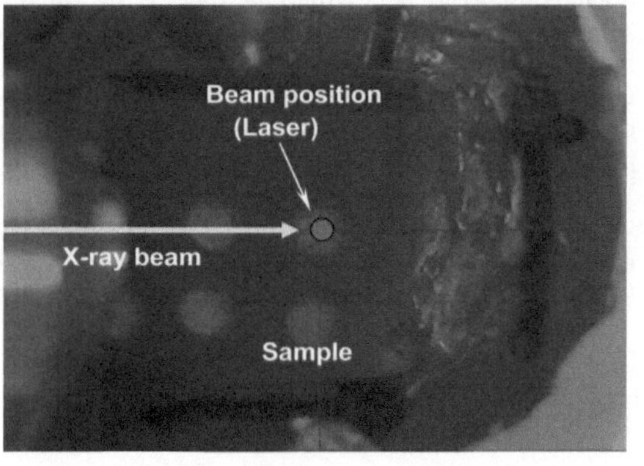

Figure 2. X-ray beam in position.

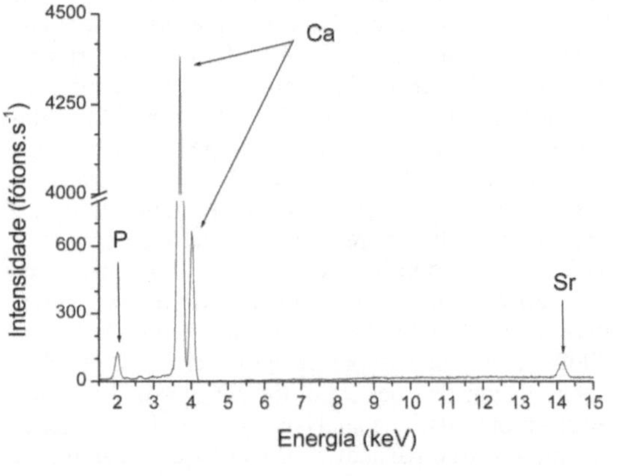

Figure 3. XRF spectrum with the peaks of the elements P and Ca discriminated.

Table 1. Mean initial count of P and Ca, standard deviation (SD) and coefficient of variation (CV) of each specimen prior to any treatment.

	Phosphorus			Calcium		
GROUP	Average	SD	CV%	Average	SD	CV%
G1	845	60	7.2	46589	891	1.9
G2	890	33	3.8	47037	1885	4.0
G3	823	19	2.3	44848	765	1.7

Table 2. Average final score of P and Ca, standard deviation (SD) and coefficient of variation (CV) of each specimen after 3 weeks of treatment.

	Phosphorus			Calcium		
GROUP	Average	SD	CV%	Average	SD	CV%
G1	805	31	3.8	44536	1344	3.0
G2	831	35	4.2	45947	168	3.5
G3	836	16	1.9	44278	652	1.5

Table 3. Third week of treatment X initial for P.

(G1)	G1 = G2 (p = 0.068)	G1 < G3 (p = 0.000)
(G2)	G2 = G1 (p = 0.068)	G2 < G3 (p = 0.000)
(G3)	G3 > G1 (p = 0.000)	G3 > G2 (p = 0.000)

suffered erosive challenge. For this challenge, each group of samples was immersed in a beaker identified in a solution of 10 ml of 2% citric acid pH 2.6 for 90 minutes (Sobral et al. 2009). Were washed with ultrapure water Milli-Q, blotted dry and then was made a new sequence of XRF measurements at the same points predefined.

Immediately after obtaining the spectra of teeth submitted to erosive challenge, each group received their corresponding treatments.

The samples were stored in separate bottles and labeled in correspondence with the respective treatment groups. Measures and XRF treatments were performed every seven days and repeated for 3 weeks.

3 RESULTS

Initially, we obtained the count of elements P and Ca interpreted from the spectrum of X-ray fluorescence, Table 1 shows the results of P and Ca standard deviation (SD) of each CP before any treatment. Table 2 shows the results of P and Ca and standard deviation (SD) of each CP after 3 weeks of treatment.

We used the Student t test to compare the means of different treatment groups with a significance level of 5%. Tables 3–4. Besides that, Bonferroni test was used for parametric comparison of means within groups of loss of Ca and P in each treatment, also with a significance level of 5%. Figures 4–5. All statistical analyzes were performed using the software "SPSS for Windows 10.0.1" (1999).

Table 4. Third week of treatment X initial for Ca.

(G1)	G1 < G2 (p = 0.029)	G1 < G3 (p = 0.009)
(G2)	G2 > G1 (p = 0.029)	G2 < G3 (p = 0.370)
(G3)	G3 > G1 (p = 0.009)	G3 > G2 (p = 0.370)

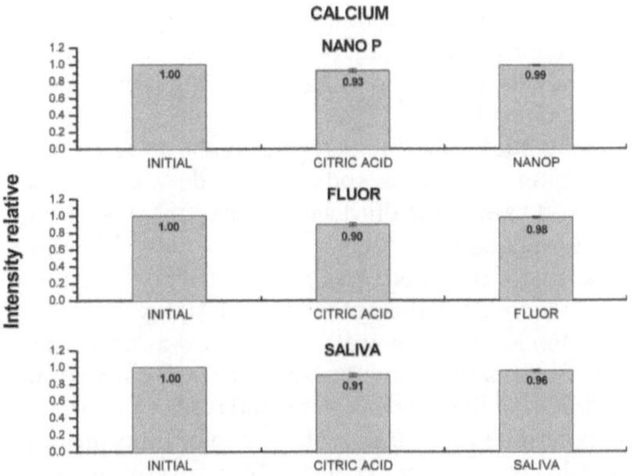

Figure 4. Relative intensity of calcium in all treatments.

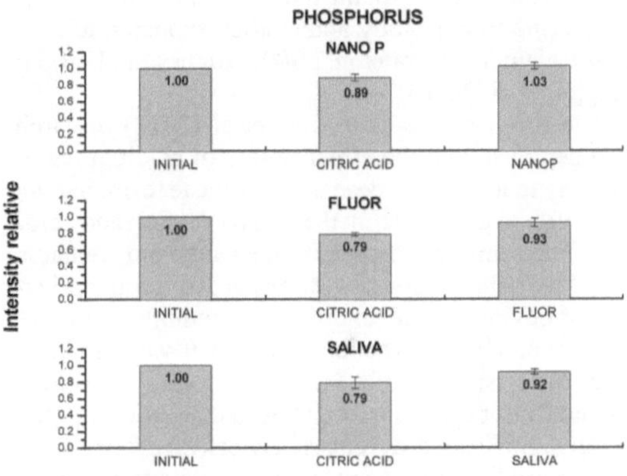

Figure 5. Relative intensity of phosphorus in all treatments.

4 DISCUSSION

The methodology for evaluating the remineralization chosen for this study was the X-ray fluorescence (XRF), a method based on the measurement of the intensities (the number of X-rays detected per unit time) of the characteristic X-rays emitted by elements constitute a sample (Klockenkamper & Bohlen, 1996) allows the evaluation of all phases of the study in the same teeth. Not being a destructive method permits the use of the same specimen at different times in the study, reducing therefore the variables.

In dentistry, the multielement analysis by X-Ray Fluorescence Energy Dispersive (EDXRF) can be used to determine changes in elemental composition for both eroded surfaces and cross sections. As can be applied for the detection deposition of active agents in therapeutic treatments on the surface of teeth

(Schlueter et al. 2009; Wiegand et al. 2009; Ganss et al. 2010).

Compared with treatment with fluorides, as some authors (Lussi et al. 2008) state that are not able to efficiently protect the growing process of erosive challenge, other conclude that there is significant improvement in the lesions caused by erosion (Hara et al. 2009; Hughes et al. 2004; Maggio et al. 2010). These controversies may be due to the use of different products and methodologies, making it difficult to compare results.

In this study, the results regarding the effect of remineralizing Gel neutral sodium fluoride was effective against P gain of the third week of treatment, showing statistical equality of means of control and of the third week. Therefore, there was partial efficacy. Since Ca did not increase sufficiently to match statistically with the initial amount (control). And there was no statistically significant difference between the control group and Fluorine in the first and second week of treatment the experiment ($p > 0.05$). The group of Fluorine only proved superior to saliva group (control) on the third week of treatment ($p < 0.05$). The acid exposure was performed only once and before the application of fluoride, which may explain the difference in efficacy of fluorine in this study and studies exposing to acid after treatment (Hara et al. 2009; Hughes et al. 2004; Maggio et al. 2010).

The result of Souza e Silva et al (2011) research also demonstrated the effectiveness of calcium nanohydroxyapatite, but in desensitizing paste form. Shown to be effective in reducing the loss by erosion and abrasion. The same folder used in this study and we had a very favorable outcome with respect to remineralization of bovine enamel exposed to a regime of erosive challenge. The Dessensibilize Nano P was effective since the first week of treatment in a gain in average Ca and P after exposure to acid. And that showed statistically significant differences between all groups since the 1st week of treatment with the average Ca What about the average P, statistical differences between the G1 and G2 since the first week and the second week compared to G4. The product also demonstrated stability in mean Ca and P maintaining the average three weeks. The manufacturer recommends at least three applications of the product with an interval of at least 3 days between each application. The result of the study confirms the effectiveness of the manufacturer's recommendations.

Finally, it is noteworthy that the erosive potential in vitro studies are overestimated and paper products are underestimated because they do not include all events intraoral (West et al. 2011).

5 CONCLUSION

It can be concluded that this methodology was effective on the measurement of de-remineralization in bovine enamel subject to erosion and their treatments in correspondence.

ACKNOWLEDGEMENTS

This work was developed with the financial support of Carlos Chagas Filho Foundation for Research Support in the State of Rio de Janeiro (FAPERJ) and National Council for Scientific and Technological Development (CNPq).

REFERENCES

Ganss C, Hardt M, Lussi A, Cocks A-K, Klimek J, Schlueter N. 2010. Mechanism of action of tin containing fluoride solutions as anti-erosive agents in dentine – an in vitro tin-uptake, tissue loss and scanning electron microscopy study. *Eur J Oral Sci* 118:376–384.

Hara, AT; Kelly, SA; Cabezas-Gonzalez, C 2009. Influence of Fluoride Availability of Dentifrices on Eroded Enamel remineralization in situ. *Caries Research* 43:57–63.

Hughes, JA; West, NX; Addy, M 2004. The protective effect of fluoride treatments against enamel erosion in vitro. *Journal of Oral Rehabilitation* 31:357–363.

Klockenkamper, R, Bohlen, A 1996. Elemental Analysis of Environmental Samples by Total Reflection Fluorescence: a Review. *X-ray Spectrom* 25:156–162.

Lachance GR, Claisse F 1995. *Quantitative X-Ray Fluorescence Analysis: Theory and Application.* 1. ed. New York: John Willey & Sons.

Lussi, A; Megert, B; Eggenberger, D; Jaeggi, T 2008. Impact of Different Toothpastes on the Prevention of Erosion. *Caries Research* 42:62–67.

Maggio, B; Guibert, RG; Mason, SC 2010. Evaluation of mouthrinse and dentifrice regimens in an in situ erosion remineralisation model. *Journal of Dentistry* 38:S37–S44.

Santos RS, Anjos MJ 2009. Análise multielementar de sangue humano de indivíduossadios e portadores de Leucemia Mielóide Crônica (LMC) através daTécnica de Fluorescência de Raios X por Reflexão Total (TXRF)usando Radiação Síncrotron. Rio de Janeiro: Instituto de Física Armando Dias Tavares Departamento de Física Aplicada e Termodinâmica, UERJ, jul 2009, 16p. Relatório técnico.

Schlueter N, Hardt M, Lussi., Engelmann F, Klimek J, Ganss C 2009. Tin-containing fluoride solutions as anti-erosive agents in enamel: an in vitro tin-uptake, tissue-loss, and scanning electron micrograph study. *Eur J Oral Sci* 117:427–434.

Sobral MAP, Lachowski KM, Rossi W, Braga SRM; Ramalho, KM 2009. Effect of Nd: YAG laser and acidulated Phosphate Fluoride on Bovine and Human Enamel Submitted to Erosion/Abrasion or Erosion Only: An in Vitro Study Preliminary. *Photomedicine and Laser Surgery* 27:709–713.

Souza e Silva, Magalhaes, AC; Buzalaf, M 2011. Effect of a New Folder with Calcium Phosphate Nanoparticles most Fluoride in erosion/abrasion of enamel and dentin in vitro. *FGMs News* 13:38–41.

Wiegand A, Waldheim E, Sener B, Magalhaes AC, Attin T 2009. Comparison of the effects of TiF 4 and NaF solutions at pH 1.2 and 3.5 on enamel erosion in vitro. *Caries Research* 43:269–277.

West, NX, Davies, M; Amaechi, BT 2011. In vitro and in situ Models for Evaluating Tooth Erosion Loss Substance. *Caries Research* 45:43–52.

Biodental Engineering II – Natal Jorge et al (Eds)
© 2014 Taylor & Francis Group, London, ISBN 978-1-138-00131-2

Analysis of a bar-implant using a meshless method

H.M.S. Duarte
Engineering Faculty of Oporto University (FEUP) Mechanical Engineering Department, Porto, Portugal

J. Belinha
Mechanical Engineering Institute (IDMEC), Porto, Portugal

L.M.J.S. Dinis & R.M. Natal Jorge
Engineering Faculty of Oporto University (FEUP) Mechanical Engineering Department, Porto, Portugal

ABSTRACT: A study of a prosthetic system consisting of two implants connected with a bar using a meshless method is presented. The results are compared with the finite element method analysis.

1 INTRODUCTION

Most fixed prostheses for partially of total edentulous patients are made of implants and a metal alloy bar connecting them and supporting the prosthetic veneering. These fixed prostheses have an important mechanical function, which consists of supporting and distributing the occlusal loads, like the ones applied during the masticatory activity. The loads induce stress paths on the prostheses and the bone tissue. It is important to obtain the right stress paths in order to assess the load transferred from the prostheses to the bone, and assure the biomechanical reliability of the prosthetic system. It is possible to conduct tests to study this reliability. However, such tests are very expensive, time consuming and they implicate the evaluation of the results transfer process to humans. In addition, it is almost impossible to predict accurately the stress or strain levels on the bone surrounding the implants. Numerical methods overcome the limitations of experimental methods, since they produce precise and reliable information about the biomechanical efficiency of the prostheses system, including bar, implants and bone response [1]. The study of multi-implant prostheses, which was studied with finite element (FEM) analysis [2], is now extended in this work to the meshless analysis.

The finite element method, as it is well-known, depends heavily on the mesh properties. When computing problems with complex and irregular geometries using the FEM, the mesh generation process is much more time consuming than the solution of the partial differential equations. To overcome the difficulty of the mesh generation, a new numerical method, meshless (or meshfree) method, has been under fast development in recent years [3, 4]. Since the field functions are approximated within an influence domain in the meshless method, as opposed to within an element in FEM, the nodes can be arbitrarily positioned inside the domain. While in FEM there is a no-overlap rule between elements, the influence domains in meshless methods may and must overlap each other. The two main categories of meshless methods are the ones that search for the weak form solution and the ones that search for the strong form solution. The first category can be divided again in two, regarding the use of approximation functions [5–8] or interpolation functions. The use of approximation functions makes difficult the imposition of the natural and essential boundary conditions, since these functions do not possess the delta Kronecker property.

To address the above problem several new meshless methods, using interpolation functions, were developed in the last few years, the Point Interpolation Method (PIM) [9, 10], the Point Assembly Method [11], the Natural Neighbour Finite Elements Method (NNFEM) [12, 13], or Natural Element Method (NEM) [14–17] and the Meshless Finite Element Method (MFEM) [18].

At this moment, one of the most popular and discussed meshless methods is the NEM. In this method, the test functions are constructed using natural neighbours interpolants [19]. This construction also uses geometrical and mathematical concepts such as the Voronoï diagrams [20] and the Delaunay tessellation [21]. The PIM uses an interpolation function based on a polynomial basis, with a simple construction and easy calculation of its derivatives. The RPIM [22, 23] is created by replacing the polynomial basis by a radial basis function (RBF). The RBF's used in these early works were the Gaussian and the multiquadric. The RBF was firstly used for data surface fitting, being later used to solve partial differential equations [24] and several engineering problems [25–28]. The RPIM uses the concept of "influence domain" instead of "global domain", which generates sparse and banded stiffness matrices, more adequate to complex geometry problems. There is however an inconvenient property of the RPIM's interpolation functions, which is the lack of compatibility. This problem is eliminated by the use of the conforming RPIM (CRPIM) [29]. Studies on these two methods showed that CRPIM can pass the standard patch tests while RPIM cannot [29, 30]. Even so, in the problems considered in the studies, the RPIM lead to satisfactory results, while being simpler and much more efficient than the CRPIM [4, 29].

One important issue to consider is the need of a background mesh for integration purposes. A meshless method is not a truly mesh free method if it relies on a background integration mesh. This multi-implant analysis is performed using the Natural Neighbour Radial Point Interpolation Method – NNRPIM [31]. Based on an unstructured set of nodes, a set of influence cells is created, using Voronï cells. After that, a node-dependent background mesh is created based on the Delaunay triangulation concept. This mesh is used in the numerical integration of the interpolation functions. While in the FEM geometrical restrictions on elements are imposed for the convergence of the method, there are no restrictions in the NNRPIM, which allows a random distribution of nodes inside the problem's domain. The interpolation functions of the NNRPIM are used in the Galerkin weak form. They are constructed in a similar process to the RPIM, with some differences that modify the method's performance. The NNRPIM is a recent developed meshless method. However, it has been extended to many fields of the computational mechanics, such as the analysis of isotropic and orthotropic plates [32], the functionally graded material plate analysis [33], the 3D shell-like approach [34, 35], the dynamic analysis of several solid-mechanic problems [36], the material non-linearity analysis [37] and the large deformation analysis [38].

2 NATURAL NEIGHBOURS AND RADIAL POINT INTERPOLATORS: A GENERAL REVIEW

The NNRPIM uses the Natural Neighbour concept [39], and these neighbours are determined using Voronoï diagrams and the Delaunay triangulation. Considering a set **N** of N distinct nodes, $N = \{n_1, n_2, \ldots, n_N\} \in \mathbb{R}^3$, the Voronoï diagram of **N** is the domain defined by **N** in sub-regions $\mathbf{V}_I$, which are closed and convex. Each of these sub-regions, called a Voronoï cell, $\mathbf{V}_I$, is related to a node, $\mathbf{n}_I$, such that any point inside the $\mathbf{V}_I$ sub-region is closer to n_I than any other node belonging to **N**. The Delaunay triangulation is then constructed by connecting the nodes whose Voronoï cells have common boundaries. By using the Voronoï diagram and the Delaunay triangulation it is possible to conclude that a Delaunary edge exists between nodes if and only if their Voronoï cells have an edge in common. The NNRPIM [31] uses the Voronoï diagram to enforce the connectivity between nodes, by creating "influence-cells", which overlap each other. There are two distinct types of influence-cells, represented in figure 1(a). The first type is called *first degree influence-cell,* and it is composed by the natural neighbours of a point of interest, $\mathbf{x}_I$. The second type is the *second degree influence-cell.* In this case, a point of interest, $\mathbf{x}_I$, searches for its neighbours, and also for the neighbours of its neighbours, being the cell composed by these two sets of nodes. The Voronoï diagram and the Delaunay triangles are used once again to construct a nodal dependent background integration mesh [31]. As shown in figure 1(b), small areas, $\mathbf{V}_I$ can be established using the referred constructions, and the intersection points, $\mathbf{P}_{Ii}$ of the neighbour edges of $\mathbf{V}_I$ can be settled. Then, the middle points, $\mathbf{M}_{Ii}$, between node I and its neighbor nodes are obtained. With these points, it is possible to divided the Voronoï cells into n quadrilateral sub-cells, $\mathbf{S}_{Ii}$, as figure 1(c) indicates. For instance the sub-cell $\mathbf{S}_{I2}$ is defined by the quadrilateral $\overline{M_{I2}\, P_{I2}\, M_{I3}\, n_I}$. Thus, a Voronoï cell, $\mathbf{V}_I$, with n neighbour nodes of the central node I has n sub-cells, $\mathbf{S}_{Ii}$, where,

$$A_{V_I} = \sum_{i=1}^{n} A_{S_{Ii}}, \quad \forall A_{S_{Ii}} \geq 0 \tag{1}$$

being A_{V_I} the Voronoï cell's area and $A_{S_{Ii}}$ the sub-cell's area. Since the set of Voronoï cells constitute a partition, without gaps, of the global domain, the

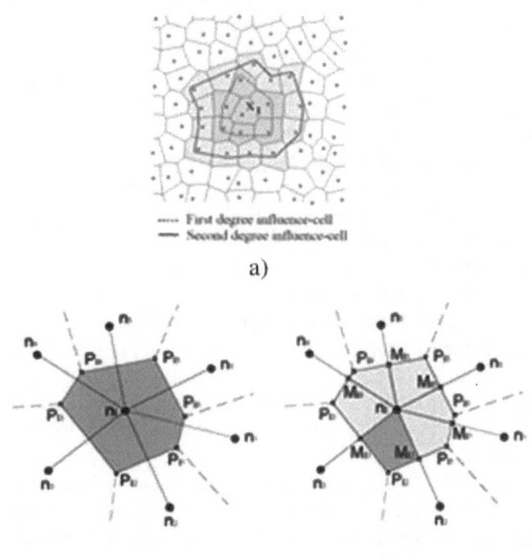

Figure 1. (a) Influence cells representation. (b) Voronoï cell and the corresponding PIi intersection points. (c) Middle points MIi and the respective generated quadrilaterals **[43]**.

set of sub-cells are also a partition, without gaps, of the global domain. This set of sub-cells, whose construction is methodically shown in [31], allows the use of several integration schemes based on the Gauss-Legendre integration.

Previous work [31] found that the "influence-cell" which produces more accurate and stable results is the second degree influence-cell, while the most efficient integration scheme is the one that uses only one quadrature point in each sub-cell. Consider a function $\mathbf{u}(\mathbf{x})$ defined in the domain Ω, which is discretized by a set of N nodes. In the NNRPIM a radial basis function is used, which passes through all nodes, though only the nodes within the influence-cell of the point of interest $\mathbf{x}_I$ have effect on $\mathbf{u}(\mathbf{x}_I)$. The value of $\mathbf{u}(\mathbf{x}_I)$ at the point of interest $\mathbf{x}_I$ is given by,

$$\mathbf{u}(\mathbf{x}_I) = \sum_{i=1}^{n} R_i(\mathbf{x}_I)\, a_i(\mathbf{x}_I) = \mathbf{R}^T(\mathbf{x}_I)\, \mathbf{a} \tag{2}$$

where $R_i(\mathbf{x}_I)$ is the radial basis function (RBF) $R^T(x_I) = \{R_1(x_I), R_2(x_I), \ldots, R_n(x_I)\}$, n is the number of nodes inside the influence-cell of $\mathbf{x}_I$ and $a_i(\mathbf{x}_I)$ are the coefficients of $R_i(\mathbf{x}_I)$, defined as $a^T(x_I) = \{a_1(x_I), a_2(x_I), \ldots, a_n(x_I)\}$ which are non-constant, varying with each point of interest $\mathbf{x}_I$. Along with the radial basis function, a polynomial basis [20] was used originally in equation (2). However, recent studies [31] found that if the polynomial basis was not used, the results would be more accurate, there would be an increase in efficiency, a decrease in computational cost and a faster convergence rate. The present work uses the Multiquadric (MC) function proposed initially by Hardy [40],

$$R(r_{Ii}) = \left(r_{Ii}^{\,2} + c^2\right)^p \tag{3}$$

where c and p are two parameters which can be optimized as shown in [31]. In this radial basis function, the variable is r_{Ii}, which represents the distance between the point of interest $\mathbf{x}_I$ and the neighbour node $\mathbf{x}_I$. This distance is simply calculated by using the Euclidean norm, $r_{Ii} = \sqrt{(x_I - x_i)^2 + (y_I - y_i)^2}$. A new equation can be written,

$$\mathbf{u}_s = \mathbf{R}_Q\, \mathbf{a} \tag{4}$$

where,

$$\mathbf{u}_s = \{u_1, u_2, \ldots, u_n\}^T \tag{5}$$

$$\mathbf{R}_Q = \begin{bmatrix} R(r_{11}) & R(r_{21}) & .. & R(r_{1n}) \\ R(r_{21}) & R(r_{22}) & .. & R(r_{2n}) \\ \vdots & \vdots & & \vdots \\ R(r_{n1}) & R(r_{n2}) & .. & R(r_{nn}) \end{bmatrix} \tag{6}$$

Since the distance between nodes does not depend on direction, i.e., $R(r_{ij}) = R(r_{ji})$, the geometric matrix $\mathbf{R}_Q$ is symmetric. By substituting in equation (2),

$$\mathbf{u}(\mathbf{x}_I) = \mathbf{R}^T(\mathbf{x}_I)\, \mathbf{R}_Q^{-1}\, \mathbf{u}_s = \varphi(\mathbf{x}_I)\mathbf{u}_s \tag{7}$$

where $\varphi(\mathbf{x})$ is the interpolation function defined as,

$$\varphi(\mathbf{x}_I) = \mathbf{R}^T(\mathbf{x}_I)\, \mathbf{R}_Q^{-1} = \{\varphi_1(\mathbf{x}_I), \varphi_2(\mathbf{x}_I), \ldots, \varphi_n(\mathbf{x}_I)\} \tag{8}$$

The partial derivative of $\varphi(\mathbf{x})$ in order to a variable ξ is defined as,

$$\varphi_{,\xi}(\mathbf{x}_I) = \mathbf{R}_{,\xi}^T(\mathbf{x}_I)\, \mathbf{R}_Q^{-1} \tag{9}$$

The partial derivatives of the MQ-RBF in order to ξ are,

$$\mathbf{R}_{,\xi}(r_{ij}) = 2p\left(r_{ij}^2 + c^2\right)^{p-1}\left(\xi_j - \xi_i\right) \tag{10}$$

Early works on the RPIM [22] prove that these interpolation functions possess the delta Kronecker property and also that the partition of unity is satisfied.

3 MODEL

The two-dimensional model, figure 2, was based on the three-dimensional model in the existent literature [2]. Small changes were performed. First, two abutment screws and metal frameworks were added, since there was no information on how the bar was connected to the implant. With this modification, the abutment screw on the right implant would come out of the bar, so the model was changed, and the right implant was lowered and leveled with the left one.

A linear elastic stress-strain relationship was considered for this study. The mechanical properties of

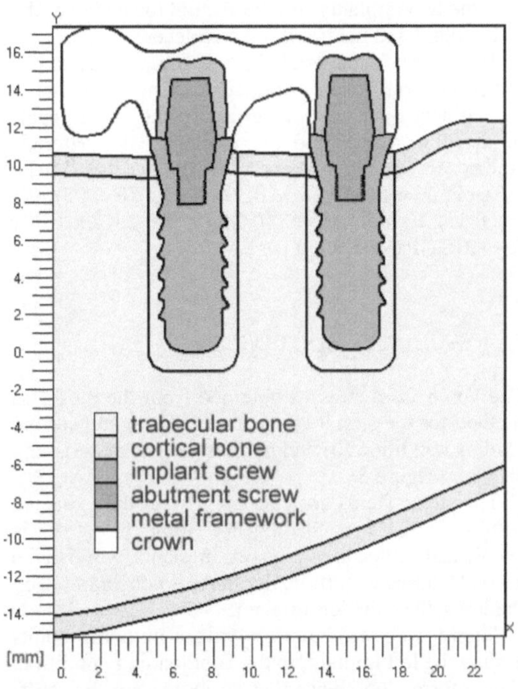

Figure 2. Complete bar-implant/mandible bone set for the two dimensional analysis.

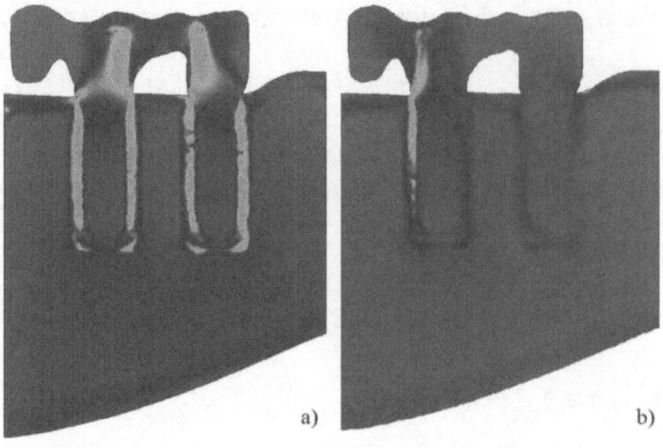

Figure 3. Stress distribution for the first loading condition (a) and second loading condition (b).

the different materials are the same as the three-dimensional model studied previously [2]. The only differences are the simplification of anisotropy on the cortical bone to isotropy, and the addition of two materials for the abutment screw (titanium) and metal framework (CoCr) [41]. For the first, a Young's modulus (E) of 110 GPa was set, with a Poisson's ratio (ν) of 0.32. The Young's modulus of the second was 220 GPa, with a Poisson's ratio of 0.30. The boundary conditions were defined as horizontal displacement blocked on both ends of the bone tissue, and vertical displacement blocked along the bottom of the cortical bone. The loading conditions were similar to the existent literature [2]. Two different cases were studied, both with parabolic forces of 150 N, the first located over the two implants and the second located over the left implant and the tip of the cantilever.

The standard material for the bar was gold [2]. Other materials were simulated in order to study the influence of these materials in the stress levels of the bone tissue and the implant. The materials studied were porcelain ($E = 61.2$ GPa, $\nu = 0.19$) [41], IV Gold ($E = 80$ GPa, $\nu = 0.33$), Silver ($E = 95$ GPa, $\nu = 0.33$), Titanium ($E = 110$ GPa, $\nu = 0.28$) and CoCr ($E = 218$ GPa, $\nu = 0.33$) [42].

4 RESULTS AND DISCUSSION

The Von Misses stresses obtained from the meshless method for the first loading condition (a) and second loading condition (b) and gold as the bar material are shown in figure 3.

The stress fields are consistent with the expected results. In the first loading condition, the stress is evenly distributed along the two implants, while in the second loading condition, the stress is concentrated on the left side of the left implant.

Figure 4 shows the stress values on some points around the left implant, in the first loading condition. This information shows that an increase in bar stiffness tends to increase the stress levels in the bone tissue and decrease these levels on the implant. The

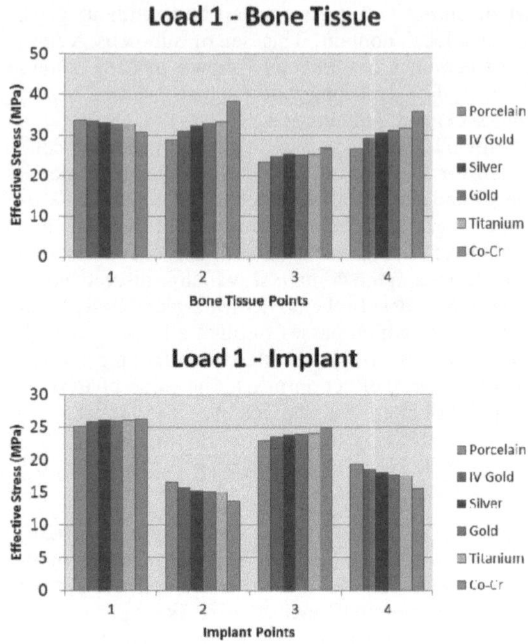

Figure 4. Effective stress values for the first loading condition on the bone tissue (top) and implant (bottom) around the left implant.

stress values on the other areas and the second loading condition are consistent with the results shown. Also, when compared with the finite element method analysis, the results have the same order of magnitude, despite the important change of 3D to 2D analysis.

5 CONCLUSIONS

The results obtained with the meshless methods are similar to the ones obtained with other numerical methods. The stress fields are smooth and according to the expected. These results also showed that a stiffer bar material induces higher stresses on the bone tissue and lower stresses on the implants.

REFERENCES

[1] Natali A.N., Pavan P.G., Numerical approach to dental biomechanics. Dental Biomechanics, (2003). p.211–239.

[2] Natali A.N., Pavan P.G., Ruggero A.L., Evaluation of stress induced in peri-implant bone tissue by misfit in multi-implant prosthesis. Dental Materials, (2006). 22: p. 388–395.

[3] Belytschko T., et al., Meshless Methods: an overview and recent developments. Computer Methods in Applied Mechanics and Engineering, (1996). 139(1): p. 3–47.

[4] Gu Y.T., Meshfree methods and their comparisons. International Journal of Computational Methods, (2005). 2(4): p. 477–515.

[5] Atluri S.N. and Zhu T., A new meshless local Petrov-Galerkin (MLPG) approach in computational mechanics. Computational Mechanics, (1998). 22(2): p. 117–127.
[6] Monaghan J.J., Smoothed Particle Hydrodynamics: Theory and Applications to Non-Spherical Stars. Monthly Notices of the Astronomical Society, (1977). 181: p. 375–389.
[7] Belytschko T., Lu Y.Y., and Gu L., Element-Free Galerkin Method. International Journal for Numerical Methods in Engineering, (1994). 37: p. 229–256.
[8] Liu W.K., Jun S., and Zhang Y.F., Reproducing Kernel Particle Methods. International Journal for Numerical Methods in Fluids, (1995). 20(6): p. 1081–1106.
[9] Liu G.R. and Gu Y.T., A Point Interpolation Method for Two-Dimensional Solids. International Journal for Numerical Methods in Engineering, (2001). 50: p. 937–951.
[10] Liu G.R., et al., A point interpolation meshfree method for static and frequency analysis of two-dimensional piezoelectric structures. Computational Mechanics, (2002). 29(6): p. 510–519.
[11] Liu G.R., A Point Assembly Method for Stress Analysis for Two-Dimensional Solids. International Journal of Solid and Structures, (2002). 39: p. 261–276.
[12] Traversoni L., Natural Neighbour Finite Elements. Int. Conf. on Hydraulic Engineering Software, Hydrosoft Proc., Computational Mechanics Publications, (1994). 2: p. 291–297.
[13] Sukumar N., Moran B., and Belytschko T., The natural element method in solid mechanics. International Journal for Numerical Methods in Engineering, (1998). 43(5): p. 839–887.
[14] Braun J. and Sambridge M., A numerical method for solving partial differential equations on highly irregular evolving grids. Nature, (1995). 376: p. 655–660.
[15] Sukumar N., et al., Natural neighbour Galerkin methods. International Journal for Numerical Methods in Engineering, (2001). 50(1): p. 1–27.
[16] Cueto E., Doblaré M., and Gracia L., Imposing essential boundary conditions in the natural element method by means of density-scaled-shapes. International Journal for Numerical Methods in Engineering, (2000). 49(4): p. 519–546.
[17] Cueto E., et al., Overview and recent advances in the Natural Neighbour Galerkin Method. Archives of Computational Methods in Engineering, (2003). 10(4): p. 307–387.
[18] Sergio R., et al., The Meshless Finite Element Method. International Journal for Numerical Methods in Engineering, (2003). 58(6): p. 893–912.
[19] Sibson R., A brief description of natural neighbor interpolation. Interpreting Multivariate Data, in V. Barnett (ed.), (Wiley, Chichester), (1981): p. 21–36.
[20] Voronoï G.M., Nouvelles applications des paramètres continus à la théorie des formes quadratiques. Deuxième Mémoire: Recherches sur les parallélloèdres primitifs, J. Reine Angew. Math., (1908). 134: p. 198–287.
[21] Delaunay B., Sur la sphére vide. A la memoire de Georges Voronoï. Izv. Akad. Nauk SSSR, Otdelenie Matematicheskih i Estestvennyh Nauk, (1934). 7: p. 793–800.
[22] Wang J.G. and Liu G.R., A Point Interpolation Meshless Method based on Radial Basis Functions. International Journal for Numerical Methods in Engineering, (2002). 54: p. 1623–1648.
[23] Wang J.G. and Liu G.R., On the Optimal Shape Parameters of Radial Basis Functions used for 2-D Meshless Methods. Computer Methods in Applied Mechanics and Engineering, (2002). 191: p. 2611–2630.
[24] Kansa E.J., A scattered data approximation scheme with applications to computational fluid-dynamics – I & II. Computers and Mathematics with Applications, (1990). 19: p. 127–161.
[25] Ferreira A.J.M., A formulation of the multiquadric radial basis function method for the analysis of laminated composite plates. Composite Structures, (2003). 59(3): p. 385–392.
[26] Ferreira A.J.M., et al., Static deformations and vibration analysis of composite and sandwich plates using a layerwise theory and multiquadrics discretizations. Engineering Analysis with Boundary Elements, (2005). 29(12): p. 1104–1114.
[27] Ferreira A.J.M., Roque C.M.C., and M. P.A.L.S., Analysis of composite plates using higher-order shear deformation theory and a finite point formulation based on the multiquadric radial basis function method. Composites Part B: Engineering, (2003). 34(7): p. 627–636.
[28] Tiago C.M. and Leitão V.M.A., Application of radial basis functions to linear and nonlinear structural analysis problems. Computers & Mathematics with Applications, (2006). 51(8): p. 1311–1334.
[29] Liu G.R., Gu Y.T., and Dai K.Y., Assessment and applications of interpolation methods for computational mechanics. International Journal for Numerical Methods in Engineering, (2004). 59: p. 1373–1379.
[30] Liu G.R., Mesh Free Methods, Moving beyond the Finite Element Method. (2002): CRC Press.
[31] Dinis L., Jorge R.N., and Belinha J., Analysis of 3D solids using the natural neighbour radial point interpolation method. Computer Methods in Applied Mechanics and Engineering, (2007). 196: p. 2009–2028.
[32] Dinis L., Jorge R.N., and Belinha J., Analysis of plates and laminates using the natural neighbour radial point interpolation method. Engineering Analysis with Boundary Elements, (2008). 32: p. 267–279.
[33] Dinis L., Jorge R.N., and Belinha J., An Unconstrained Third-Order Plate Theory applied to Functionally Graded Plates using a Meshless Method. Mechanics of Advanced Materials and Structures, (2010). 17: p. 1–26.
[34] Dinis L., Jorge R.N., and Belinha J., A 3D Shell-Like approach using a Natural Neighbour Meshless Method: isotropic and orthotropic thin structures. Composite Structures, (2009)(doi:10.1016/j.compstruct.2009.10.014).
[35] Dinis L., Jorge R.N., and Belinha J., Composite Laminated Plates: A 3D natural neighbour radial point interpolation method approach. Journal of Sandwich Structures and Materials, (2010). 12(2): p. 119–138.
[36] Dinis L., Jorge R.N., and Belinha J., The Natural Neighbour Radial Point Interpolation Method: Dynamic Applications. Engeneering Computations, (2009). 26(8): p. 911–949.
[37] Dinis L., Jorge R.N., and Belinha J., Radial Natural Neighbours Interpolators: 2D and 3D Elastic and Elastoplastic Applications, in Progress on Meshless Methods – Computational Methods in Applied Sciences, Ferreira A.J.M., et al., Editors. (2008), Springer.
[38] Dinis L., Jorge R.N., and Belinha J., Large Deformation Applications with the Radial Natural Neighbours

Interpolators. Computer Modelling in Engineering and Sciences, (2009). 44(1): p. 1–34.
[39] Sibson R., A vector identity for the Dirichlet tesselation. Mathematical Proceedings of the Cambridge Philosophical Society, (1980). 87: p. 151–155.
[40] Hardy R.L., Theory and applications of the multiquadrics – Biharmonic method (20 years of discovery 1968–1988). Computers and Mathematics with Applications, (1990). 19: p. 127–161.
[41] Kayabasi O., Yuzbasıoglu E., Erzincanli F., Static, dynamic and fatigue behaviors of dental implant using finite element method. Advances in Engineering Software, (2006). 37: p. 649–658.
[42] Spazzin A.O., Santos M.B.F., Sobrinho L.C., Consani R.L.X., Mesquita M.F., Effects of Horizontal Misfit and Bar Framework Material on the Stress Distribution of an Overdenture-Retaining Bar System: A 3D Finite Element Analysis. Journal of Prosthodontics, (2011). 20: p. 517–522.
[43] Dinis L., Jorge R.N., and Belinha J., Bone remodelling optimization using the Natural Neighbour Radial Point Interpolation Method. 2nd International Conference on Engineering Optimization, Lisbon 2010.

Biodental Engineering II – Natal Jorge et al (Eds)
© 2014 Taylor & Francis Group, London, ISBN 978-1-138-00131-2

Analysis of dental implant using a meshless method

J. Rafael Andrade & J. Belinha
Mechanical Engineering Institute (IDMEC), Porto, Portugal

L.M.J.S. Dinis & R.M. Natal Jorge
Engineering Faculty of Oporto University (FEUP), Mechanical Engineering Department, Porto, Portugal

ABSTRACT: The present work uses a radial interpolation meshless method, the "Natural Neighbour Radial Point Interpolation Method", in order to perform an elastic-static analysis of a dental implant application in the bone.

1 INTRODUCTION

Nowadays, a significant portion of the computational mechanics scientific community is focused on solving partial differential equations (PDEs) using numerical methods, such as "Finite Element Method" (FEM). This popular numerical method consists of dividing the problem in small elements and using shape functions in order to obtain field variables. The influence domain is defined by the elements which can not overlap each other. When an element is manifestly distorted, the shape functions obtained show a poor quality, affecting the results. In the computation of problems with irregular geometries, mesh generation is more time-consuming than the actual solution of the PDEs. Taking in consideration these disadvantages, meshless methods emerge, using nodes random distributed along the domain and field functions approximated within an influence domain rather than an element. In opposition to the FEM, the influence domains may and must overlap each other.

In the last few years, several meshless methods were developed [2, 3]. There are approximant meshless methods [4–7] and interpolant meshless methods. Using approximations functions instead of interpolation functions has a disadvantage: the lack of delta Kronecker property, which increases the difficulty to impose of the essential and natural boundary conditions. In order to avoid the mentioned problem, several new meshless methods, using interpolation functions, were developed: Point Interpolation Method (PIM) [8, 9], the Point Assembly Method [10], the Natural Neighbour Finite Elements Method (NNFEM) [11, 12], or Natural Element Method (NEM) [13–16] and the Meshless Finite Element Method (MFEM) [17]. At the moment, the NEM stands out as the most popular and discussed meshless method. In the NEM the trials and test functions are constructed using natural neighbour interpolants [18] based on the Voronoï diagrams [19] and the Delaunay tessellation [20]. In the PIM it is used polynomial basis interpolation functions, its construction is simple and its derivatives are easily obtained. The Radial Point Interpolation Method (RPIM) [21, 22] is generated, replacing the polynomial basis by radial basis functions (RBF). In the recent works, the used RBFs were Gaussian and the multiquadric radial basis functions. The RBF was originally used for data surface fitting, and later the RBF was used for solving partial differential equations [23] and to solve several engineering problems [24–27]. RPIM allows to generate sparse and banded stiffness matrices, because it uses the concept of "influence domain" rather than "global domain". This topic is more adequate to complex geometry problems.

Another relevant subject is the necessity of a background mesh for integration purposes. Actually meshless method depending on a secondary background integration method, consequently it is not a truly mesh free method.

In the present work the Natural Neighbour Radial Point Interpolation Method – NNRPIM [28] – is used to numerically analyze dental implants. Using Voronoï diagrams, a set of influence cells are constructed departing from an unstructured set of nodes. The Delaunay triangulation concept is used to create a node-dependent background mesh used in the numerical integration of the NNRPIM interpolation functions. Its interpolation functions use in the Galerkin weak form and are created in an analogous process to the RPIM, with some adjustments that adapt the method's performance. In the NNRPIM there are not imposed geometrical restrictions for the convergence of the method, which permits a random node distribution for the discretized problem. Although the NNRPIM is a recent developed meshless method it has been extended to many fields of the computational mechanics, such as the analysis of isotropic and orthotropic plates [29], the functionally graded material plate analysis [30], the 3D shell-like approach [31, 32], the dynamic analysis of several solid-mechanic problems [33], the material non-linearity analysis [34] and the large deformation analysis [35].

Recently meshless methods started to enter the biomechanics field. In the work of Doblaré [36] a meshless method was extended to the bone tissue remodelling and hyperelasticity. In the work of Belinha [37, 38] a bone remodelling algorithm with meshless methods was applied to the femoral bone and the calcaneus bone. The Smooth Particle Hydrodynamics (SPH) was recently applied to analyse the blood behaviour [39].

In present work it is analysed a dental implant using a meshless method. Regarding this subject, there are only works using FEM, addressing the dental implant analysis [40] and studying the influence of the materials on the stress distribution in bone [41, 42].

2 NNRPIM

In NNRPIM natural neighbour nodes are established using Voronoï diagrams and the Delaunay triangulation. Consider a set of n distinct nodes, the Voronoï diagram results from a division of the domain in sub-regions closed and convex, also called "Voronoï cells". Any point belonging to a sub-region is closer from a certain node than any other, causing an association with the referred node. The Delaunay triangulation promotes the connection of the nodes whose Voronoï cells have common boundaries, creating a Delaunay edge. This edge exists between two nodes if and only if their Voronoï cells share a common edge. This concept is used in the NNRPIM [28] to create the "influence-cells", where the nodal connectivity is applied with overlapping of influence domains. Two types of influence-cells are created using this concept, as shown in Figure 1. In the first case, a point of interest searches for its neighbour nodes using the Natural Neighbour Voronoï construction and establish the first degree influence-cell. In the second case, a point of interest searches its natural neighbours, just like the first one, but in addition, all those natural neighbours search their own natural neighbours, making a larger influence-cell (second degree influence-cell).

The NNRPIM uses the Voronoï concept and Delaunay triangulation in order to construct a nodal dependent background integration mesh [28].

In the NNRPIM the test function passes through all nodes using a radial basis function (RBF), and only the nodes within the influence-cell of the point of interest affects the function. In early works, it considered a polynomial basis [22] to obtain the test function, however it was recently found [28] that removing the polynomial basis from the formulation leads to more accurate results, higher efficiency, lower computational cost and faster convergence rates. In the RBF the variable is the distance between the central node and the neighbour node.

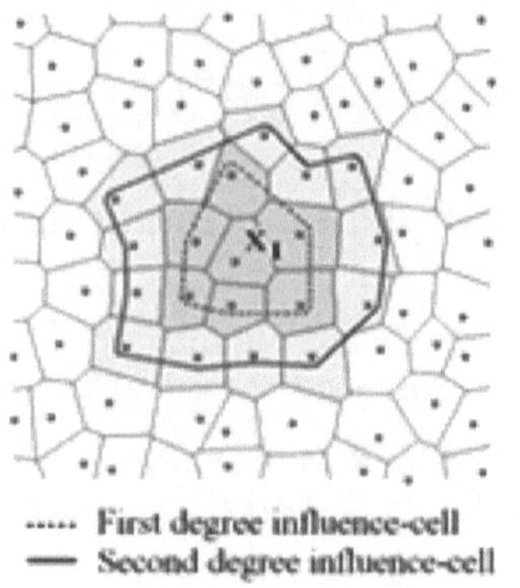

Figure 1. First and second degree influence-cells [1].

The present work uses the Multiquadratic (MQ) function proposed originally by Hardy [43]:

$$R(r_{Ii}) = \left(r_{Ii}^{2} + c^{2}\right)^{p} \quad (1)$$

where c and p are two parameters which can be optimized as shown in [28]. Recent works on the RPIM [22] show that these interpolation functions possess the delta Kronecker property and also the partition of unity is satisfied.

3 NUMERICAL MODEL

3.1 *Model*

A two-dimensional model was constructed for the analysis, considering the three-dimensional geometry suggested in [44]. As shown in Figure 2, the model is composed of: occlusal material, metal framework, abutment and implant screw, cortical and trabecular bone. The model main dimensions are represented too in Figure 2. A bone block, 24 mm high and 10 mm wide, representing the mandibular section, was modelled.

Several interest points were selected and they are represented in the Figure 3.

The boundary conditions were determined avoiding x and y displacement in the boundary nodes of bone, as exemplified in Figure 4(a). The established loading conditions were a 114.5 N vertical load and a 23.4 N horizontal load. These loads were distributed by 6 nodes, as shown in Figure 4(a). The model was constructed using a preprocessing software (FEMAP) and the obtained nodal mesh has 4597 nodes (Figure 4(b)).

3.2 *Material cases*

In this work, a titanium alloy is used for the implant and abutment screws and a cobalt-chromium alloy for the metal framework. For the bone study, different combinations of bone properties were selected and they represent diverse possibilities of bone behaviour. For the occlusal material study several materials are used

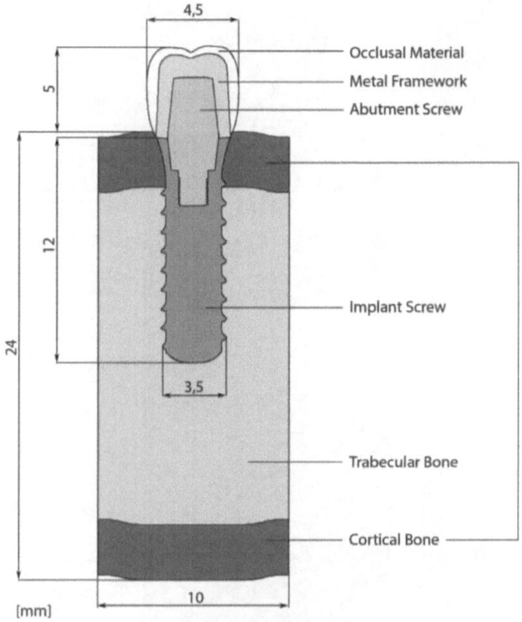

Figure 2. Dental implant bidimensional model.

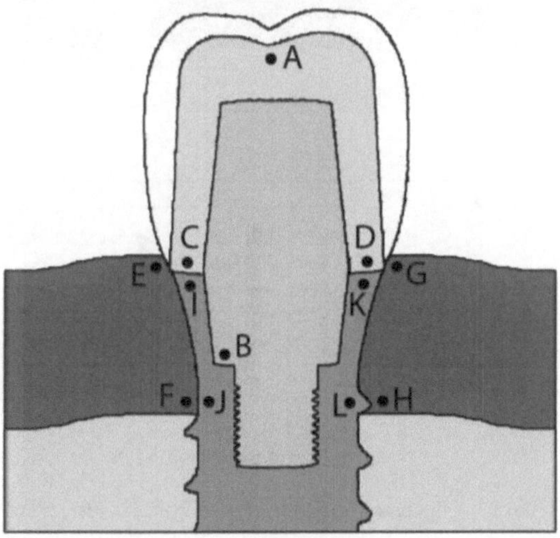

Figure 3. Selected interest points.

for the occlusal material, such as feldspathic porcelain, gold alloy, ceramic veneering, resin and hybrid composite. All used materials are represented with linear isotropic material models. The mechanical properties of the materials used in this study are shown in Table 1.

4 RESULTS

4.1 *Model validation*

Using some of the mechanical properties in the Table 1, the results were consistent with the FEM work [47]. In the Figure 5, the stress distribution is represented.

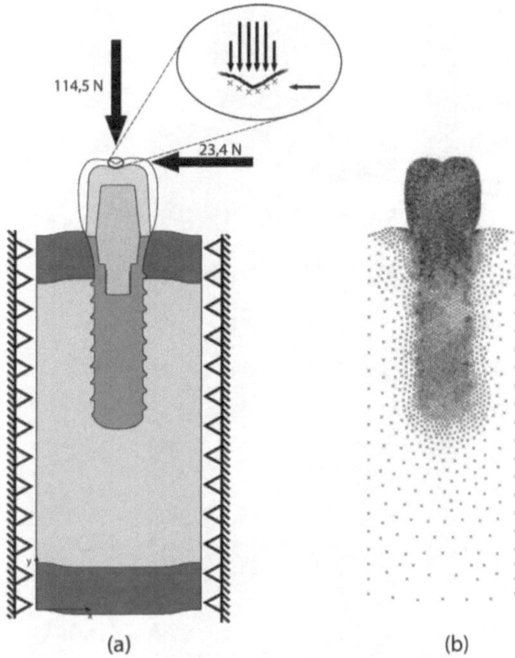

Figure 4. Boundary and loading conditions; (b) Obtained nodal mesh.

Table 1. Material mechanical properties.

Material	Young Modulus MPa	Poisson Ratio	Ref.
Titanium	110000	0.32	[44]
Cobalt-Chromium	220000	0.30	[44]
Resin	2700	0.35	[40]
Hybrid Composite	22000	0.19	[45]
Feldspathic Porcelain	61200	0.19	[44]
Ceramic Veneering	70000	0.20	[46]
Gold	100000	0.33	[47]

As shown in the Figure 6, the obtained Von Mises stress in the point A of the metal framework was 115 MPa (bibliographic reference – 114 MPa) and in the point B of the abutment screw was 113 MPa (bibliographic reference – 112 MPa). This small difference could be result of three-dimensional to two-dimensional approximation.

4.2 *Bone study*

The properties of the different bone cases are represented in the Table 2 and the expected stress map for the case 2 is shown in the Figure 7.

A higher level of cortical bone stiffness provides lower effective stresses in the cortical bone (Figure 8) and higher stresses in the implant.

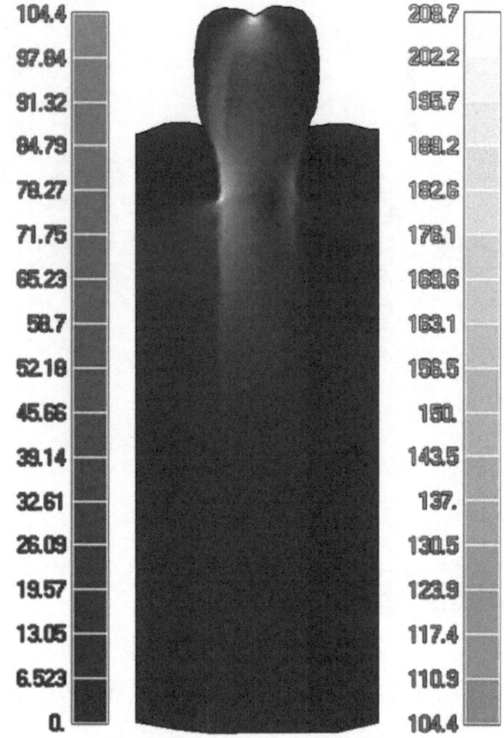

Figure 5. Model validation stress map.

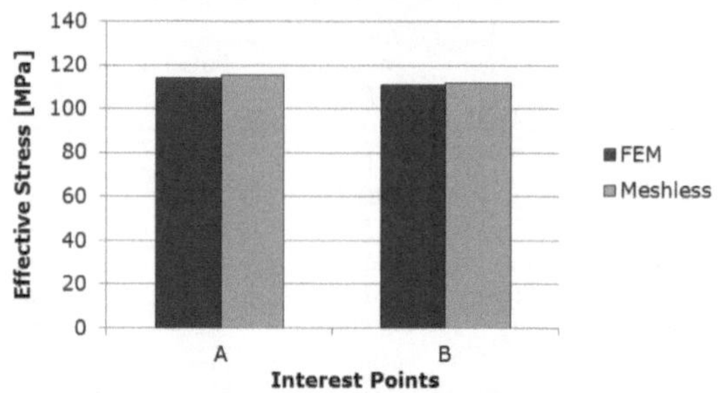

Figure 6. Effective stress in points A and B.

Table 2. Mechanical properties of bone cases.

Case	Cortical Bone Young Modulus MPa	Trabecular Bone Young Modulus MPa	Ref.
1	10000	250	[46]
2	11500	2130	[44]
3	13400	790	[40]
4	13700	1000	[48]
5	14800	1850	[45]

4.3 *Occlusal material study*

The stress distribution for the gold case is represented in the Figure 9.

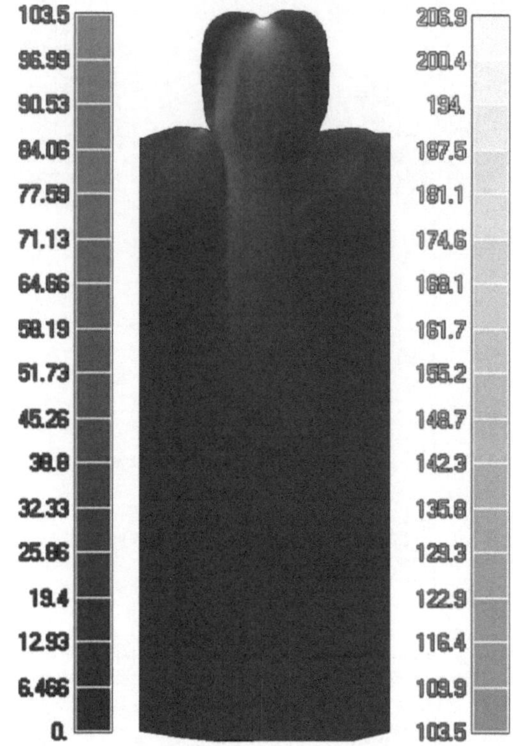

Figure 7. Case 2 stress map.

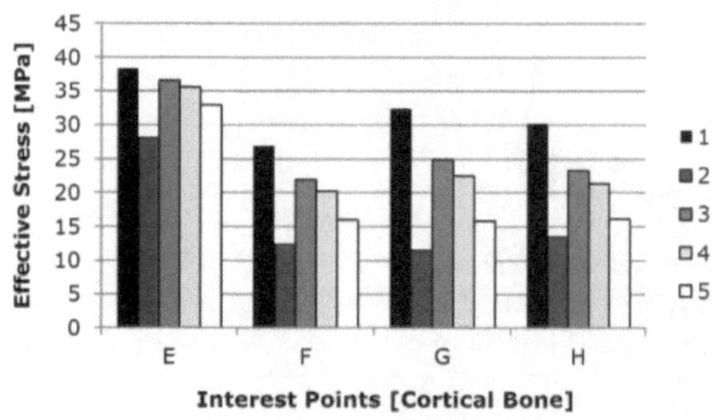

Figure 8. Effective stress of the cortical bone interest points.

A higher level of occlusal material stiffness provides lower effective stresses in the implant, in the abutment, in the metal framework and in the cortical bone (Figure 10).

5 CONCLUSIONS AND FUTURE WORKS

The obtained NNRPIM results permit to gauge that meshless methods are a suitable numerical tool to analyse the biomechanical behaviour of dental prostheses with similar results to FEM. Permitting in the near future the inclusion of more complex assumptions, such the material inelasticity, the large deformations, and transient analysis.

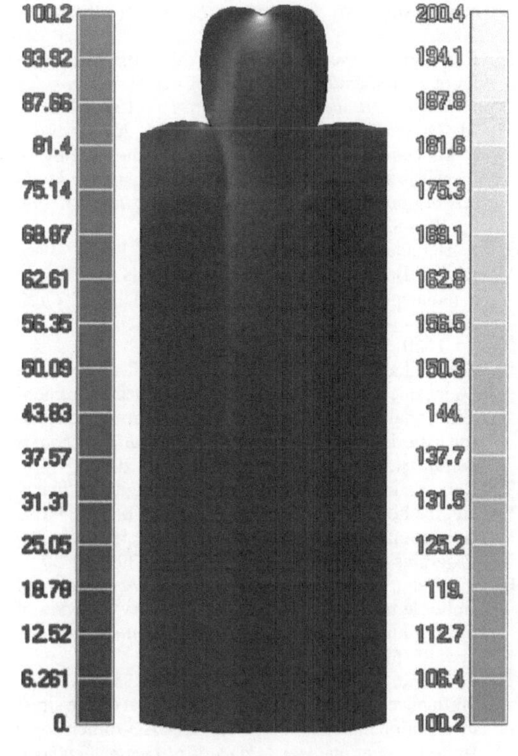

Figure 9. Gold case stress map.

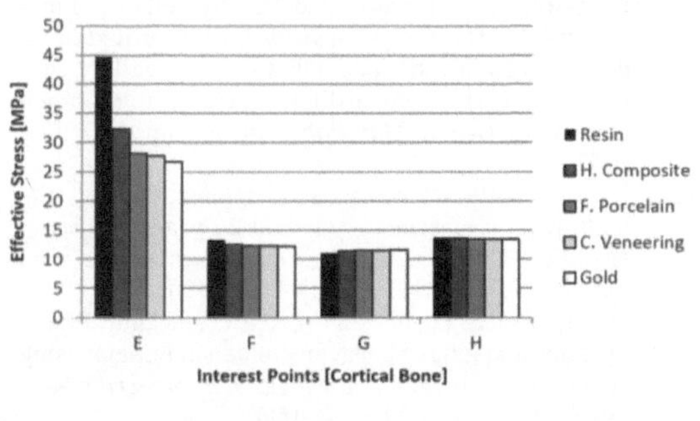

Figure 10. Effective stress of the cortical bone interest points.

ACKNOWLEDGEMENTS

The authors truly acknowledge the funding provided by Ministério da Ciência, Tecnologia e Ensino Superior – Fundação para a Ciência e a Tecnologia (Portugal), under grant SFRH/BPD/75072/2010, and by FEDER/FSE, under grant PTDC/EME-TME/098050/2008.

REFERENCES

[1] L. M. J. S. Dinis, R. M. N. Jorge, and J. Belinha, "Bone remodelling optimization using the Natural Neighbour Radial Point Interpolation Method," in *2nd International Conference on Engineering Optimization*, Lisbon, 2010.

[2] T. Belytschko, Y. Krongauz, D. Organ, M. Fleming, and P. Krysl, "Meshless methods: An overview and recent developments," *Computer Methods in Applied Mechanics and Engineering,* vol. 139, pp. 3–47, 1996.

[3] Gu Y.T., "Meshfree methods and their comparisons," *International Journal of Computational Methods,* vol. 2, pp. 477–515, (2005).

[4] S. N. Atluri and T. Zhu, "A new Meshless Local Petrov-Galerkin (MLPG) approach in computational mechanics," *Computational Mechanics,* vol. 22, pp. 117–127, 1998.

[5] Monaghan J.J., "Smoothed Particle Hydrodynamics: Theory and Applications to Non-Spherical Stars," *Monthly Notices of the Astronomical Society,* vol. 181, pp. 375–389, (1977).

[6] Belytschko T., Lu Y.Y., and Gu L., "Element-Free Galerkin Method," *International Journal for Numerical Methods in Engineering,* vol. 37, pp. 229–256, (1994).

[7] Liu W.K., Jun S., and Zhang Y.F., "Reproducing Kernel Particle Methods," *International Journal for Numerical Methods in Fluids,* vol. 20, pp. 1081–1106, (1995).

[8] G. R. Liu and Y. T. Gu, "A point interpolation method for two-dimensional solids," *International Journal for Numerical Methods in Engineering,* vol. 50, pp. 937–951, 2001.

[9] G. R. Liu, K. Y. Dai, K. M. Lim, and Y. T. Gu, "A point interpolation mesh free method for static and frequency analysis of two-dimensional piezoelectric structures," *Computational Mechanics,* vol. 29, pp. 510–519, 2002.

[10] G. R. Liu, "A point assembly method for stress analysis for two-dimensional solids," *International Journal of Solids and Structures,* vol. 39, pp. 261–276, 2001.

[11] L. Traversoni, "Natural neighbour finite elements," 1994, pp. 291–297.

[12] N. Sukumar, B. Moran, and T. Belytschko, "The natural element method in solid mechanics," *International Journal for Numerical Methods in Engineering,* vol. 43, pp. 839–887, 1998.

[13] J. Braun and M. Sambridge, "A numerical method for solving partial differential equations on highly irregular evolving grids," *Nature,* vol. 376, pp. 655–660, 1995.

[14] N. Sukumar, B. Moran, A. Y. Semenov, and V. V. Belikov, "Natural neighbour Galerkin methods," *International Journal for Numerical Methods in Engineering,* vol. 50, pp. 1–27, 2000.

[15] Cueto E., Sukumar N., Calvo B., Cegoñino J., and Doblaré M., "Overview and recent advances in the Natural Neighbour Galerkin Method," *Archives of Computational Methods in Engineering,* vol. 10, pp. 307–387, (2003).

[16] E. Cueto, M. Doblaré, and L. Gracia, "Imposing essential boundary conditions in the natural element method by means of density-scaled α-shapes," *International Journal for Numerical Methods in Engineering,* vol. 49, pp. 519–546, 2000.

[17] Sergio R., Idelsohn S., Oñate E., Calvo N., and Del Pin F., "The Meshless Finite Element Method," *International Journal for Numerical Methods in Engineering,* vol. 58, pp. 893–912, (2003).

[18] R. Sibson, "A brief description of natural neighbour interpolation," *Interpreting Multivariate Data,* pp. 21–36, 1981.

[19] G. Voronoi, "Nouvelles applications des paramètres continus à la théorie des formes quadratiques," *J. Reine Angew. Math.*, vol. 134, pp. 198–287, 1908.

[20] B. Delaunay, "Sur la sphere vide," *Bull. Acad. Sci. USSR*, vol. 7, pp. 793–800, 1934.

[21] J. G. Wang and G. R. Liu, "On the optimal shape parameters of radial basis functions used for 2-D meshless methods," *Computer Methods in Applied Mechanics and Engineering*, vol. 191, pp. 2611–2630, 2002.

[22] J. G. Wang and G. R. Liu, "A point interpolation meshless method based on radial basis functions," *International Journal for Numerical Methods in Engineering*, vol. 54, pp. 1623–1648, 2002.

[23] Kansa E.J., "A scattered data approximation scheme with applications to computational fluid-dynamics – I & II," *Computers and Mathematics withApplications*, vol. 19, pp. 127–161, (1990).

[24] Ferreira A.J.M. , "A formulation of the multiquadric radial basis function method for the analysis of laminated composite plates," *Composite Structures*, vol. 59, pp. 385–392, (2003).

[25] A. J. M. Ferreira, C. M. C. Roque, R. M. N. Jorge, and E. J. Kansa, "Static deformations and vibration analysis of composite and sandwich plates using a layerwise theory and multiquadrics discretizations," *Engineering Analysis with Boundary Elements*, vol. 29, pp. 1104–1114, 2005.

[26] A. J. M. Ferreira, C. M. C. Roque, and P. A. L. S. Martins, "Analysis of composite plates using higher-order shear deformation theory and a finite point formulation based on the multiquadric radial basis function method," *Composites Part B: Engineering*, vol. 34, pp. 627–636, 2003.

[27] C. M. Tiago and V. M. A. Leitão, "Application of radial basis functions to linear and nonlinear structural analysis problems," *Computers and Mathematics with Applications*, vol. 51, pp. 1311–1334, 2006.

[28] L. M. J. S. Dinis, R. M. Natal Jorge, and J. Belinha, "Analysis of 3D solids using the natural neighbour radial point interpolation method," *Computer Methods in Applied Mechanics and Engineering*, vol. 196, pp. 2009–2028, 2007.

[29] L. M. J. S. Dinis, R. M. Natal Jorge, and J. Belinha, "Analysis of plates and laminates using the natural neighbour radial point interpolation method," *Engineering Analysis with Boundary Elements*, vol. 32, pp. 267–279, 2008.

[30] L. M. J. S. Dinis, R. M. N. Jorge, and J. Belinha, "An unconstrained third-order plate theory applied to functionally graded plates using a meshless method," *Mechanics of Advanced Materials and Structures*, vol. 17, pp. 108–133, 2010.

[31] L. M. J. S. Dinis, R. M. N. Jorge, and J. Belinha, "A 3D shell-like approach using a natural neighbour meshless method: Isotropic and orthotropic thin structures," *Composite Structures*, vol. 92, pp. 1132–1142, 2010.

[32] L. M. J. S. Dinis, R. M. Jorge, and J. Belinha, "Composite laminated plates: A 3D natural neighbor radial point interpolation method approach," *Journal of Sandwich Structures and Materials*, vol. 12, pp. 119–138, 2010.

[33] L. M. J. S. Dinis, R. M. Natal Jorge, and J. Belinha, "The natural neighbour radial point interpolation method: Dynamic applications," *Engineering Computations (Swansea, Wales)*, vol. 26, pp. 911–949, 2009.

[34] R. M. N. J. Lúcia M. J. S. Dinis, Jorge Belinha, *Radial Natural Neighbours Interpolators: 2D and 3D Elastic and Elastoplastic Applications*: Springer Netherlands, 2008.

[35] R. Sibson, "A vector identity for the Dirichlet tesselation," *Mathematical Proceedings of the Cambridge Philosophical Society*, vol. 87, pp. 151–155, 1980.

[36] M. Doblaré, E. Cueto, B. Calvo, M. A. Martínez, J. M. Garcia, and J. Cegoñino, "On the employ of meshless methods in biomechanics," *Computer Methods in Applied Mechanics and Engineering*, vol. 194, pp. 801–821, 2005.

[37] J. Belinha, R. M. Natal Jorge, and L. M. J. S. Dinis, "Bone tissue remodelling analysis considering a radial point interpolator meshless method," *Engineering Analysis with Boundary Elements*, vol. 36, pp. 1660–1670, 2012.

[38] J. Belinha, R. M. N. Jorge, and L. M. J. S. Dinis, "A meshless microscale bone tissue trabecular remodelling analysis considering a new anisotropic bone tissue material law," *Computer Methods in Biomechanics and Biomedical Engineering*, pp. 1–15, 2012.

[39] K. i. Tsubota, S. Wada, and T. Yamaguchi, "Particle method for computer simulation of red blood cell motion in blood flow," *Computer Methods and Programs in Biomedicine*, vol. 83, pp. 139–146, 2006.

[40] J. P. Geng, K. B. C. Tan, and G. R. Liu, "Application of finite element analysis in implant dentistry: A review of the literature," *Journal of Prosthetic Dentistry*, vol. 85, pp. 585–598, 2001.

[41] G. Meriç, E. Erkmen, A. Kurt, Y. Tunç, and A. Eser, "Influence of prosthesis type and material on the stress distribution in bone around implants: A 3-dimensional finite element analysis," *Journal of Dental Sciences*, vol. 6, pp. 25–32, 2011.

[42] R. Sorrentino, R. Aversa, V. Ferro, T. Auriemma, F. Zarone, M. Ferrari, and A. Apicella, "Three-dimensional finite element analysis of strain and stress distributions in endodontically treated maxillary central incisors restored with diferent post, core and crown materials," *Dental Materials*, vol. 23, pp. 983–993, 2007.

[43] R. L. Hardy, "Theory and applications of the multiquadric-biharmonic method 20 years of discovery 1968–1988," *Computers and Mathematics with Applications*, vol. 19, pp. 163–208, 1990.

[44] O. Kayaba°i, E. Yüzbasioglu, and F. Erzincanli, "Static, dynamic and fatigue behaviors of dental implant using finite element method," *Advances in Engineering Software*, vol. 37, pp. 649–658, 2006.

[45] G. Meriç, E. Erkmen, A. Kurt, A. Eser, and G. Çelik, "Biomechanical evaluation of a fiber-reinforced composite prosthesis supported by implants with and without a microthread collar design," *Journal of Dental Sciences*, vol. 5, pp. 201–208, 2010.

[46] D. Lin, Q. Li, W. Li, and M. Swain, "Dental implant induced bone remodeling and associated algorithms," *Journal of the Mechanical Behavior of Biomedical Materials*, vol. 2, pp. 410–432, 2009.

[47] D. Lin, Q. Li, W. Li, N. Duckmanton, and M. Swain, "Mandibular bone remodeling induced by dental implant," *Journal of Biomechanics*, vol. 43, pp. 287–293, 2010.

[48] D. Bozkaya, S. Muftu, and A. Muftu, "Evaluation of load transfer characteristics of five different implants in compact bone at different load levels by finite elements analysis," *Journal of Prosthetic Dentistry*, vol. 92, pp. 523–530, 2004.

Biodental Engineering II – Natal Jorge et al (Eds)
© 2014 Taylor & Francis Group, London, ISBN 978-1-138-00131-2

Mandible bone tissue remodelling analysis using a new numerical approach

J. Belinha
Mechanical Engineering Institute (IDMEC), Porto, Portugal

L.M.J.S. Dinis & R.M. Natal Jorge
Engineering Faculty of Oporto University (FEUP), Mechanical Engineering Department, Porto, Portugal

ABSTRACT: Based on deformation energy methods a topology optimization model was developed for predicting bone density distribution on the mandible bone due the insertion of dental implants. The bone structure is assumed to be a self-optimizing anisotropic biological material which maximizes its own structural stiffness. A recently developed mathematical law for the biologic behaviour of the bone anisotropic material is assumed, based on experimental data available in the literature. This mathematical law permits to correlate the bone density with the obtained level of stress. The numerical method used in the analysis is the Natural Neighbour Radial Point Interpolator Method (NNRPIM), an efficient and flexible meshless method, presenting various advantages in the topologic analysis comparing with other numerical methods such as the Finite Element Method.

1 INTRODUCTION

The bone tissue is a live regenerating and adapting tissue. During life the bone tissue continuously experience reinforce and resorption phenomenon, adapting the internal microstructure and the external shape to the surrounding stress conditions [1]. The first to suggest that there was a direct relation between the bone micro microstructure and the applied external mechanical load was Julius Wolff. The Wolff's Law [2] established that trabecular (or cancellous) bone tends to be aligned with the principal stress directions. In the attempt to write new mathematical laws that explain the bone remodelling mechanism many other models have been developed. The "Theory of Adaptive Elasticity" [3] was probably the first complete consistent model, in which the authors assumed that strain controls the variation of bone apparent density, which is defined as mass per bulk volume of porous tissue, and consequently the bone elastic properties. Many further isotropic models have follow [4–6]. Initially these models developed for predicting trabecular architecture were based on the hypothesis that cancellous bone is a self-optimizing biological material seeking to maximize its own structural design [4, 7, 8]. The relationship between the bone mass and the local strain values in the bone tissue was obtained by minimizing the local strain-energy density (SDE), the objective remodelling function. More recently others have developed anisotropic models [9, 10], which are more close to reality as have been widely observed and measured experimentally [11, 12].

Many experimental studies show that the bone mechanical properties depend on the bone composition and on the bone porosity (directly related with the bone density) [11, 13–17]. In this work the bone properties are approximated with a new law, which is based in the experimental curve obtained in the work of Zioupos [18] and the Lotz law [19]. The bone process of microstructural change is known as "bone remodelling" process, which can be divided in two distinguishable processes, as "internal remodelling", where only the change in the distribution of the material properties is considered, or as "external remodelling", in which the analyses changes the external geometry. Bone remodelling, that has been extensively studied with finite element (FEM) analysis [4, 20–24].

The FEM, as it is well-known, depends strongly on the mesh properties. However, to compute problems with irregular complex geometries by using these methods, mesh generation is a far more time consuming and expensive task than the actual solution of the partial differential equations (PDEs). Considering the difficulty of FEM in the mesh generation, a new numerical method, meshless method (also called meshfree method), has been under fast development in recent years [25, 26]. In the meshless methods the nodes can be arbitrarily distributed, since the field functions are approximated within an influence domain rather than in an element. As opposed to the no-overlap rule between elements in the FEM, in meshless methods the influence domains may and must overlap each other. Meshless methods can be classified in two categories, a first category that pursues the weak form solution and another that seeks the strong form solution. In the first category the meshless methods can be once more divided, the ones that use approximation functions [27–30] and others that use interpolation functions. An immediate consequence of using approximation functions instead of interpolation functions is the lack of the delta Kronecker property, which makes more difficult the imposition of the essential and natural boundary conditions.

To address the above problem several new meshless methods, using interpolation functions, were developed in the last few years, the Point Interpolation Method (PIM) [31, 32], the Point Assembly Method [33], the Natural Neighbour Finite Elements Method (NNFEM) [34, 35], or Natural Element Method (NEM) [36–39] and the Meshless Finite Element Method (MFEM) [40].

The NEM is at the moment, possibly, one of the most popular and discussed meshless method. In the NEM the trial and test functions are constructed using natural neighbour interpolants [41], and its construction relies on geometrical and mathematical concepts such as the Voronoï diagrams [42] and the Delaunay tessellation [43]. In the PIM the interpolation function is obtained based on a polynomial basis, its construction is simple and its derivatives are easily obtained. Substituting the polynomial basis by radial basis function (RBF) the Radial Point Interpolation Method (RPIM) [44, 45] is created. In these early works, the used RBFs were the Gaussian and the multiquadric radial basis functions. The RBF was firstly used for data surface fitting, and later the RBF was used for solving partial differential equations [46] and to solve several engineering problems [47–50]. However the RPIM uses, unlike Kansa's algorithm, the concept of "influence domain" instead of "global domain", generating sparse and banded stiffness matrices, more adequate to complex geometry problems. An inconvenient property of the RPIMs interpolation functions is the lack of compatibility, which is achieved using the conforming RPIM (CRPIM) [51]. Studies on CRPIM and RPIM have concluded that CRPIM can exactly pass the standard patch tests and the RPIM can not [51, 52]. However, for the problems considered in the studies, the RPIM lead to satisfactory results, was also convergent, simpler and much more efficient than the CRPIM [26, 51].

Another important issue is the need of a background mesh for integration purposes. In fact a meshless method is not a truly mesh free method, if it relies on a secondary background integration mesh. Nevertheless the general idea [52] is that truly meshless methods, methods that do not require any mesh at all, are less stable and less accurate.

In this bone remodelling analysis is performed resorting to the Natural Neighbour Radial Point Interpolation Method – NNRPIM [53]. Resorting to Voronoï cells, a set of influence cells are created departing from an unstructured set of nodes. The Delaunay triangulation concept is used to create a node-dependent background mesh used in the numerical integration of the NNRPIM interpolation functions. Unlike the FEM, where geometrical restrictions on elements are imposed for the convergence of the method, in the NNRPIM there are no such restrictions, which permits a random node distribution for the discretized problem. The NNRPIM interpolation functions, used in the Galerkin weak form, are constructed in a similar process to the RPIM, with some differences that modify the method's performance. Although the NNRPIM is a recent developed meshless method it has been extended to many fields of the computational mechanics, such as the analysis of isotropic and orthotropic plates [54], the functionally graded material plate analysis [55], the 3D shell-like approach [56, 57], the dynamic analysis of several solid-mechanic problems [58], the material non-linearity analysis [59] and the large deformation analysis [60].

More recently the NNRPIM was extended to the bone tissue remodelling analysis. A SED based remodelling algorithm combined with the NNRPIM was proposed in [61] to predict the trabecular bone architecture. The success of the approach permitted to obtain results very close with the clinical cases [62] of the femur bone and the calcaneus bone internal trabecular structure.

2 NNRPIM: A GENERAL REVIEW

The Natural Neighbour concept [63] is used in the NNRPIM, where natural neighbour nodes are determined using the Voronoï diagrams and the Delaunay triangulation. Consider a set **N** of N distinct nodes $N = \{n_1, n_2, \ldots, n_N\} \in \mathbb{R}^3$, the Voronoï diagram of **N** is the partition of the domain defined by **N** in sub-regions V_I, closed and convex. Each sub-region V_I is associated with the node I, n_I, in a way that any point in the interior of the V_I is closer to n_I than any other node n_J, where $n_J \in N$ $(J \neq I)$. The sub-regions V_k are defined as "Voronoï cells" which form the Voronoï diagram, $k = 1, \ldots, N$. The Delaunay triangulation is constructed by connecting the nodes whose Voronoï cells have common boundaries. The relation between the Voronoï diagram and the Delaunay triangulation implies that a Delaunay edge exists between two nodes in the plane if and only if their Voronoï cells share a common edge. The NNRPIM [53] uses the Voronoï diagram to create the "influence-cells", where overlap enforces the connectivity between the nodes in **N**. The two distinct types of influence-cells presented in figure 1(a) are defined as: (1) A point of interest, $\mathbf{x}_I$, searches for its neighbour nodes following the Natural Neighbour Voronoï construction. Thus the *first degree influence-cell* is composed by these first natural neighbours; (2) A point of interest, $\mathbf{x}_I$, searches for its neighbour nodes, in the same manner as in the *first degree influence-cell*. Then, based on a previous construction of the Voronoï diagram for the node mesh, the natural neighbours of the first natural neighbours of $\mathbf{x}_I$ are added to the influence-cell. Thus the *second*

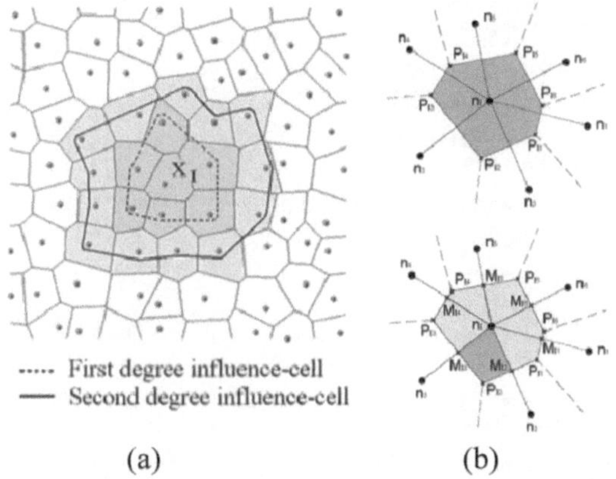

Figure 1. (a) Influence cells representation, (b) Voronoï cell and the corresponding PIi intersection points and Middle points MIi and the respective generated quadrilaterals.

degree influence-cell is composed by these sets of natural neighbours. The duality between the Voronoï cells and the Delaunay triangles is used in order to construct a nodal dependent background integration mesh [53] Using the above referred constructions small areas are established. Then, with the construction of the Voronoï cells, V_I, the intersection points, P_{Ii}, of the neighbour edges of V_I can be settled, figure 1(b). Afterwards the middle points, M_{Ii}, between node I and its neighbour nodes are obtained. Thus the Voronoï cells are divided in n quadrilateral sub-cells, S_{Ii}, as figure 1(b) indicates. For instance the sub-cell S_{I2} is defined by the quadrilateral $\overline{M_{I2}\,P_{I2}\,M_{I3}\,n_I}$. Any Voronoï cell, V_I, with n neighbour nodes of the central node I has n sub-cells, S_{Ii}, where,

$$A_{V_I} = \sum_{i=1}^{n} A_{S_{Ii}},\ \forall A_{S_{Ii}} \geq 0 \tag{1}$$

being A_{V_I} the Voronoï cell area and $A_{S_{Ii}}$ the subcell area. If the set of Voronoï cells are a partition, without gaps, of the global domain then, the set of subcells are also a partition, without gaps, of the global domain. Using these sub-cells, which are constructed as it is methodically shown in [53], several integration schemes based on the Gauss-Legendre numerical integration can be obtained.

In [53] was found that the more efficient integration scheme is the one that uses only one quadrature point in each sub-cell and that the type of "influence-cell" that produces more accurate and stable results is the second degree influence-cell. Consider a function $\mathbf{u}(\mathbf{x})$ defined in the domain Ω, which is discretized by a set of N nodes. In the NNRPIM the function $\mathbf{u}(\mathbf{x})$ passes through all nodes using a radial basis function. It is assumed that only the nodes within the influence-cell of the point of interest $\mathbf{x}_I$ have effect on $\mathbf{u}(\mathbf{x}_I)$. The value of function $\mathbf{u}(\mathbf{x}_I)$ at the point of interest $\mathbf{x}_I$ is obtained by,

$$\mathbf{u}(\mathbf{x}_I) = \sum_{i=1}^{n} R_i(\mathbf{x}_I)\, a_i(\mathbf{x}_I) = \mathbf{R}^T(\mathbf{x}_I)\, \mathbf{a} \tag{2}$$

here $R_i(\mathbf{x}_I)$ is the radial basis function (RBF) $R^T(\mathbf{x}_I) = \{R_1(\mathbf{x}_I), R_2(\mathbf{x}_I), \ldots, R_n(\mathbf{x}_I)\}$, n is the number of nodes inside the influence-cell of $\mathbf{x}_I$. The coefficients $a_i(\mathbf{x}_I)$ are non constant coefficients of $R_i(\mathbf{x}_I)$, defined as $\mathbf{a}^T(\mathbf{x}_I) = \{a_1(\mathbf{x}_I), a_2(\mathbf{x}_I), \ldots, a_n(\mathbf{x}_I)\}$. Originally the Radial Point Interpolator functions, in addition to the RBF, used a polynomial basis [44] in equation (2), however it was recently found [53] that the removal of the polynomial basis from the formulation conducts to more accurate results and to an increase of efficiency, lower computational cost and faster convergence rates. In the RBF the variable is the distance r_{Ii} between the relevant node $\mathbf{x}_I$ and the neighbour node $\mathbf{x}_i$, $r_{Ii} = \sqrt{(x_I - x_i)^2 + (y_I - y_i)^2}$. The present work uses the Multiquadric (MQ) function proposed initially by Hardy [64],

$$R(r_{Ii}) = \left(r_{Ii}^{\ 2} + c^2\right)^p \tag{3}$$

where c and p are two parameters which can be optimized as it can be found in [64]. Therefore a new equation can be written,

$$\mathbf{u}_s = \mathbf{R}_Q\ \mathbf{a} \tag{4}$$

where,

$$\mathbf{u}_s = \{u_1, u_2, \ldots, u_n\}^T \tag{5}$$

$$\mathbf{R}_Q = \begin{bmatrix} R(r_{11}) & R(r_{21}) & .. & R(r_{1n}) \\ R(r_{21}) & R(r_{22}) & .. & R(r_{2n}) \\ \vdots & \vdots & & \vdots \\ R(r_{n1}) & R(r_{n2}) & .. & R(r_{nn}) \end{bmatrix} \tag{6}$$

It must be noted that the geometric matrix $\mathbf{R}_Q$ is a symmetric matrix because the distance is direction independent, i.e., $R(r_{ij}) = R(r_{ji})$. By substituting in equation (2),

$$\mathbf{u}(\mathbf{x}_I) = \mathbf{R}^T(\mathbf{x}_I)\ \mathbf{R}_Q^{-1}\ \mathbf{u}_s = \varphi(\mathbf{x}_I)\mathbf{u}_s \tag{7}$$

where $\varphi(\mathbf{x})$ is the interpolation function defined as,

$$\begin{aligned}\varphi(\mathbf{x}_I) &= \mathbf{R}^T(\mathbf{x}_I)\ \mathbf{R}_Q^{-1} = \\ &= \{\varphi_1(\mathbf{x}_I), \varphi_2(\mathbf{x}_I), \ldots, \varphi_n(\mathbf{x}_I)\}\end{aligned} \tag{8}$$

The partial derivative of $\varphi(\mathbf{x})$ in order to a variable ξ is defined as

$$\varphi_{,\xi}(\mathbf{x}_I) = \mathbf{R}_{,\xi}^T(\mathbf{x}_I)\ \mathbf{R}_Q^{-1} \tag{9}$$

The partial derivatives of the MQ-RBF in order to ξ are

$$\mathbf{R}_{,\xi}(r_{ij}) = 2p\left(r_{ij}^2 + c^2\right)^{p-1}\left(\xi_j - \xi_i\right) \tag{10}$$

Early works on the RPIM [44] prove that these interpolation functions possess the delta Kronecker property and also that the partition of unity is satisfied.

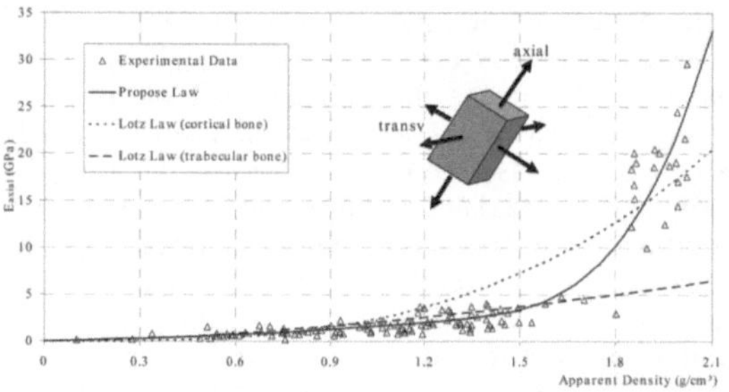

Figure 2. Elasticity Modulus from the apparent density correlation.

3 MATERIAL LAW

The recent experimental work of Zioupos [18] reinforces the idea that the bone apparent density is an important bone property, which influences directly the mechanical properties of the bone tissue. Through apparent density measurements, this experimental study was able to objectively isolate the bone tissue in the trabecular and cortical form. The results obtained by Zioupos, figure 2, show that the relation between the bone apparent density and the bone elasticity modulus is a curve with a boomerang shape, instead a monotonic function.

The Zioupos experimental work shows that the mathematical law governing the trabecular bone is the same governing the cortical bone. Following Zioupos conclusions it was determined an unified curve for both bone structures (trabecular and cortical), figure 2. The proposed curve [61, 62] presents a 95% correlation with Zioupos experimental data.

4 REMODELLING ALGORITHM

The remodelling algorithm considered in the architectural optimization analysis of bone tissue with the NNRPIM is an adaptation of Carter's remodelling algorithm [20]. It is based on the assumption that the adaptation of bony tissue responds mainly to mechanical stimulus, acting as driving forces in the remodelling process, which can be suitably described by stress and/or strain measures. The local density and material orientation is dependent on the stress/strain field caused by the mechanical load. A forward Euler scheme is implemented, resulting in the iterative remodelling process illustrated in figure 3.

5 MODEL

The efficiency of the proposed algorithm was validated with the analysis of a transversal section of the manbible bone, in which was inserted a dental implant, figure 4. The essential and natural boundary conditions are presented in figure 5.

The imposed boundary conditions follow the suggestion in the literature. The remodelling analysis

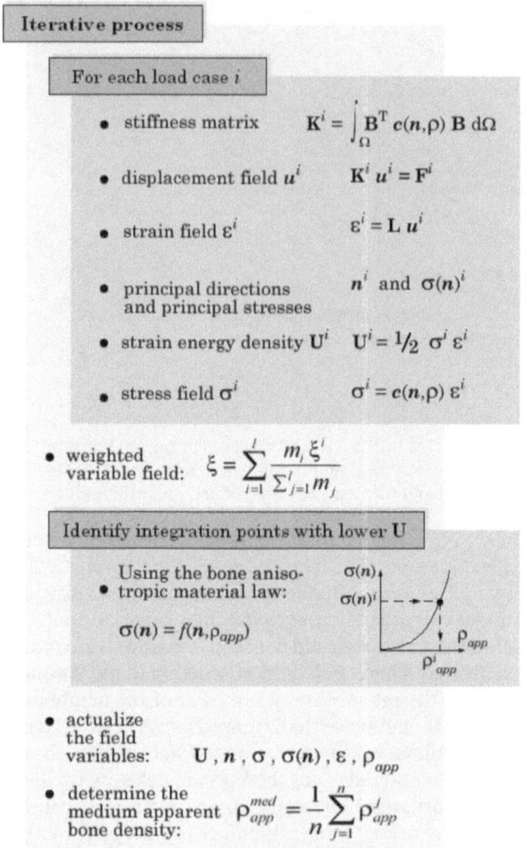

Figure 3. Bone remodelling algorithm.

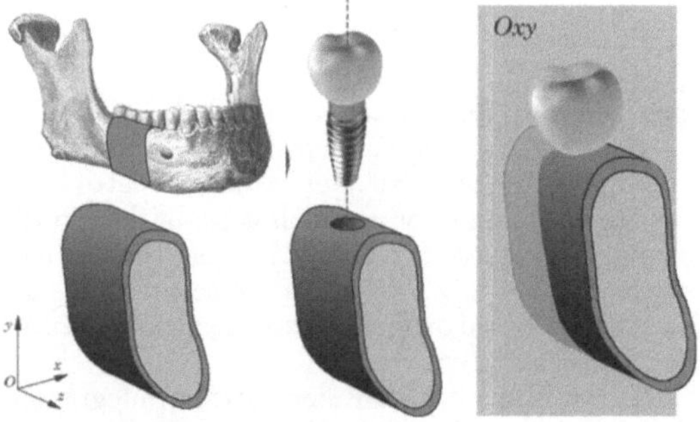

Figure 4. Studied model.

results, figure 6, show that obtained trabecular architecture is very similar with the clinical cases and other numerical approaches.

6 CONCLUSIONS

This work the Natural Neighbour Radial Point Interpolation Method (NNRPIM) was extended to the bone remodelling analysis of the mandible bone due the insertion of dental implants. The results validate the

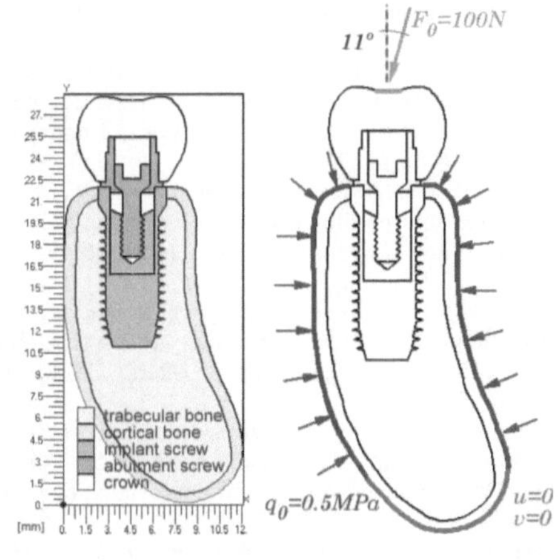

Figure 5. Final 2D model.

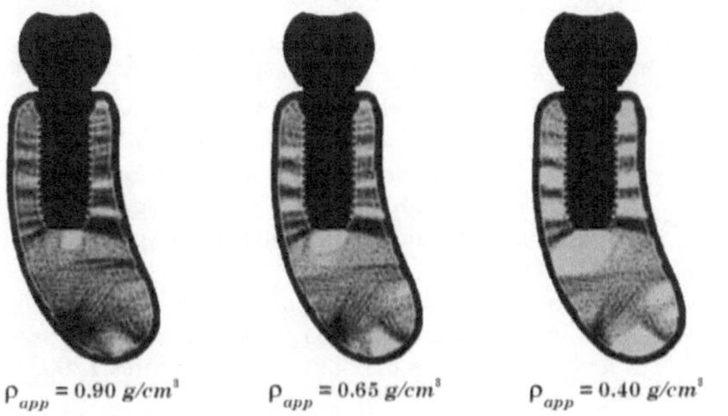

Figure 6. Mandible remodelling.

proposed bone remodelling algorithm, which can be useful, in the near future, to predict the correct loads that should be applied in the dental implant, in order to maximize the mandible bone density in the implant vicinity.

ACKNOWLEDGEMENTS

The authors truly acknowledge the funding provided by Ministério da Ciência, Tecnologia e Ensino Superior – Fundação para a Ciência e a Tecnologia (Portugal), under grant SFRH/BPD/75072/2010, and by FEDER/FSE, under grant PTDC/EME-TME/098050/2008.

REFERENCES

[1] van der Meulen M.C.H. and Huiskes R., *Why mechanobiology?: A survey article.* Journal of Biomechanics, (2002). **35**(4): p. 401–414.

[2] Wolff J., *The Law of Bone Remodeling (Das Gesetzder Transformationder Knochen, Hirschwald,1892).* (1986), Berlin Heidelberg New York: Springer.

[3] Cowin S.C. and Hegedus D.H., *Bone remodeling I: A theory of adaptive elasticity.* Journal of Elasticity, (1976). **6**: p. 313–326.

[4] Huiskes R., Weinans H., Grootenboer H.J., Dalstra M., Fudala B., and Sloof T.J.J.H., *Adaptive bone-remodeling theory applied to prosthetic-design analysis.* Journal of Biomechanics, (1987). **20**(11–12): p. 1135–1150.

[5] Carter D.R., Orr T.E., and Fyhrie D.P., *Relationship between loadingt history and femoral cancellous bone architecture.* Journal of Biomechanics, (1989). **22**(3): p. 231–244.

[6] Beaupré G.S., Orr T.E., and Carter D.R., *An approach for timedependent bone modelling and remodelling. Theoretical development.* Journal of Orthopaedic Research, (1990). **8**(5): p. 651–661.

[7] Pettermann H., Reiter T., and Rammerstorfer F.G., *Computational simulation of internal bone remodeling.* Archives in Computational Methods in Engineering, (1997). **4**(4): p. 295–323.

[8] Prendergast P.J., *Finite element models in tissue mechanics and orthopaedic implant design.* Clinical Biomechanics, (1997). **12**(6): p. 343–366.

[9] Doblaré M. and García J.M., *Anisotropic bone remodelling model based on a continuum damage-repair theory.* Journal of Biomechanics, (2002). **35**(1): p. 1–17.

[10] Jacobs C.R., Simo J.C., Beaupré G.S., and Carter D.R., *Adaptive bone remodeling incorporating simultaneous density and anisotropy considerations.* Journal of Biomechanics, (1997). **30**(6): p. 603–613.

[11] Carter D.R. and Hayes W.C., *The compressive behavior of bone as a two phase porous structure.* Journal of Bone and Joint Surgery, (1977). **59**(A): p. 954–962.

[12] Cowin S.C., *Optimisation of the strain energy density in linear anisotropic elasticity.* Journal of Elasticity, (1994). **34**: p. 45–68.

[13] Carter D.R. and Spengler D.M., *Mechanical properties and composition of cortical bone.* Clinical Orthopaedics and Related Research, (1978). **135**: p. 192–217.

[14] Gibson L.J., *The mechanical behaviour of cancellous bone.* Journal of Biomechanics, (1985). **18**: p. 317–328.

[15] Goldstein S.A., *The mechanical properties of trabecular bone: dependence on anatomic location and function.* Journal of Biomechanics, (1987). **20**: p. 1055–1061.

[16] Rice J.C., Cowin S.C., and Bowman J.A., *On the dependence of the elasticity and strength of cancellous bone on apparent density.* Journal of Biomechanics, (1988). **21**(2): p. 155–168.

[17] Martin R.B., *Determinants of the mechanical properties of bones.* Journal of Biomechanics, (1991). **24**(1): p. 79–88.

[18] Zioupos P., Cook R.B., and Hutchinsonc J.R., *Some basic relationships between density values in cancellous and cortical bone.* Journal of Biomechanics, (2008). **41**: p. 1961–1968.

[19] Lotz J.C., Gerhart T.N., and Hayes W.C., *Mechanical properties of metaphyseal bone in the proximal femur.* Journal of Biomechanics, (1991). **24**(5): p. 317–329.

[20] Carter D.R., Fyhrie D.P., and Whalen R.T., *Trabecular bone density and loading history: regulation of connective tissue biology by mechanical energy.* Journal of Biomechanics, (1987). **20**(8): p. 785–794.

[21] Beaupré G.S., Orr T.E., and Carter D.R., *An approach for timedependent bone modelling and remodelling. A preliminary remodelling simulation.* Journal of Orthopaedic Research, (1990). **8**(5): p. 662–670.

[22] Weinans H., Huiskes R., and Grootenboer H.J., *The behaviour of adaptive bone-remodelling simulation models.* Journal of Biomechanics, (1992). **25**(12): p. 1425–1441.

[23] Jacobs C.R., Levenston M.E., Beaupre G.S., Simo J.C., and Carter D.R., *Numerical instabilities in bone remodelling simulations: the advantages of a node-based finite element approach.* Journal of Biomechanics, (1995). **28**(4): p. 449–459.

[24] Rossi J.M. and Wendling-Mansuy S., *A topology optimization based model of bone adaptation.* Computer Methods in Biomechanics and Biomedical Engineering, (2007). **10**(6): p. 419–427.

[25] Belytschko T., Krongauz Y., Organ D., Fleming M., and Krysl P., *Meshless Methods: an overview and recent developments.* Computer Methods in Applied Mechanics and Engineering, (1996). **139**(1): p. 3–47.

[26] Gu Y.T., *Meshfree methods and their comparisons.* International Journal of Computational Methods, (2005). **2**(4): p. 477–515.

[27] Atluri S.N. and Zhu T., *A new meshless local Petrov-Galerkin (MLPG) approach in computational mechanics.* Computational Mechanics, (1998). **22**(2): p. 117–127.

[28] Monaghan J.J., *Smoothed Particle Hydrodynamics: Theory and Applications to Non-Spherical Stars.* Monthly Notices of the Astronomical Society, (1977). **181**: p. 375–389.

[29] Belytschko T., Lu Y.Y., and Gu L., *Element-Free Galerkin Method.* International Journal for Numerical Methods in Engineering, (1994). **37**: p. 229–256.

[30] Liu W.K., Jun S., and Zhang Y.F., *Reproducing Kernel Particle Methods.* International Journal for Numerical Methods in Fluids, (1995). **20**(6): p. 1081–1106.

[31] Liu G.R. and Gu Y.T., *A Point Interpolation Method for Two-Dimensional Solids.* International Journal for Numerical Methods in Engineering, (2001). **50**: p. 937–951.

[32] Liu G.R., Dai K.Y., Lim K.M., and Gu Y.T., *A point interpolation meshfree method for static and frequency analysis of two-dimensional piezoelectric structures.* Computational Mechanics, (2002). **29**(6): p. 510–519.

[33] Liu G.R., *A Point Assembly Method for Stress Analysis for Two-Dimensional Solids.* International Journal of Solid and Structures, (2002). **39**: p. 261–276.

[34] Traversoni L., *Natural Neighbour Finite Elements.* Int. Conf. on Hydraulic Engineering Software, Hydrosoft Proc., Computational Mechanics Publications, (1994). **2**: p. 291–297.

[35] Sukumar N., Moran B., and Belytschko T., *The natural element method in solid mechanics.* International Journal for Numerical Methods in Engineering, (1998). **43**(5): p. 839–887.

[36] Braun J. and Sambridge M., *A numerical method for solving partial differential equations on highly irregular evolving grids.* Nature, (1995). **376**: p. 655–660.

[37] Sukumar N., Moran B., Semenov A.Y., and Belikov V.V., *Natural neighbour Galerkin methods.* International Journal for Numerical Methods in Engineering, (2001). **50**(1): p. 1–27.

[38] Cueto E., Doblaré M., and Gracia L., *Imposing essential boundary conditions in the natural element method by means of density-scaled-shapes.* International Journal for Numerical Methods in Engineering, (2000). **49**(4): p. 519–546.

[39] Cueto E., Sukumar N., Calvo B., Cegoñino J., and Doblaré M., *Overview and recent advances in the Natural Neighbour Galerkin Method.* Archives of Computational Methods in Engineering, (2003). **10**(4): p. 307–387.

[40] Sergio R., Idelsohn S., Oñate E., Calvo N., and Del Pin F., *The Meshless Finite Element Method.* International Journal for Numerical Methods in Engineering, (2003). **58**(6): p. 893–912.

[41] Sibson R., *A brief description of natural neighbor interpolation.* Interpreting Multivariate Data, in V. Barnett (ed.), (Wiley, Chichester), (1981): p. 21–36.

[42] Voronoï G.M., *Nouvelles applications des paramètres continus à la théorie des formes quadratiques.* Deuxième Mémoire: Recherches sur les parallélloèdres primitifs, J. Reine Angew. Math., (1908). **134**: p. 198–287.

[43] Delaunay B., *Sur la sphére vide. A la memoire de Georges Voronoï.* Izv. Akad. Nauk SSSR, Otdelenie Matematicheskih i Estestvennyh Nauk, (1934). **7**: p. 793–800.

[44] Wang J.G. and Liu G.R., *A Point Interpolation Meshless Method based on Radial Basis Functions.* International Journal for Numerical Methods in Engineering, (2002). **54**: p. 1623–1648.

[45] Wang J.G. and Liu G.R., *On the Optimal Shape Parameters of Radial Basis Functions used for 2-D Meshless Methods.* Computer Methods in Applied Mechanics and Engineering, (2002). **191**: p. 2611–2630.

[46] Kansa E.J., *A scattered data approximation scheme with applications to computational fluid-dynamics – I & II.* Computers and Mathematics with Applications, (1990). **19**: p. 127–161.

[47] Ferreira A.J.M., *A formulation of the multiquadric radial basis function method for the analysis of laminated composite plates.* Composite Structures, (2003). **59**(3): p. 385–392.

[48] Ferreira A.J.M., Roque C.M.C., Jorge R.M.N., and Kansa E.J., *Static deformations and vibration analysis of composite and sandwich plates using a layerwise theory and multiquadrics discretizations.* Engineering Analysis with Boundary Elements, (2005). **29**(12): p. 1104–1114.

[49] Ferreira A.J.M., Roque C.M.C., and M. P.A.L.S., *Analysis of composite plates using higher-order shear deformation theory and a finite point formulation based on the multiquadric radial basis function method.* Composites Part B: Engineering, (2003). **34**(7): p. 627–636.

[50] Tiago C.M. and Leitão V.M.A., *Application of radial basis functions to linear and nonlinear structural analysis problems.* Computers & Mathematics with Applications, (2006). **51**(8): p. 1311–1334.

[51] Liu G.R., Gu Y.T., and Dai K.Y., *Assessment and applications of interpolation methods for computational mechanics.* International Journal for Numerical Methods in Engineering, (2004). **59**: p. 1373–1379.

[52] Liu G.R., *Mesh Free Methods, Moving beyond the Finite Element Method.* (2002): CRC Press.

[53] Dinis L., Jorge R.N., and Belinha J., *Analysis of 3D solids using the natural neighbour radial point interpolation method.* Computer Methods in Applied Mechanics and Engineering, (2007). **196**: p. 2009–2028.

[54] Dinis L., Jorge R.N., and Belinha J., *Analysis of plates and laminates using the natural neighbour radial point interpolation method.* Engineering Analysis with Boundary Elements, (2008). **32**: p. 267–279.

[55] Dinis L., Jorge R.N., and Belinha J., *An Unconstrained Third-Order Plate Theory applied to Functionally Graded Plates using a Meshless Method.*

Mechanics of Advanced Materials and Structures, (2010). **17**: p. 1–26.
[56] Dinis L., Jorge R.N., and Belinha J., *A 3D Shell-Like approach using a Natural Neighbour Meshless Method: isotropic and orthotropic thin structures.* Composite Structures, (2009)(doi:10.1016/j.compstruct.2009.10.014).
[57] Dinis L., Jorge R.N., and Belinha J., *Composite Laminated Plates: A 3D natural neighbour radial point interpolation method approach.* Journal of Sandwich Structures and Materials, (2010). **12**(2): p. 119–138.
[58] Dinis L., Jorge R.N., and Belinha J., *The Natural Neighbour Radial Point Interpolation Method: Dynamic Applications.* Engeneering Computations, (2009). **26**(8): p. 911–949.
[59] Dinis L., Jorge R.N., and Belinha J., *Radial Natural Neighbours Interpolators: 2D and 3D Elastic and Elastoplastic Applications*, in *Progress on Meshless Methods – Computational Methods in Applied Sciences*, Ferreira A.J.M., et al., Editors. (2008), Springer.
[60] Dinis L., Jorge R.N., and Belinha J., *Large Deformation Applications with the Radial Natural Neighbours Interpolators.* Computer Modelling in Engineering and Sciences, (2009). **44**(1): p. 1–34.
[61] Belinha J., Jorge R.M.N., and Dinis L.M.J.S., *A meshless microscale bone tissue trabecular remodelling analysis considering a new anisotropic bone tissue material law.* Computer Methods in Biomechanics and Biomedical Engineering, 2012: p. 10.1080/10255842.2012.654783.
[62] Belinha J., Jorge R.M.N., and Dinis L.M.J.S., *Bone tissue remodelling analysis considering a radial point interpolator meshless method.* Engineering Analysis with Boundary Elements, 2012: p. http://dx.doi.org/10.1016/j.enganabound.2012.05.009.
[63] Sibson R., *A vector identity for the Dirichlet tesselation.* Mathematical Proceedings of the Cambridge Philosophical Society, (1980). **87**: p. 151–155.
[64] Hardy R.L., *Theory and applications of the multiquadrics – Biharmonic method (20 years of discovery 1968–1988).* Computers and Mathematics with Applications, (1990). **19**: p. 127–161.

Biodental Engineering II – Natal Jorge et al (Eds)
© 2014 Taylor & Francis Group, London, ISBN 978-1-138-00131-2

A meshless method analysis of maxillary central incisor

S.F. Moreira
Engineering Faculty of Oporto University (FEUP), Mechanical Engineering Department, Porto, Portugal

J. Belinha
Mechanical Engineering Institute (IDMEC), Porto, Portugal

L.M.J.S. Dinis & R.M. Natal Jorge
Engineering Faculty of Oporto University (FEUP), Mechanical Engineering Department, Porto, Portugal

1 INTRODUCTION

The meshless methods [1] have been stated as a numerical alternative to the Finite Element Methods (FEM) [2], allowing to solve and analyze problems with complex geometries with a less computing time [1, 3]. Distinct of FEM, in meshless methods the domain of the problem is discretized in a nodal mesh and the nodal connectivity is obtained by influence domains which, unlike the elements in FEM, may and should overlap. In fact, it is this overlap and the choice of the influence domains that allow meshless methods to achieve good results, even with very irregular nodal meshes. In this work it is intended to analyze the behavior of an innovative meshless method in the elastostatic analysis of the maxillary central incisor. In order to do that, a two dimensional model, obtained based on the literature [4], was used. In this case, the numerical method used for the bone tissue remodeling analysis is the Natural Neighbour Radial Point Interpolator Method (NNRPIM), [5, 6], an efficient and flexible meshless method, presenting various numerical advantages when compared with other numerical methods such as the Finite Element Methods (FEM), and presenting a stress field more accurate and smooth when compared with the FEM [5].

2 RESULTS AND DISCUSSION

The computational model used in this work, represented in Figure 1, was obtained with the data available in the literature from a computerized axial tomography (CAT) scan performed by Poiate et al. [4]. With the CAT scan it was possible the segmentation of the anatomic structure, allowing this way the extraction of the upper central incisor model.

After the model definition it was possible to proceed to the construction of the nodal mesh. In this case it was constructed a nodal mesh with 4387 nodes. The essential and natural boundary conditions represented in Figure 2 were imposed in the computational model.

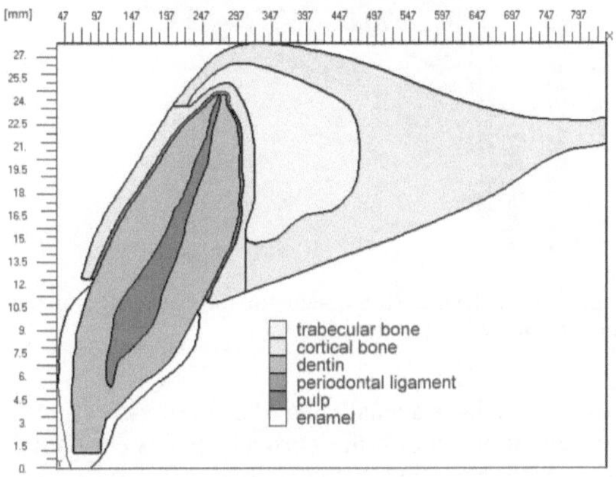

Figure 1. Complete maxillary central incisive set for the two dimensional analysis.

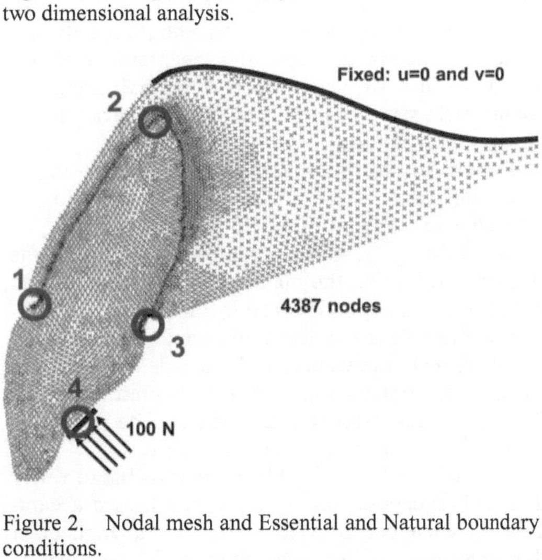

Figure 2. Nodal mesh and Essential and Natural boundary conditions.

The 100 N load was applied in the incisor inner surface with a 45 degree angle.

In Figure 2 it is also shown the four regions where the analysis was centered. Note that in the case of the

Table 1. Mechanical properties of the anatomical structures.

Anatomical Structure	Young's Modulus E (GPa)	Poisson's Ratio
Pulp	0.02	0.45
Dentin	18.60	0.31
Enamel	41.00	0.30
Trabecular Bone	1.37	0.30
Cortical Bone	13.70	0.30
Periodontal ligament	0.0689	0.45

Table 2. Stress results obtained for the first stage of the analysis of the central incisor.

Stress σ_{11}	FEM	NNRPIM	Error (%)
Region 1	18.40	19.96	8.50
Region 2	33.80	29.98	11.30
Region 3	68.50	134.01	95.64
Region 4	123.00	123.71	0.58

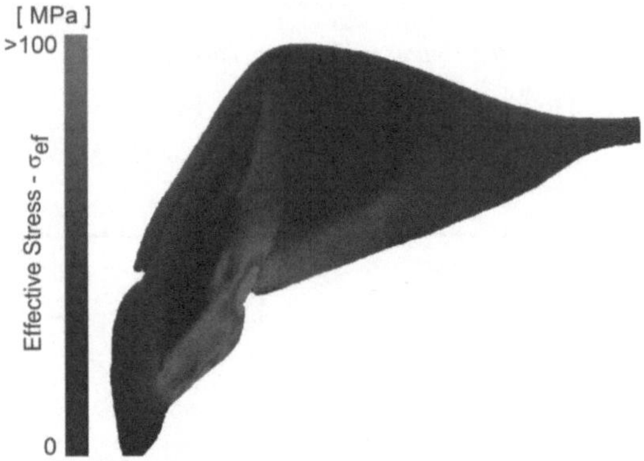

Figure 3. Effective stress field for the first stage of the analysis of the central incisor.

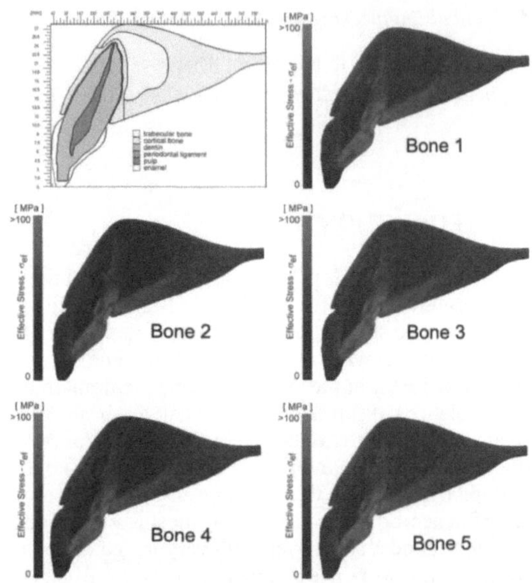

Figure 4. Effective stress field considering five different materials for the cortical and the trabecular bone.

region 1 we have a small area of a compressive stress concentration among the cortical bone, periodontal ligament and dentin structures. Region 3 is very similar to region 1, however, instead of a compressive area we have a small area of tensile stress. Region 2 is also a small area of tensile stress concentration but now, among the dentin structure and the periodontal ligament. At last, we have region 4, a small area of a compressive stress concentration among the dentin ant the enamel structures.

The model analysis involves three distinct stages. Next, each one of the stages is described and the respective results are presented.

In a first stage, the two dimensional model was studied considering the material properties indicated in Poiate et al., [4], referenced in Table 1.

The effective stress distribution map obtained with the NNRPIM is presented in Figure 3. The effective stress results obtained in each interest point indicated in Figure 2 are presented in Table 2. The NNRPIM results are compared with the FEM results.

From the analysis of Table 2 it is possible to verify that with exception for region 3, results are acceptable. In what concerns to region 3, the high error that appeared may be associated to the fact that in that region exists a convex boundary, which reveals a numerical problem not fully solved in the present analysis.

The second stage of the analysis consisted in considering five distinct cases of material properties of for the cortical and the trabecular bone. For that, it was made a bibliographic search [4, 7–10]. With the five distinct material cases for bone tissue material properties selected, the model was analyzed with the NNRPIM for each material case. In Figure 4 are presented the obtained effective stress maps obtained for each analysis.

Observing the results it is possible to visualize the similarity between the distinct obtained effective stress fields. However, a more careful examination of the results allow to conclude that it is Bone Case 2 that presents a higher stress values for Regions 1, 3 and 4. Therefore, in the next stage only the Bone Case 2 material properties are considered for the cortical and trabecular bone tissue material properties.

The third stage of the analysis consisted in the study of the inclusion of restorative materials for the enamel, with the objective of determine which material lead to the most homogeneous stress field. The restorative material properties were obtained in the literature, Table 3, [11]. Recall we are considering the cortical bone and trabecular bone properties that introduce higher stresses in the second stage of the analysis, that is, in the Bone Case 2. In Figure 5 are presented the effective stress maps for the distinct analysis. After

Table 3. Mechanical properties of the restorative materials considered.

Crown Material	Young's Modulus E (GPa)	Poisson's Ratio
Feldspathic Ceramics	69.0000	0.3000
Gradia flow	7.4000	0.2200
Gradia forte	13.0000	0.2200
Natural Enamel	41.0000	0.3000

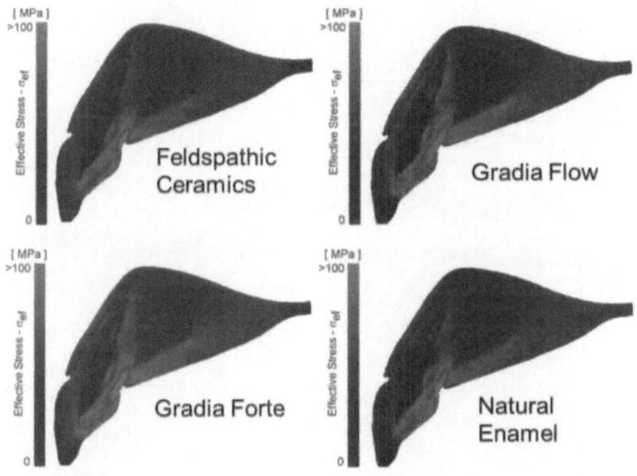

Figure 5. Effective stress field considering different materials for the enamel crown.

studying the obtained results it was concluded that using materials with a lower Young Modulus, as is the case of Gradia Flow and Gradia Forte, leads to a lower stress level in regions 1, 3 and 4. Using materials with higher Young Modulus like Feldspathic Ceramics and the Natural Enamel, considered in the first stage of this analysis, leads to lower values of the effective stress in the region 2.

3 CONCLUSIONS

The results obtained with the NNRPIM shown that meshless methods are a suitable numerical tool to analyse the biomechanical behaviour of dental structures, permitting in the near future the inclusion of more complex assumptions, such the material inelasticity in the periodontal ligament, for example, the large deformations and transient analysis.

However, it is necessary, in a future work, to improve the meshless method nodal connectivity imposition procedure, in order to overcome the numerical problems when convex boundaries are considered.

ACKNOWLEDGEMENT

The authors truly acknowledge the funding provided by Ministério da Ciência, Tecnologia e Ensino Superior – Fundação para a Ciência e a Tecnologia (Portugal), under grant SFRH/BPD/75072/2010, and by FEDER/FSE, under grant PTDC/EME-TME/098050/2008.

REFERENCES

[1] T. Belytschko, Y. Krongauz, D. Organ, M. Fleming, P. Krysl, "Meshless Methods: an overview and recent developments," Computer Methods in Applied Mechanics and Engineering, vol. 139, pp. 3–47, (1996).

[2] B. Nayroles, G. Touzot, and P. Villon, "Generalizing the Finite Element Method: Diffuse Approximation and Diffuse Elements," Computational Mechanics, vol. 10, pp. 307–318, (1992).

[3] Y. T. Gu, "Meshfree methods and their comparisons," International Journal of Computational Methods, vol. 2(4), pp. 477–515, 2005.

[4] I. A. V. P. Poiate, A. B. Vasconcellos, M. Mori, and E. P. Jr., "2D and 3D finite element analysis of central incisor generated by computerized tomography," Computer Methods and Programs in Biomedicine, vol. 104, pp. 292–299, 2011.

[5] L. M. J. S. Dinis, R. M. Natal Jorge, and J. Belinha, "Analysis of 3D solids using the natural neighbour radial point interpolation method," Computer Methods in Applied Mechanics and Engineering, vol. 196, pp. 2009–2028, 2007.

[6] J. Belinha, R. M. N. Jorge, and L. M. J. S. Dinis, "Bone tissue remodelling analysis considering a radial point interpolator meshless method," Engineering Analysis with Boundary Elements, vol. 36(11), pp. 1660–1670, 2012.

[7] L. Baggi, I. Cappelloni, F. Maceri, and G. Vairo, "Stress-based performance evaluation of osseointegrated dental implants by finite-element simulation," Simulation Modelling Practice and Theory, vol. 16, pp. 971–987, 2008.

[8] G. Meriç, E. Erkmen, A. Kurt, A. Eser, and G. Çelik, "Biomechanical evaluation of a fiber-reinforced composite prosthesis supported by implants with and without a microthread collar design," Journal of Dental Sciences, vol. 5, pp. 201–208, 2010.

[9] G. Meriç, E. Erkmen, A. Kurt, Y. Tunç, and A. Eser, "Influence of prosthesis type and material on the stress distribution in bone around implants: A 3-dimensional finite element analysis," Journal of Dental Sciences, vol. 6, pp. 25–32, 2011.

[10] J. Yang and H.-J. Xiang, "A three-dimensional finite element study on the biomechanical behaviour of an FGBM dental implant in surrounding bone," Journal of Biomechanics, pp. 2377–2385, 2007.

[11] R. Sorrentino, R. Aversa, V. Ferro, T. Auriemma, F. Zarone, M. Ferrari, and A. Apicella, "Three-dimensional finite element analysis of strain and stress distributions in endodontically treated maxillary central incisors restores with different post, core and crown materials," Dental Materials, vol. 23, pp. 983–993, 2007.

Biodental Engineering II – Natal Jorge et al (Eds)
© 2014 Taylor & Francis Group, London, ISBN 978-1-138-00131-2

Effects of Hydrogen Peroxide on the inorganic composition of bovine enamel

R.F. Moreira & F.S. Calazans
University of Rio de Janeiro State, Odontology College, Dentistry Department, Rio de Janeiro, RJ. Brazil

R.S. Santos & M.J. dos Anjos
University of Rio de Janeiro State, Physics Institute, Laboratory of Thermodynamics and Applied Physics, Rio de Janeiro, RJ. Brazil

J.T. de Assis
University of Rio de Janeiro State, Multii-technical Institute, Nova Friburgo, RJ. Brazil

M.S. Miranda
University of Rio de Janeiro State, Odontology College, Coordinator of the Coctorate Course in Odontology/Dentistry, Rio de Janeiro, RJ. Brazil

ABSTRACT: Hydrogen Peroxide is a bleaching agent that is capable of oxidizing a wide range of colored organic materials, causing discoloration and hence bleaching of the substrate, but some authors have reported the occurrence of side effects related to bleaching of the tooth structure, such as changes in superficial morphology. In this experiment, 6 bovine incisors were used, and each tooth was initially evaluated six times in different areas to obtain the count of phosphorus and calcium, as interpreted from a range of X-Ray Fluorescence. The teeth were randomly divided into two groups: both groups were submitted to bleaching in the office with hydrogen peroxide 38%, once a week for three weeks. Group 1 was stored in distilled water, and group 2 was stored in artificial saliva between the sessions. The measurements were repeated every seven days before the bleaching treatment, and changes in mineral levels were recorded in the same manner and area. The bleaching was unable to demineralize the enamel.

1 INTRODUCTION

Bleaching therapy has become a more common procedure in dentistry since it was described in 1989 [1]. However, concerns have arisen simultaneously about the biological effects of its use, mainly due to the ability thereof to demineralize tissues and to soften them [2].

The bleaching agents are composed of hydrogen peroxide (HP) or carbamide peroxide (CP), whereas the latter decomposes into urea and hydrogen peroxide (HP). Hydrogen Peroxide (HP) is an oxidizing agent that is capable of oxidizing organic macromolecules, which have a chromogenic potential. The result of this process is a destruction of the long organic chains into colorless short chains [3–5].

Bleaching at home is a method by which the patient fills a custom-designed tray with bleaching material, using carbamide peroxide from 10% to 22% and hydrogen peroxide from 5% to 11%. Furthermore, in the office one can use carbamide peroxide from 35% to 37% and hydrogen peroxide from 20% to 38%.

Some authors have described the occurrence of several side effects related to bleaching of the tooth structure and different restorative materials, such as increased roughness, decreased hardness and changes in superficial morphology [6, 7, 8]. However other *in vitro* and *in vivo* studies have shown that carbamide peroxide and hydrogen peroxide have potent antimicrobial effects against certain bacterial species that are present in the oral cavity, demonstrating that various aspects of oral health improve when solutions containing peroxides are used [9–12].

Scanning electron microscopy (SEM) is a rapid and convenient method for qualitatively analyzing the surface morphology of enamel specimens following bleaching [13]. On the other hand, energy dispersive spectrometry (EDS) provides a specific method for determining the concentration of chemical elements on the substratum. But these methods are destructive and hence it is impossible to compare results in the same sample with which the first analyses were done. By using Energy Dispersive X-Ray Fluorescence (EDXRF) method, one can do some scans in the same sample and position.

The aim of this study was to measure the levels of inorganic elements *in vitro* by using EDXRF to determine changes in chemical composition of bovine enamel by using hydrogen peroxide 38% (Opalescence Xtra Boost. Ultradent, USA) in the office.

2 MATERIALS AND METHODS

Six central upper bovine incisors were stored in 0.1% thymol solution at room temperature before use. Teeth with any visible cracks or hypoplastic defects were excluded.

These were cleaned and sectioned at the cement enamel line, fixed in epoxy resin and standardized by the planning area, using sandpaper (400, 600 and 1200 grit) and polishing paste 0.1 μm. The enamel surfaces were examined with a light microscope with magnification of ×50, for any defects on the surface after finishing.

Each tooth was initially evaluated six times in different areas to obtain the counts of phosphorus (P) and calcium (Ca) as interpreted from a range of X-Ray Fluorescence obtained by Artax 800 (Figure 1). ARTAX is an EDXRF spectrometer designed to meet the specific needs of nondestructive elemental analysis. ARTAX is suitable for multielement analysis of Sodium to Uranium. The experimental conditions used were Molybdenum X-ray target, 30 kV, 100 μA and spatial resolution of 500 μm. The coordinates of each scan were saved, using images obtained by the ARTAX camera to repeat the next scans on the same position.

In XRF analysis, a source of X-rays irradiates a sample. When an atom absorbs the source X-rays, the incident radiation can dislodge electrons from the innermost shells of the atom, creating vacancies. Electrons from outer shells will fill the inner shell vacancy void emit X-ray photons. Each atom has specific energy levels, so the emitted radiation is characteristic of that atom. By measuring the intensity of the emitted energies it is possible to quantify how much of a particular element is present in a sample (Figure 2) (XRF fingerprint) [14].

The teeth were randomly divided into two groups: both groups were submitted to bleaching in the office with hydrogen peroxide 38% (Opalescence Xtra Boost. Ultradent, USA), which was prepared and used following the manufacturer's instruction, once a week for three weeks. Group 1 (G1) was stored in distilled water and group 2 (G2) was stored in artificial saliva at 35°C between the sessions (Table 1).

After this process the measurements were repeated every seven days before the bleaching treatment (Figure 3), and changes in mineral levels were recorded in the same manner and area. The data were analyzed using Bonferroni and Student's t-tests ($\alpha = 0.05$).

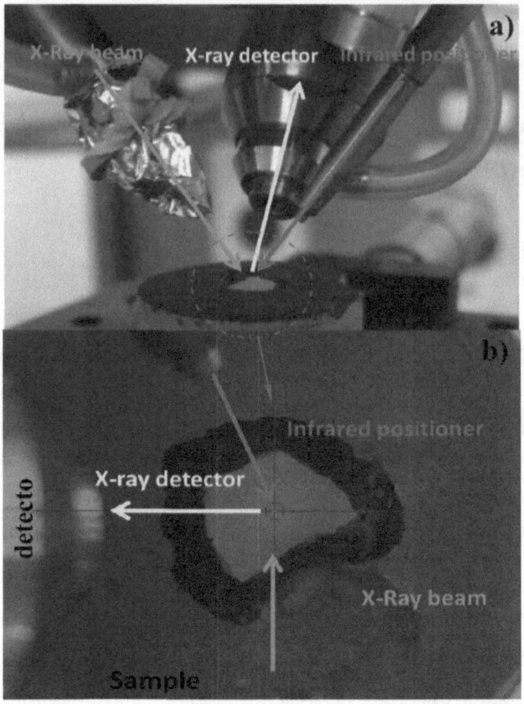

Figure 1. Image obtained by ARTAX. a) ARTAX setup, b) image obtained by CCD camera, 500 × 582 pixels.

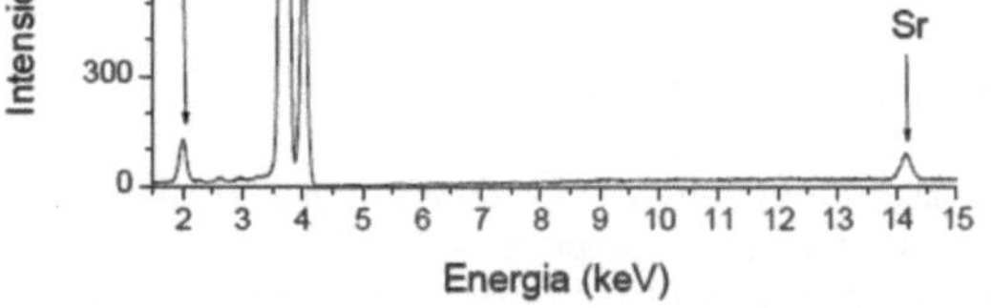

Figure 2. Spectrum obtained by X-Ray Fluorescence in bovine enamel.

Table 1. The samples distribution.

	Sample	Scans/Sample	Stored
Group 1	3	6	Destilled water
Group 2	3	6	Artificial salivar

3 RESULTS

Along with the results of the scans, the mean counts of phosphorous and calcium were obtained in both groups.

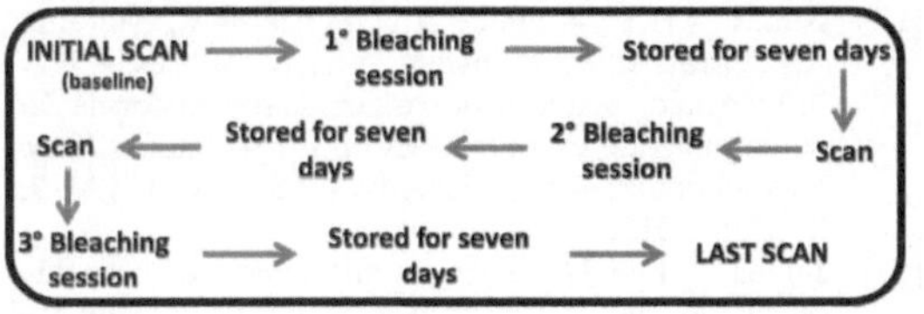

Figure 3. Schematic representation of the sequence used in the study.

Table 2. Compare the relation Group 1 scans/Baseline.

Group 1						
Baseline/	1° scan		2° scan		3° scan	
Scan	Ca	P	Ca	P	Ca	P
Sample 1	1.00	0.88	1.01	1.04	0.97	0.91
Sample 2	0.99	0.93	1.01	0.99	1.01	1.02
Sample 3	1.00	1.00	0.98	1.02	0.97	0.98
Average	0.99	0.94	1.00	1.01	0.99	0.97
a)Sdt. Dev.	0.00	0.06	1.01	0.02	0.05	0.02
b)CV (%)	0.3	6.3	1.5	2.2	2.5	5.7

a)Standard Deviation, b)Coefficient of Variation

Table 3. Compare the relation of Group 2 scans/Baseline.

Group 2						
Baseline/	1° scan		2° scan		3° scan	
Scan	Ca	P	Ca	P	Ca	P
Sample 1	0.97	0.95	0.99	1.00	0.96	0.92
Sample 2	0.97	0.95	1.01	1.05	0.99	1.00
Sample 3	0.99	1.06	1.02	1.10	0.98	1.02
Average	0.98	0.99	1.01	1.05	0.98	0.98
a)Sdt. Dev.	0.01	0.06	0.01	0.05	0.02	0.06
b)CV (%)	0.9	6.4	1.4	4.8	1.8	5.7

a)Standard Deviation, b)Coefficient of Variation

Table 4. Compare the relation 3° scan of both groups/ baseline.

	Group 1		Group 2	
3° Scan/Baseline	Ca	P	Ca	P
Sample 1	0.97	0.91	0.96	0.92
Sample 2	1.01	1.02	0.99	1.00
Sample 3	0.97	0.98	0.98	1.02
Average	0.99	0.97	0.98	0.98
a)Sdt. Dev.	0.02	0.05	0.02	0.06
b)CV (%)	2.5	5.3	1.8	5.7

a)Standard Deviation, b)Coefficient of Variation

The mean of each scan was compared with the baseline (first scan), and between the groups to analyze and to compare the demineralization (Tables 2, 3 and 4).

The results don't show significantly differences between the initial point and the others data obtained and the groups.

4 DISCUSSION

In order to analyze the concentration of inorganic elements and to quantify enamel demineralization by the bleaching agent, some authors use energy dispersive spectrometry (EDS), because it is a rapid and convenient method [13]. But this is a destructive technique, hence it is necessary to exclude the sample after the scan, and due to this fact it is impossible to do other analyses in the same sample, and consequently the comparison is questionable.

The present trail was done by the X-Ray Fluorescence (XRF) method, as this can scan and quantify the inorganic elements present on enamel surfaces without excluding the sample that has been scanned Hence this characteristic makes it possible to measure on the same areas several times, therefore reducing the variables.

The count of phosphorous and calcium was interpreted by X-Ray Fluorescence to show the loss of inorganic structures from bovine enamel after the use of an office bleaching agent. In dental research, the levels of mineral content in enamel and dentin are a good indication of the demineralization [15].

The study simulated oral conditions by storing the teeth in artificial saliva between the bleaching sessions, but this can interfere in results and in knowing the real effect of peroxide on enamel, because saliva has a remineralization property. Thus another group was added, in which the sample was stored in distilled water, which does not interfere with the results.

Although studies about the effects of bleaching on morphological changes to tooth tissue are contradictory, it is generally agreed that peroxides can alter tooth mineral content, increase enamel roughness and decrease the surface microhardness [13, 15–20].

However, this paper does not show the demineralizer potential of hydrogen peroxide (38%). The differences between the results obtained and the literature can be explained by the method chosen and the non-existence of a protocol for this study.

The present result is more reliable than the others, because a nondestructive technique (EDXRF) was used, the same sample can be used at different moments of treatments [15], and teeth were stored in saliva and distilled water in order to evaluate the real effect of hydrogen peroxide on enamel, thereby reducing the variables.

5 CONCLUSION

Under these experimental conditions *in vitro*, bleaching with hydrogen peroxide 38% was not able to demineralize the bovine enamel.

There are not significant statistical differences between the groups.

Further analysis of enamel surface could be performed in order to evaluate the surface topography changes in organic content and the influence on mechanical properties.

REFERENCES

[1] Haywood, V. B., Heymann, H. O. Nightguard vital bleaching. Quintessence Int. 1989; 20 (3): 173–6.

[2] Haywood, V. B., Heymann, H. O. Nightguard vital bleaching: How safe is it? Quintessence Int. 1991; 22 (7): 515–23.

[3] Seghi RR, Denry I (1992) Effects of external bleaching on indentation and abrasion characteristics of human enamel in vitro. J Dent Res 71:1340–1344.

[4] Goldberg M, Grootveld M, Lynch E (2010) Undesirable and adverse effects of tooth whitening products: a review. Clin Oral Investig 14:1–10.

[5] Wiegand A, Vollmer D, Foitzik M, Attin R, Attin T (2005) Efficacy of different whitening modalities on bovine enamel and dentin. Clin Oral Investig 9:91–97.

[6] Attin T, Kocabiyik M, Buchalla W, Hannig C, Becker K. Susceptibility of enamel surfaces to demineralization after application of fluoridated carbamide peroxide gels. Caries Res. 2003;37(2):93–9.

[7] Lewistein I, Fuhrer N, Churaru N, Cardash H. Effect of different peroxide bleaching regimens and subsequent fluoridation on the hardness of human enamel and dentin. J Prosthet Dent. 2004;92:337–42.

[8] Hairu Nizan H.R., Lim C.T., Cheng H. K., Yap A. U.J. Nanoindentation study of human premolar subjected to bleaching agent. *Journal of Biomechanics*. 2005; 38: 2204–11.

[9] Napimoga, M. H., De Oliveira, R., Reis, A. F. *et al.* In vitro antimicrobial activity of peroxide-based bleaching agents. Quintessence Int. 2007; 38 (6): e329–33.

[10] Zinner, D. D., Duany, L. F., Chilton, N. W. Controlled study of the clinical effectiveness of a new oxygen gel on plaque, oral debrisand gingival inflammation. Pharmacol Ther Dent 197O; 1: 7–15, apud Haywood, V. B., Heymann, H. O. Nightguard vital bleaching: how safe is it? Quintessence Int. 1991; 22 (7): 515–23.

[11] Shipman, B., Cohen, E., Kaslick, R. S. The effect of a urea peroxidegel on plaque deposits and gingival status. Periodontol. 1971; 42: 283–5. Apud Haywood, V. B., Heymann, H. O. Nightguard vital bleaching: how safe is it? Quintessence Int. 1991; 22 (7): 515–23.

[12] Nunes, V.H.S., Andrade A.O., Vilar, R.V., Moreira, R.F., Hirata Jr, R., Monnerat, A.F., Carvalhaes, R.F. A influência do peróxido de carbamida sobre a formação de colônias de estreptococos do grupo mutans. Rev. bras. odontol., Rio de Janeiro, v. 68, n. 1, p. 124–7, jan./jun. 2011.

[13] Joiner A. (2007) Review of the effects of peroxide on enamel and dentine properties Journal of Dentistry 35(12) 889–896.

[14] Klockenkamper, R. *et al. X-ray Spectrom.*, **25,** 156–162, 1996.

[15] Poorni S., Kumar, R.A., Shankar, P., Indira, R., Ramachandran, S. Effect of 10% sodium ascorbate on the calcium: Phosphorus radio of enamel bleached with 35% hydrogen peroxide: An *in vitro* quantitative energy-dispersive X-Ray analysis. Comtemp. Clin. Dent. 2010. Oct–Dec; 1(4): 223–226.

[16] Basting, R.T., Amaral, F.L.B., França, F.M.G., Flório, F.M. Clinical comparative study of the effectiveness of and tooth sensitivity to 10% and 20% carbamide peroxide home-use and 35% and 38% hydrogen peroxide in-office bleaching materials containing desensitizing agents. Operative Dentistry, 2012, 37–4.

[17] Cakir, F.Y., Korkmaz, Y., Firat, E., Oztas, S.S., Gurgan, S. Chemical analysis of enamel and dentin following the application of three different at-home bleaching system. Operative Dentistry, 2011, 36-5, 529–536.

[18] Souza, R.O.A, Lombardo, G.H.L., Pereira, S.M.B., Zamboni, S.C., Valera, M.C., Araújo, M.A.M., Özcan, M. Analysis of tooth enamel after excessive bleaching: A study using scanning eléctron microscopy and energy dispersive x-ray spectroscopy. The International Journal of Prosthodontics, 2010, 23(1), 29–32.

[19] Khoroushi, M., Mazaheri, H., Manoochehri. Effect of CPP-ACP application on flexural strength of bleached enamel and dentin complex. Operative Dentistry, 2011, 36–4, 372–379.

[20] Gjorgiesvka, E., Nicholson, J.W. Prevention of enamel demineralization after tooth bleaching by bioactive glass incorporated into toothpaste. Australian Dental Journal, 2011, 56: 193–200.

Biodental Engineering II – Natal Jorge et al (Eds)
© 2014 Taylor & Francis Group, London, ISBN 978-1-138-00131-2

Analysis of failure cobalt-chromiun alloy for partial removable dental prostheses

C.P.S. Porto
Doutoranda do Programa de Pós-Graduação em Ciência e Engenharia dos Materiais (P^2 CEM), Universidade Federal de Sergipe (UFS), Professora do Curso de Odontologia da Universidade Tiradentes (UNIT), Aracaju, Sergipe, Brasil

E.A. Monteiro
Graduando do P^2 CEM, UFS, Aracaju, Sergipe, Brasil

P.G.A. Borges
Mestranda do P^2 CEM, UFS, Aracaju, Sergipe, Brasil

M.A.R. Nunes
Professor do Curso de Odontologia da UNIT, Aracaju, Sergipe, Brasil

S. Griza
Professor doutor do P^2 CEM, UFS, Aracaju, Sergipe, Brasil

ABSTRACT: Two Partial Removable Dental Prosthesis (PRDP) fractured after in continuous use. The analysed material is a metallic CoCrMo alloy, prepared by investment casting. The failure analysis was performed using the Scanning Electron Microscope (SEM) in order to characterize the fracture and to identify crack initiation. EDS microprobe was carried out aiming the material confirmation. Then the metallographic analysis was performed to the highlight microstructural aspects associated with the fracture process. The fracture was predominantly interdendritic with fatigue striations and was encouraged by the existence of microstructural defects arised from investment casting process.

We conducted a study of a case and analysis of a casting of a two partially removable PRDP, which was broken prematurely after a few years of continuous use.

The analysed material was a metal alloy consisting primarily of: 60% Co, 29% Cr, 6.2% Mo, used in dentistry for making PRDPs. These prostheses were made through the technique by investment casting, in order to restore the lost dental elements, re-establishing function (mastication and phonation) and aesthetics.

The technique of investment casting also known as investment casting produces articles weighing more than 5 kg, complex shape, better surface finish, and generally no smaller tolerances male. Parts are produced from alloys of aluminium, nickel, magnesium, copper, beryllium copper, silicon bronze, brass silicon-alloy heat-resistant than the common steel and stainless steel. This process is very effective in producing small parts and apparently unfeasible for other processes (for complex shapes and cost) (Centro Federal de Educação Tecnológica de Santa Catarina 2007).

There are two ways to melt a PRDP: through the model or on the model. The casting through the model is a technique that saves time, but increases the risk of porosity at the entrance of cone injection. The casting on the model is safer, in this case is placed on the feeder base model.

The casting is performed within a ring of casting made with the same coating of refractory model preheated slowly in an electric programmable furnace to a temperature of 1000°C to 1050°C. The leakage of the liquid metal into the mold performed through a centrifuge, where the metal is cast by the centrifugal force generated by rotation, and under pressure helps the metal fill small sections and keep a good contact between the metal and mold (Allsop & Kennedy 1983).

For Strickland & Sturdevant (1959) among the factors that can cause faults or defects in metallic structures has the alloy composition, its handling and method of manufacture of feed channel. Other authors also mention the coating composition, the temperature of the alloy and cast, the alloy casting technique, either by use of the torch, induction or electrical devices (Todescan 1960, Phillips 1993).

For many years gold alloys were a choise material of to manufacture metallic structures of PRDP.

However, due to the high cost of gold, new alternative alloys were developed to replace it. With the advancement of knowledge about the alloys and with the need to reduce costs, came the alternative alloys. At the beginning were developed by changing the proportions of noble and non-noble metals and later, without the presence of noble metals in their composition. From the 30 s, the cobalt-chromium alloys have assumed a growing use and currently become the election in the manufacture of metal structures of PRDP. The advantages of using these alloys for dental castings are associated with the fact that they are light (low density), resistant to corrosion and provide greater resistance to deflection in structural dimensions smaller due to its high modulus of elasticity (Anusavice, 1998), furthermore, they are biocompatible with tissues per implant possess good castability and low cost (Chao et al. 1988, Hulterström & Nilsson 1991).

Despite the clinical success of Co-Cr alloys, they have some unfavourable properties such as low fatigue limit and low ductility and are responsible for a large number of clinical failure, especially the loss of retaining clips (Giampaolo et al. 1991a, b, Mjör & Christensen 1993).

The retention of PRDP is usually achieved by the use of extra coronal retainers (staples). These Retentive clasp arms must be capable of flexing and returning to original form and should satisfactorily retain prosthesis. In addition, claps should not unduly stress abutment teeth or be permanently distorted during service (Ali et al. 2001).

As the dentures are fabricated on a metallic structure their life may be compromised due to the defects resulting from the casting process. Among the casting defects can be highlighted the presence of porosities and shrinkage (Bowman 1970, Ben-Hur et al. 1991). Among the most common complaints by patients who use the clip removable partial dentures, are prominent losses of elasticity of the clip, or a fracture. In 1965, Bates presented a study that attributed the fatigue failure to structural changes as porosity or cracks. Anderson (1972) strengthens the fractured components of a PRDP can be attributed to the presence of inclusions as eutectoids rainfall, large crystalline grains or fatigue failure. Studies that aid in the detection of faults are important reasons for the evolution of the design of removable partial dentures, once the flaw causes discomfort, possible inflammatory processes in the patient and the need for repair or replacement procedure.

This study sought to define the factors that caused the fracture of a removable partial denture. To this end, we used the following techniques: analysis of low magnifying increase, analysis by optical microscopy (OM) and scanning electron microscope (SEM), where the analyses were performed fracture, observation of the microstructure of the material and the qualitative composition of alloy and Vickers microhardness test to verify whether this corresponded to the values provided by the manufacturer of the alloy.

1 MATERIALS AND METHODS

Analyses of failure are usually performed through macroscopic and microscopic observations, where it is possible to determine various characteristics of the material, including the determination of causes of fractures, premature wear and other types of failures.

The first performed analysis is macroscopic, using low magnification glass. Then the samples are observed in optical microscopy (OM), if necessary, and finally use the SEM, which characterise microscopic analysis. The SEM plays an important role in the study of failures due to its high resolution, depth of focus and use of analytical resources, which allow performing in situ microanalysis or chemical mapping of the sample surface.

1.1 *Analysis of fracture in low rise*

The broken pieces were cut using a precision cutting machine. Then, there was a clean fracture with detergent solution and a soft bristle brush so as not to damage the fractured surface. Macroscopic observation was performed in magnifier (Zeiss Stemi 2000C) in order to visualize the macroscopic aspects of the fracture and the surface conditions of the parts adjacent to the fracture plane.

1.2 *Analysis by Scanning Electron Microscopy and EDS*

The fracture surfaces were analysed by scanning electron microscopy (JEOL JCM 5700) to verify the micromechanics of fracture. Microprobe analysis was performed by energy dispersive (EDS) to determine the relative content of the major constituents of the alloys.

1.3 *Microstructural analysis*

After analysing failures held sample preparation for metallography in order to verify the conditions microstructure of the materials. To this end, samples were cut previously built to observe a metallographic plane parallel to the fracture. Then the specimens were polished with sandpaper water (100, 200, 400, 600 and 1200) and finally polished with a felt disc with diamond paste to particle size, 6 μm, 3 μm and 1 μm.

Subsequently the samples were analysed by an optical microscope (Zeiss Axioscope A1), provided as polished and after etching to reveal their microstructures. Chemical attacks were performed as recommended ASM Handbook (2004) using a solution consisting of: 15 ml distilled water, 15 ml of glacial acetic acid, 60 ml of 32% HCl and 15 ml 65% HNO_3. This solution was aged for one hour and then the sample was dipped for a period between 10 and 30 seconds.

1.4 *Test of microhardness*

Were performed microhardness test to ascertain the hardness of parts and then confront with the data

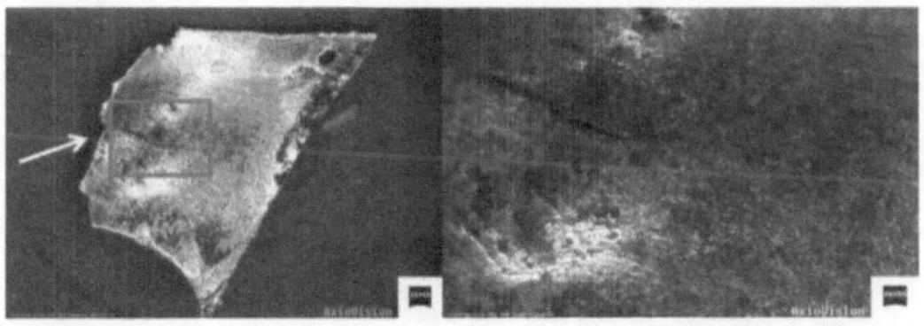

Figure 1. Left image shows a section cut for analysis, and the arrow shows the fracture plane. The image to the right shows in detail the surface defects found: cracks and porosities.

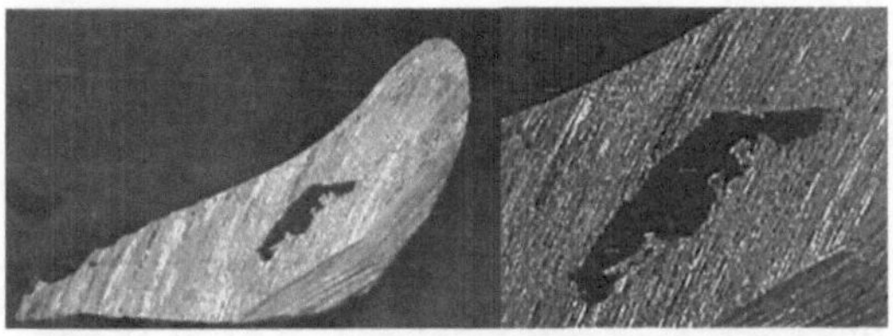

Figure 2. Images of the lower cut plane, with a large internal defect.

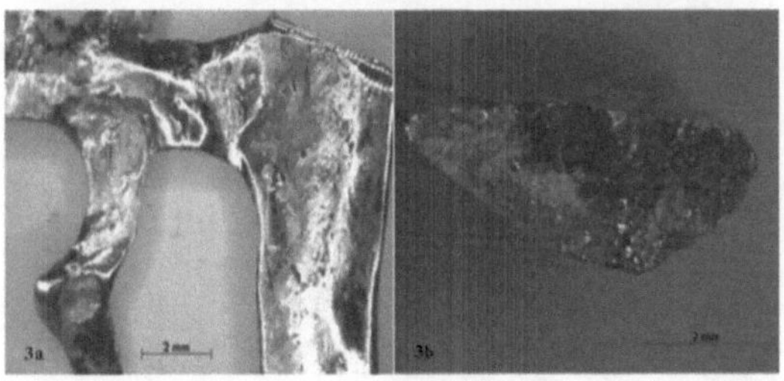

Figure 3. a, b. Magnifying images of the analysed material.

provided by the manufacturer. This test was conducted using a microhardness tester (Shimadzu Micro Hardeness Tester – HMV) with a load of 200 g (1961N – HV0, 2) for 15 seconds. There were five random measurements on sample embedded.

2 RESULTS AND DISCUSSION

2.1 *Analysis of fracture in low rise*

The fracture surface seen in low-rise had a rough exterior, typical fracture in coarse grain materials. An image held on the side wall part showed evidence of surfacing defects as pores and cracks on the surface (Fig. 1). The observation of the fracture plane of the lower part of the piece cut for analysis showed the presence of a large internal defect (Fig. 2). This plan was later prepared for metallography.

For sample 2 can be observed the presence of shrinkage characteristic of precision casting process, the surface is rough in appearance, Figure 3a, b.

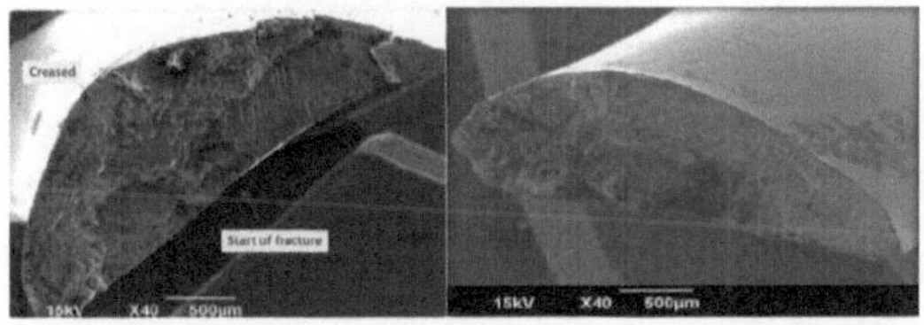

Figure 4. Appearance of fracture. This fracture was predominantly interdendritic.

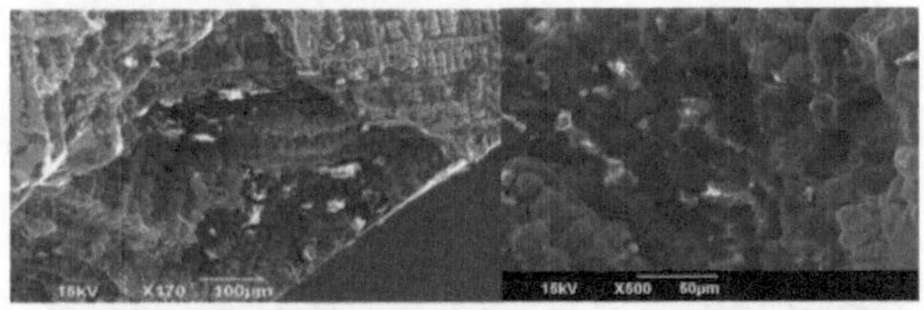

Figure 5. Image in an increase of the fracture initiation region, where pores are observed (shrinkage).

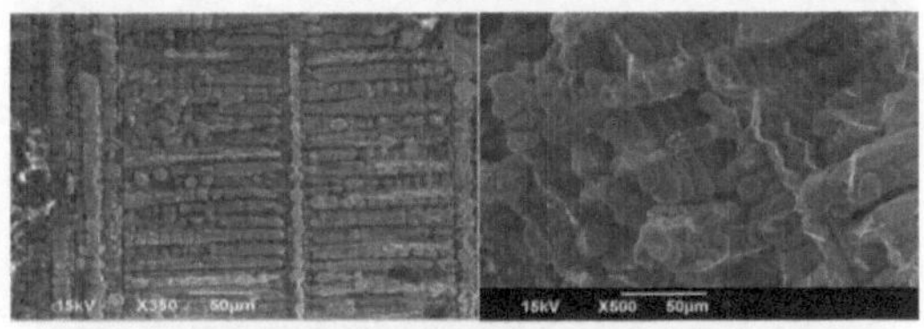

Figure 6. The image of interdendritic separation.

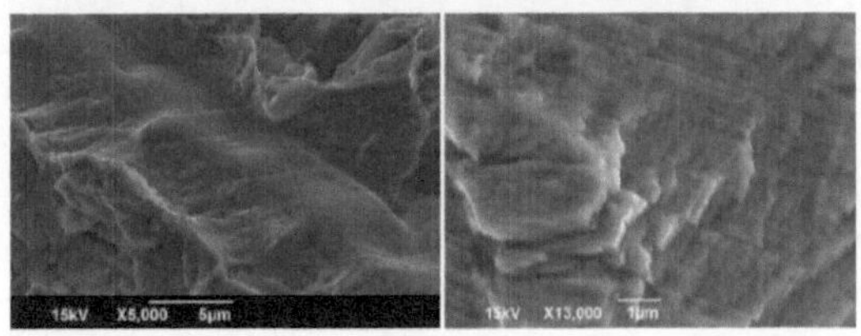

Figure 7. Fatigue striations aspects.

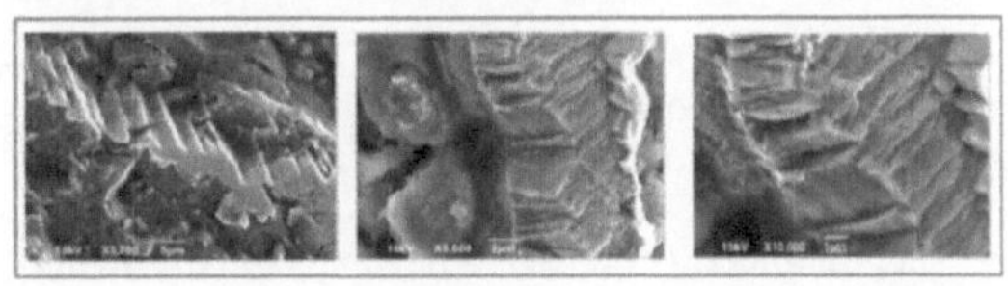

Figure 8. Fractography showing rebounds fatigue characteristic of Co-Cr alloys, found the fracture.

2.2 *Analysis by Scanning Electron Microscopy and EDS*

The fracture surface obtained in the electron microscope shows an aspect of interdendritic fracture and crushes in some regions (Fig. 4). In greater increase was observed a region containing pores (Fig. 5), which was identified as the beginning region of the fracture. This region coincides with that where surface defects were observed (as viewed in Figs. 1–3). The predominant mechanism of fracture consists of interdendritic separation (Fig. 6). Were also observed regions that showes streaks and unevenness characteristic of fatigue failure (Figs. 7, 8). The grooves are

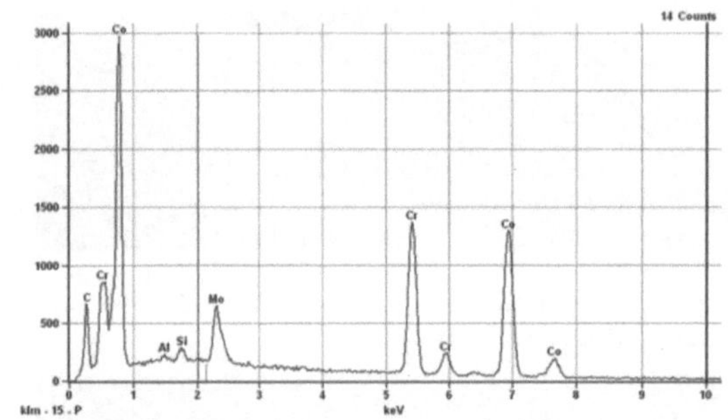

Figure 9. Test result by EDS microprobe, showing characteristic peaks for Co, Cr and Mo.

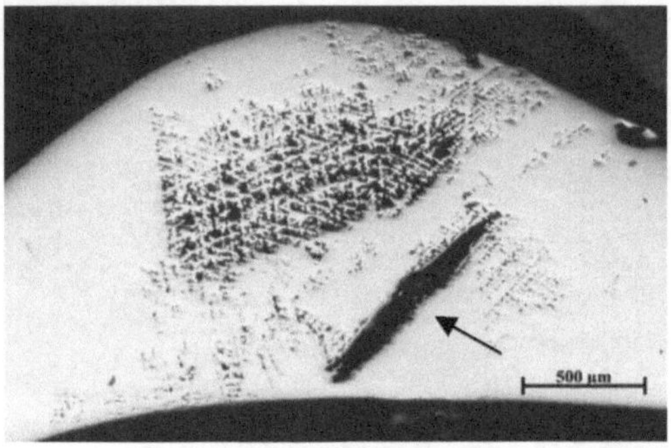

Figure 10. Microstructure showing a great lack of fusion defect (arrow), and generalized shrinkage.

arranged to indicate the direction of propagation of the fracture from the region identified as the beginning of the fault. The microprobe analysis in SDS shows characteristic peaks at Co, Cr, Mo (Fig. 9).

2.3 *Microstructural analysis*

The microstructural analysis below magnifying and without attack shows the formation of a defect of lack of fusion associated with the fracture initiation region and a large amount of shrinkage dispersed in the section piece (Fig. 10). The analysis following attack indicated the typical microstructure of alloy Cr-Mo-Co, consisting of matrix cobalt-rich solid solution containing dispersed carbides in grain boundaries dendritic, besides particulate inclusions (Fig. 11). In the sample 02 can be observed the presence of shrinkage without attack (Fig. 12). After etching in the shrinkage greenish tint was observed, the presence of carbides long and thick, and the matrix with the highest cobalt percentage (Fig. 13).

2.4 *Microhardness*

In this study was compared the values of Vickers hardness provided by the manufacturer and performed in the laboratory. Found the average value of 364.8 HV, and standard deviation of 5.12, with a coefficient of variation of 26.2. Since the value provided by

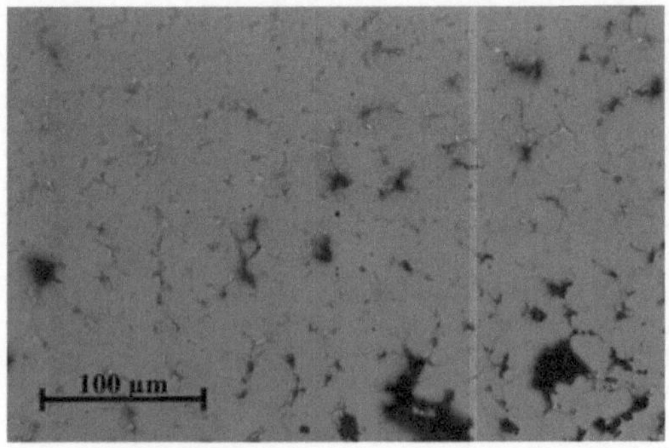

Figure 11. Carbides (gray phase) in cobalt-rich matrix, typical of alloy Cr-Co-Mo.

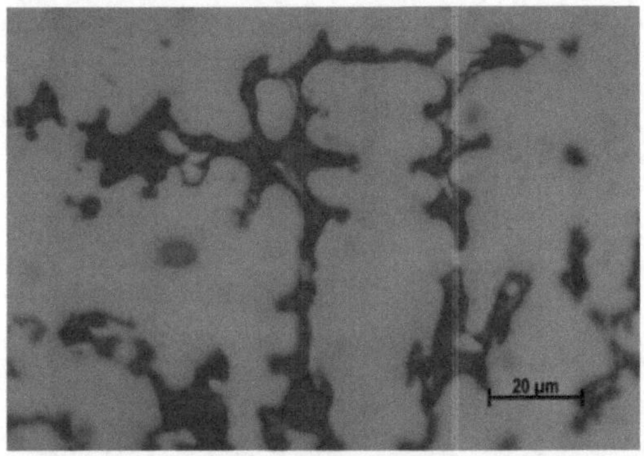

Figure 12. Microstructure before attack.

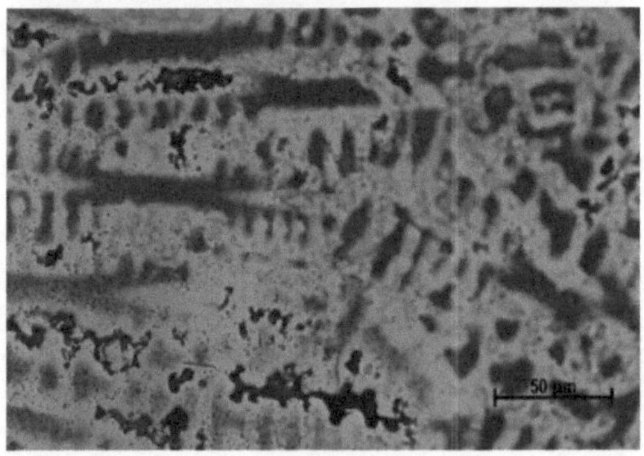

Figure 13. Microstructure after attack.

the manufacturer was 473 HV. For a second sample five measurements were taken, totalling an average of 418 HV and a standard deviation of 4.21. According to ASTM F75-12, the value of 418 HV is not in the range of 25–35 HRc, but this value is not a criterion for rejection.

3 DISCUSSION

The fact alloys Co-Cr-Mo being high temperature resistant determines a greater difficulty in processing, so that the most frequently used process for the manufacture of the component is a casting. By having a high melting point, these alloys are often liquefied by a flame torch with gas and air. Whichever casting method, a skilled operator is necessary because any negligence in the process can cause severe damage to the properties of metals or lead you to failure (Craig & Powers 2004).

Was found that the failure is related to microstructural defects and inclusions from the manufacturing process by casting part. Found internal defects by the initiation region of the fracture, characterized by lack of fusion, inclusions shrinkage and particles.

The shrinkage caused during the solidification of the material can be obtained from a wrong calculation of the size of the feed channels for low pressure or low temperature heating.

The literature reports that microstructural defects like pores, cracks, inclusions, produced before or after the manufacturing process can lead to material failure (Bates 1965, Bowman 1970, Anderson 1972, Ben-Hur et al. 1991).

Failures due to casting are frequently reported. Iwana (1985) found that the clips were fractured in PRDP casting errors, which was later confirmed in Dental Advisor (1989) attributed the failures to foundries prostheses inappropriate or project failure.

According to Rodrigues (2005) methods of casting affect in the microstructure, the microhardness and porosity level. According Vallittu & Miettinen (1996), Mahmoud et al. (2005), Ramamoorthi & Al Khuraif (2011) fatigue resistance is an important factor in the durability of dental materials. In the case study, the fatigue fracture occurred due to defects in material. This fact was ratified by the presence of striations in the fracture.

4 CONCLUSIONS

This study was devoted to identifying the factors that led to the premature fracture of two removable partial denture. Analyses indicated that the failures were due to fatigue. Defects arising from the casting process as lack of fusion, inclusions and a large amount of shrinkage found along the flaw initiation region.

REFERENCES

Ali, M., Waters, N.E., Nairn, R.I., West, F., Sherriff, M. 2001. A laboratory investigation of the role of guide planes in the retention of cast cobalt-chromium alloy partial denture frameworks. *Journal of Dentistry* 29: 291–299.

Allsop, D.F. & Kennedy, D. 1983. *Pressure Diecasting – Part 2; The Technology of the Casting and the Die*, Oxford: Pergamon Press.

Anderson, J.N. 1972. *Applied Dental Materials*. 4ª ed. Oxford: Blackwell Scientific Publications.

Anusavice, K.J. 1998. *Phillips: Materiais Dentários*. 10ª ed. Rio de Janeiro: Guanabara Koogan.

ASM Handbook. 2004. Metallography and Microstructures. In: *ASM International,* v.9.Materials Park. OH.

ASTM F75-12 *Standard Specification for Cobalt-28 Chromium-6 Molybdenum alloy casting and casting alloy for surgical implants* (UNS R30075).

Bates, J.F. 1965. Studies related to the fracture of partial dentures. *Brazil Dental Journal* 118(12): 532–537.

Ben-Hur, Z., Aviv, I., Maharshak, F.C. 1991. Factors affecting displacement of free-end saddle removable partial dentures. *Quintessence International* 22 (1): 23–27.

Bowman, J.F. 1970. Removable partial prosthodontics: comparison surveys–1964 and 1969. *Journal Dentistry Education* 97: 34–93.

Centro Federal de Educação Tecnológica de Santa Catarina; curso técnico de mecânica industrial; Prof. Eng. Mec. Norberto Moro; Téc. Mec. André Paegle Auras; Florianópolis – 2007.

Chao, Y., Zarb, G.A., Judes H. 1988. A study into the use of chromiumcobalt alloy for constructing the framework for osteointegrated prostheses. *Clinical Materials*. 3: 309–15.

Craig, R.G & Powers, J.M. 2004. *Materiais dentários restauradores*. 11ª ed. São Paulo: Santos.

Dental Advisor. 1989. *Removable partial denture* 6(4): 1–8.

Giampaolo, E.T., Leonardi, P., Cucci, A.L.M., Fuller, J.B. 1991a. Grampos de retenção para prótese parcial removível. Análise da resistência à flexão em função degrampos, ligas e técnicas de fusão. *Revista de Odontologia da UNESP* 20.

Giampaolo, E.T., Leonardi, P., Cucci, A.L.M., Fuller, J.B. 1991b. Análise da resistência à flexão de grampos de retenção em prótese parcial removível. Efeito da interação grampos, ligas e técnicas de fusão. *Revista de Odontologia da UNESP* 20.

Hulterström, M. & Nilsson, U. 1991. Cobalt-Chromium as a framework material in implant supported fixed prostheses – a preliminary report. *International Journal Oral Maxillofac Implants* 6(4): 475–80.

Iwana, C.Y. 1985. *Verificação de deformação e fratura de grampos circunferenciais em ligas de cromo-cobalto*. M.Sc. – Faculdade de Odontologia, Universidade de São Paulo, São Paulo.

Mahmoud, A., Wakabayashi, N., Takahashi, H, Ohyama, T. 2005. Deflection fatigue of Ti-6Al- 7Nb, Co-Cr, and gold alloy cast clasps. *Journal Prosthetic Dentistry* 93: 183–8.

Mjör, I.A., Christensen, G.J. 1993.Assessment of local side effects of casting alloys. *Quintessence International* 24: 343–51.

Phillips, R.W. 1993. *Skinner Materiais Dentários*. Trad. de Júlio Jorge D'Albuquerque Lossio. 9ª ed. Rio de Janeiro: Guanabara Koogan.

Ramamoorthi, M. & Al Khuraif, A.A. 2011. A comparative evaluation of fatigue behavior of removable partial denture alloys with and without heat treatment. *International Journal of Dental Clinics* 3(1): 14–17.

Rodrigues, R.C.S. 2005. *Estudo comparativo de dois métodos utilizados na fundição*. Tese (Livre Docência em Prótese Dentária), Faculdade de Farmácia e Odontologia, Universidade de São Paulo, São Paulo.

Strickland, W.D. & Sturdevant, C.M. 1959. Porosity in full cast crown. *Journal American Dental Association* 58: 69–78.

Todescan, R. 1960. *Contribuição ao estudo da porosidade nos aparelhos parciais móveis*. Tese (Livre Docência em Prótese Dentária). Faculdade de Farmácia e Odontologia, Universidade de São Paulo, São Paulo.

Vallittu, P.K. & Miettinen T. 1996. Duration of induction melting of cobalt-chromium alloy and its effect on resistance to deflection fatigue of cast denture clasps. *Journal Prosthetic Dentistry* 75: 322–6.

Biodental Engineering II – Natal Jorge et al (Eds)
© 2014 Taylor & Francis Group, London, ISBN 978-1-138-00131-2

Stress distribution in a zirconia one-piece dental implant

A. Correia & J.C. Reis Campos
Faculty of Dental Medicine of the University of Porto, Portugal; Institute of Mechanical Engineering and Industrial Management (INEGI)

P. Couto Viana
Dr. Manuel Neves Dental Clinic, Porto, Portugal

Z. Kovacs
DentalMaia Dental Lab

N.V. Ramos & M. Vaz
Laboratory of Optics and Experimental Mechanics – Faculty of Engineering of the University of Porto, Portugal; Institute of Mechanical Engineering and Industrial Management (INEGI)

ABSTRACT: The aim of this research was to perform a numerical stress analysis in a zirconia dental implant virtually inserted in a maxilla bone. A zirconia one-piece dental implant was scanned with a CAD-CAM dental system and a 3D geometry .stl file was exported and processed into a numerical model to perform a simulation with finite elements. A qualitative analysis was performed using unitary load in a vertical and oblique direction. Results of the stress analysis with FEM showed that the highest stresses are located in the abutment of the implant when a vertical load is applied and when an oblique load is used there is also a stress concentration on the implant but this time in the surface opposed to the load. Therefore, it seems that there is not an increased risk of implant failure, when compared to traditional titanium implants.

1 INTRODUCTION

Nowadays, all-ceramic dental prostheses are increasingly applied in the dental practice, mostly due to its superior aesthetics and to the higher mechanical properties obtained for these materials.

When an edentulous space exist, the dentist has the possibility to replace the dental roots by dental implants, which are usually made in titanium, a material proved to have outstanding biological and mechanical properties in the oral cavity.

However, some occurrences of titanium allergy, and the desire to avoid metals in the oral cavity, mostly due to biological and aesthetic reasons, lead to the development of zirconia implants [e.g. Ceraroot® Barcelona).

Using these ceramic implants, all-ceramic dental rehabilitations (implant and prosthesis) became possible.

Although some studies reveal high clinical success-rates (Oliva 2010) we have no knowledge of studies on the stress distribution on zirconia implants (Chang 2012).

As so, the aim of this research was to perform a numerical stress analysis in a zirconia dental implant virtually inserted in a maxilla bone submitted to vertical and oblique loads.

2 MATERIAL AND METHODS

A zirconia one-piece (implant + abutment) dental implant (Ceraroot® Barcelona) was scanned with the CAD-CAM dental system Zirconzahn (® Zirconzahn, Italy) available in DentalMaia Dental Lab (Castelo da Maia, Portugal).

The 3D geometry .stl file generated was exported and processed with Solidworks (®Dassault Systèmes, France) in the Laboratory of Optics and Experimental Mechanics (LOME) of the Faculty of Engineering of the University of Porto (FEUP), Portugal (Figure 1).

This CAD software allowed building a numerical model used to perform a simulation with finite elements. For that the zirconia implant was placed in a bone cube with an outer cortical layer and an inner trabecular bone layer as it can be seen in Figure 2. The implant was virtually placed according to the manufacturer instructions to place this type of dental implants in the maxillary bone, being the neck of the implant in the cortical bone and the root part in the trabecular bone.

Then, the Ansys software (®Ansys, PA, USA) was selected to build-up a 3D mesh to analyse the stress distribution with the finite element method (FEM).

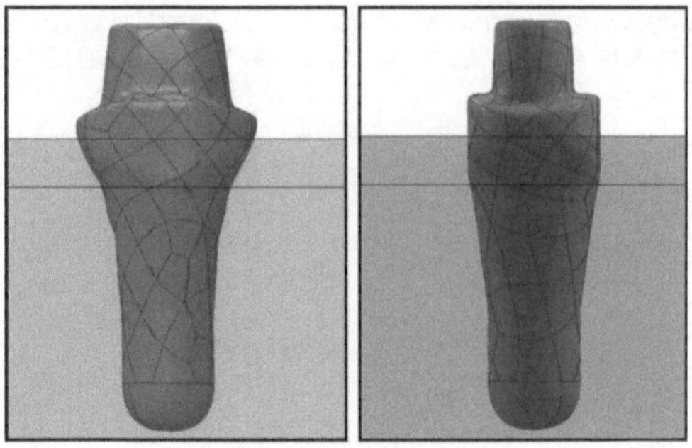

Figure 1. Computer aided design of a zirconia one-piece implant.

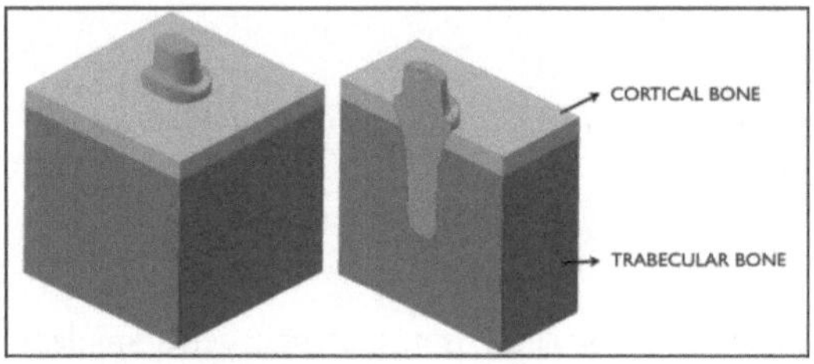

Figure 2. Computer aided design of a zirconia one-piece implant placed in a bone cube simulating an outer cortical layer and an inner trabecular bone.

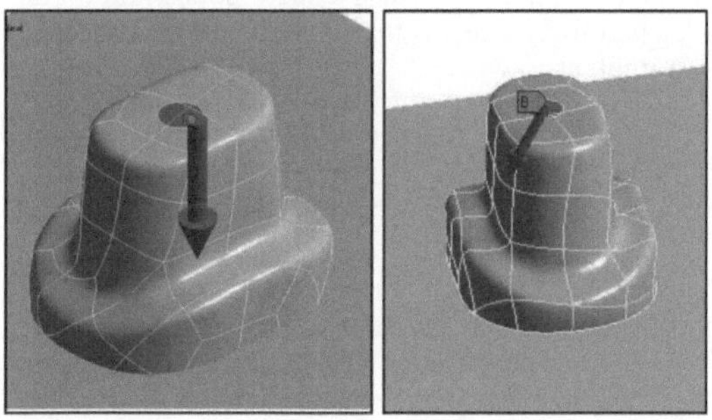

Figure 3. Direction of the load applied on the zirconia implant. Left – vertical load; Right – oblique load.

A qualitative analysis was performed using unitary load in a vertical and oblique direction (Figure 3). These loads were selected to allow further simulations of different values. The boundary conditions of this simulation included a rigid connection of the interface implant-bone.

3 RESULTS

As the load due to mastication depends on the individual it was decided to perform a qualitative analysis using unit loads.

Results of the stress analysis with FEM showed that the highest stresses are located in the abutment of the one-piece zirconia implant when a vertical load is applied (Figure 4).

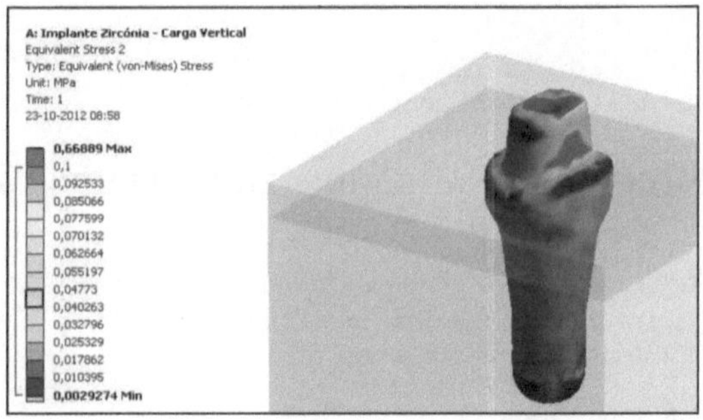

Figure 4. Finite element analysis of the simulation with a vertical 1 N load. Representation of 3D distribution of the von Mises equivalent stress.

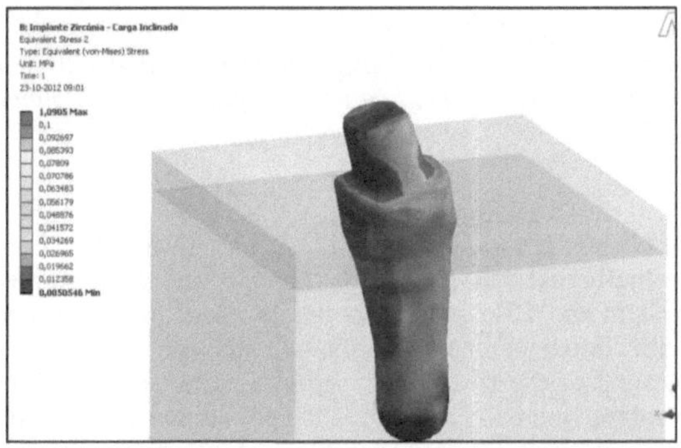

Figure 5. Finite element analyses of the simulation with an oblique 1 N load. Representation of 3D distribution of the von Mises equivalent stress.

When an oblique load is used there is also a stress concentration on the implant, this time in the surface opposed to the load (Figure 5).

4 DISCUSSION

In our 3D FEM model it has been observed that when a vertical load is applied (Figure 4), stresses are mostly located in the abutment part (supraosseous) of the implant. Lower stresses are located in the intraosseous part of the implant.

These results are different from the ones described by other authors (Eskitascioglu 2004). In this study about a one-piece dental implant in titanium, this author reported that the highest stresses were concentrated at the neck of the implant. Probably this difference is related to the shape/geometry of the implant. The model used by Eskitascioglu was a traditional cylindrical implant. The model select for the present work is shaped more like a real human tooth with a larger neck, which probably allows a better stress distribution when a vertical load is applied.

However, when an oblique load is applied there are higher stresses, not only in the abutment but also in the root part of the implant, in the opposite side of the applied load. These stresses are higher (Figure 5) than those that occur with a vertical load.

The aim of placing a dental implant in the oral cavity is to replace a natural tooth that has been lost. So, the stress behavior of a dental implant should be similar to a natural tooth or, at least, it should resist the loads that occur in the oral cavity.

The behavior of this implant with an oblique load is different from the stress distribution verified by other authors (Hasegawa 2010) with natural teeth. According to this author, when an oblique load is applied on a natural tooth stresses do not extend beyond the enamel-dentin junction which is, in a healthy tooth, in the bone/tooth transition.

Although this stress behavior is different from a natural tooth it must also be considered in the evaluation of the mechanical performance of this implant. In this work a unitary load has been applied to allow the simulation of other load values similar to those that occur in the oral cavity. If an extreme load situation of 500 N in the oral cavity is considered, the highest von Mises stress values obtained are approximately 335 MPa (0.67*500). When an oblique load is applied the maximum stress values are higher and may reach 545 Mpa (1.09*500). Though these values are high, they are below the fracture strength of zirconia that is around 900–1200 MPa.

5 CONCLUSIONS

It is possible to state that this one-piece zirconia implant may withstand high load values similar to those that can occur in the oral cavity. Therefore, it seems that there is not an increased risk of implant failure, when compared to traditional titanium implants.

REFERENCES

Chang CL, Chen CS, Yeung TC & Hsu ML. 2012. Biomechanical effect of a zirconia dental implant-crown system: a three-dimensional finite element analysis. Int J Oral Maxillofac Implants, 27: e49–57.

Eskitascioglu G, Usumez A, Sevimay M, Soykan E & Unsal E. 2004. The influence of occlusal loading location on stresses transferred to implant-supported prostheses and supporting bone: A three-dimensional finite element study. J Prosthet Dent, 91: 144–50.

Hasegawa A, Shinya A, Nakasone Y, Lassila LV, Vallitu PK & Shinya A. 2010. Development of a 3D CAD/FEM analysis system for natural teeth and jaw bone constructed from x-ray CT images. Int J Biomater, 2010: 1–7.

Oliva J, Oliva X & Oliva JD. 2010. Five-year Success Rate of 831 Consecutively Placed Zirconia Dental Implants in Humans: A Comparison of Three Different Rough Surfaces. Int J Oral Maxillofac Implants, 25: 336–44.

Biodental Engineering II – Natal Jorge et al (Eds)
© 2014 Taylor & Francis Group, London, ISBN 978-1-138-00131-2

Clinical records in removable prosthodontics: Paper vs computorized format

A. Cunha
Dentist, External Collaborator of the Faculty of Dental Medicine of the University of Porto (FMDUP), Portugal

A. Correia, J.C. Reis Campos & M.H. Figueiral
Department of Removable Prosthodontics, FMDUP, Portugal
Researcher of the Institute of Mechanical Engineering and Industrial Management (INEGI), Porto, Portugal

J. Fonseca
Invited Assistant Professor in the Department of Health Information and Decision Science,
Faculty of Medicine of the University of Porto (FMUP), Portugal

ABSTRACT: Oral-health clinical records in a computorized format are increasingly being adopted in dental schools with the objective to improve office efficiency and operations, diagnosis and treatment and patient communication and perception. However, computer pacient records only cover the information of paper-based records partially. The aim of this research was to evaluate the contents of paper-based clinical records of a dental medicine specialty (removable prosthodontics), of national and foreing dental schools, in order to develop a Baseline Prosthodontic Record (BPR), and compare it to the school's records in paper and in an electronic format. The data recorded allowed us to establish a Baseline Prosthodontic Record with 14 categories and 266 parameters distributed by these same categories. A review of the paper and the electronic-based records with the BPR shows that the former contains, on average, 49.5% of the parameters of the BPR, while the latter contains only 26.7%.

1 INTRODUCTION

Oral-health clinical records in a computorized format are increasingly being adopted in dental schools with the objective to improve office efficiency and operations, diagnosis and treatment and patient communication and perception. However, the computer pacient records only cover the information of paper-based records partially (Schleyer et al. 2007 & Acharya et al. 2010). According to Thyvalikakath (2008) the quality of e-records is low, with 28% of fields fail to be filled and 30% are filled with errors.

The poor usability of electronic records, the lack of efficiency and user satisfaction with the system, the time-consuming learning curve for its use in the dental office, and the cross-infection problems are examples of barriers and disadvantages that may affect the quality of the electronic record (Schleyer et al. 2006, 2007).

1.1 *Electronic oral health records in dental schools*

Dental Schools play a major role in the development of the dentist skills to achieve a correct and complete clinical record. Nowadays it is known that the university clinics are changing the paradigm of clinical records by implementing a computerized format. However, it is disturbing to realize that literature regarding this issue is rather scarce.

Atkinson (2002) mentioned various functions for the e-oral health records, mostly related to quality indicators, university dental clinic population (medical and dental history), data to support clinical decisions and clinical management. However, this e-oral health records are integrated in practice management systems primarily developed by dental companies for the private dental practice, and its use in a university dental clinic requires major specifications to this particular environment. In the study of 2002, Atkinson concluded that the e-records were not adapted to the needs of a university clinic.

1.2 *Aim*

The aim of this research was to evaluate the contents of paper-based clinical records of a dental medicine specialty (removable prosthodontics), of national and foreing dental schools, in order to develop a Baseline Prosthodontic Record (BPR), and compare it to the school's records in paper and in an electronic format.

2 MATERIAL AND METHODS

Dental schools in the Iberian Peninsula, and dental institutions that have exchange programs with the Faculty of Dental Medicine of the University of

Porto (FMDUP) were contacted in order to share their removable prosthodontics paper-based oral health records for this research. Four dental schools [2 from Portugal (DS1 = FMDUP; DS2), and 2 from Spain (DS3 and DS4) answer our request and their paper records were analyzed. All the data fields present were recorded and categorized, in order to create a Baseline Prosthodontic Record. This record was then compared to the paper-based records analyzed and to the electronic oral-health record Newsoft DS 9®, academic version, available in FMDUP, to verify which parameters were included in the BDR.

3 RESULTS

The data recorded in the different university clinical records allowed us to establish a Baseline Prosthodontic Record with 14 categories (numbered from I to XIV) and 266 parameters distributed by these same categories (Table 1). Data from Table I indicate that categories I, IV, IX, XII, XIII and XIV are not covered by all records, and this occurs in more that one record for categories IX and XII. Records from DS-1 cover 64.7% of the BPR parameters, DS-2 49.6%, DS-3 48.9% and DS-4 34.6%.

Regarding the electronic clinical record Newsoft DS9®, Table 2 shows that this does not include the categories VII (Occlusion and TMJ), VIII (Study models analysis Models) and X (Discussion and Prognosis) and has only 26.7% of the parameters of the BPR.

As seen through Tables 1 and 2 the categories that are present in all records are "II – Aim of the visit; III – Medical History; V – Extra-oral Exam; VI – Intra-oral exam and XI – Treatment Plan.

A review of the paper and the electronic-based records with the BPR shows that the former contains, on average, 49.5% of the parameters of the BPR, while the latter contains only 26.7%. (Table 1 and Table 2).

Table 1. Parameters included in the Removable Prosthodontic Clinical Records of different dental schools and in the *Baseline Prosthodontic Record* created.

	DS1	DS2	DS3	DS4	BPR
I – Patient Identification	10	–	4	9	**10**
II – Aim of the visit	1	0	0	0	**1**
III – Medical History	35	6	39	8	**41**
IV – Dental History	20	5	3	–	**24**
V – Extra-oral exam	6	5	7	10	**16**
VI – Intra-oral exam	47	87	26	19	**104**
VII – Oclusion and TMJ	16	16	21	22	**22**
VIII – Models analysis	19	2	10	10	**19**
IX – Medical exams	–	2	–	7	**7**
X – Discussion/Prognosis	11	9	13	7	**15**
XI – Treatment Plan	7	0	7	0	**7**
XII – Treatment Budget	0	–	–	–	**0**
XIII – Treatment Sequence	0	–	0	0	**0**
XIV – Progress Notes	0	–	0	0	**0**
TOTAL	172	132	130	92	**266**

– absent category; 0 category present, but with no parameters

Table 2. Parameters included in the e-record available in FMDUP and in the *Baseline Prosthodontic Record* created.

	Newsoft DS9®	BPR
I – Patient Identification	9	**10**
II – Aim of the visit	0	**1**
III – Medical History	29	**41**
IV – Dental History	8	**24**
V – Extra-oral exam	4	**16**
VI – Intra-oral exam	19	**104**
VII – Oclusion and TMJ	–	**22**
VIII – Models analysis	–	**19**
IX – Medical exams	2	**7**
X – Discussion / Prognosis	–	**15**
XI – Treatment Plan	0	**7**
XII – Treatment Budget	0	**0**
XIII – Treatment Sequence	0	**0**
XIV – Progress Notes	0	**0**
TOTAL	**71**	**266**

– absent category; 0 category present, but with no parameters

4 CONCLUSIONS

The development of a BPR has as main objective the creation of an information model that allows the recording of the patient's clinical data in a standard and structured format so that the dentist can establish the right decisions and provide the best oral health care to their patients (Schleyer et al. 2007 & Acharya et al. 2010). As the Baseline Dental Record of Schleyer (2007), the BPR of this study can not be regarded as the "gold standard" for removable prosthodontics records, but rather as a model for its development following the 'tower of achievment in medical informatics' by C. Friedman (1995).

The ideal process for the development of a Baseline Prosthodontic Records should pass through the establishment of a consensus by a Delphy methodology, based on the individual experience of several experts in the area.

It is essential a deep analysis of the paper records for a subsquent application in a e-format. The implementation of BPR in an electronic form should be studied by applying usability testing and heuristic evaluation of its functioning (Thyvalikakath, 2008).

Although the limitations of this research, it may be concluded that the electronic clinical records, in the Removable Prosthodontics specialty, is not yet sufficient adapted to the university environment, since it is incomplete when compared to the BPR and to the paper-based records.

The Baseline Prosthodontic Record should not be seen as a standard model in clinical records in Prosthodontics, but it must serve as a basis for the study of a clinical electronic record dedicated to Prosthodontics.

REFERENCES

Acharya A et al. 2010: The Realities of eHealth. Advances in Health Informatics Conference (AHIC); Apr 28–30; University of Waterloo, Kitchener, Ontario.

Atkinson JC & Zeller GG & Shah C. 2002. Electronic patient records for dental school clinics: more than paperless systems. Journal of dental education 66:634–42.

Friedman CP. 1995. Where's the science in medical informatics? J Am Med Inform Assoc 2:65–7.

Schleyer T & Spallek H & Hernandez P. 2007. A qualitative investigation of the content of dental paper-based and computer-based patient record formats. J Am Med Inform Assoc 14:515–26.

Schleyer TK et al. 2006. Clinical computing in general dentistry. J Am Med Inform Assoc 13:344–52.

Schleyer TK. 2007. Assessing software usability through heuristic evaluation. J Am Dent Assoc 138:211–2.

Schleyer TK & Thyvalikakath TP & Hong J. 2007. What is user-centered design? J Am Dent Assoc 138:1081–2.

Thyvalikakath TP et al. 2008. A usability evaluation of four commercial dental computer-based patient record systems. J Am Dent Assoc 139:1632–42.

Biodental Engineering II – Natal Jorge et al (Eds)
© 2014 Taylor & Francis Group, London, ISBN 978-1-138-00131-2

Development of a thematic learning object for removable partial denture teaching

Susana Alves
GILT, ISEP, Oporto, Portugal

Maria Helena Figueiral & André Correia
FMDUP, Oporto, Portugal

António Vieira de Castro
GILT, ISEP, Oporto, Portugal

ABSTRACT: Health professionals constantly need to improve its education with continuing education. However these courses are costly, not only for participants, but also to the institutions due the absence of health professional available work to participate on physical courses. According with Castro (Castro et al., 2011) it is necessary to find new teaching and learning methods in the health area, with the development of actual, innovative and appealing digital resources that could be used in different learning activities. Learning Management Systems (LMS), Learning Objects and Thematic repositories of digital contents are some concepts linked together with the purpose to create a new global model of teaching and learning. The Faculty of Dental Medicine of the University of Porto (FMDUP), particularly, professors of Removable Prosthodontics pretends to implement a thematic Learning Object to support the teaching of Removable Partial Denture. This paper will describe a work in progress to achieve this goal.

1 INTRODUCTION

One of the biggest challenges of the University of Porto and, particularly, of the Faculty of Dental Medicine (FMDUP), is the use of new technologies to support a more flexible and distributed education to their students (theoretical, theoretical-practical and practical) and also mechanisms that could help student's evaluation assignments.

Professors of the Removable Prosthodontics are constantly improving their teaching methods by using new technologies, in order to reach the students easily, clearly and in a motivating way.

The team involved in this research, composed by multimedia specialists of the Superior Institute of Engineering of Oporto (ISEP) and the professors of Removable Prosthodontics of the FMDUP, intends to analyze the possibility of adopting new technological tools and methods that may centralize in Learning Object information organized according the pedagogical needs of the discipline of removable partial denture.

During this work some traditional student's manuals, delivered in paper, will be integrated on this digital educational resource.

Some other resources will be created as videos, animations, images (photos and diagrams) and immersive manipulation of molds. All contents will be organized in a sequence with a pedagogical purpose.

2 THE DISCIPLINE OF PPR II (PARTIAL PROSTHESIS REMOVABLE SECOND)

Partial Prosthesis Removable II is a discipline from the 1st semester of 4th year of the Master degree in Dental Medicine at FMDUP. During its operation classes are divided on theoretical and practical lessons. Week after week, one hour theoretical and two practical hours where students must develop their skills, both practical and theoretical, to proceed to the oral rehabilitation of the partially edentulous patient, resorting to the use of a removable prosthesis.

To support their teaching activity PPRII professors have an presently and e-learning open-source platform (Moodle) where they available their educational digital resources.

For now, they are using electronic presentations, and a few videos and also a procedural manual composed by static text and still images.

On the practical classes its usual a physical demonstration by a specialist (prosthetic). After, students must practice and create their own molds.

The main problem is related with the absence of a student during this demonstration and understands how he could learn if he misses this kind of activity. Also it was identified a second problem that is related with the weak field of view of some of these students as shown on the figure 1.

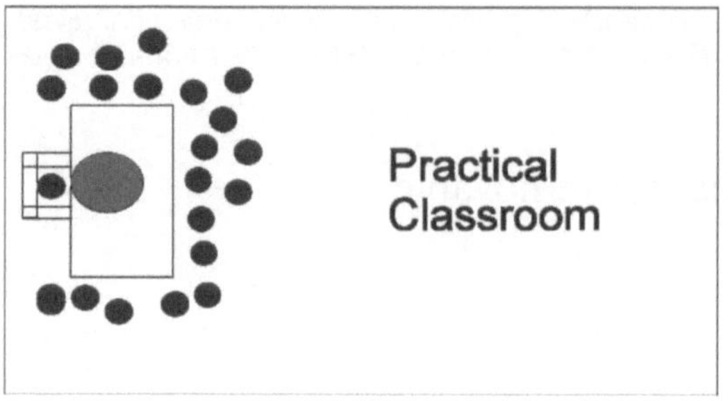

Figure 1. Students during a physical demonstration.

As we can see in scheme of figure 1, it is often difficult to correctly display the demonstration for the student mainly due to its positioning resulting in a weak field of view of the same.

In this sense we consider to be necessary to find alternative mechanisms that allow the student a proper learning. The video could be one of the technologies to be used to document and preserve these moments.

The analysis of other technologies to support learning in this area leads us to an detailed analysis related technologies with the potential to support education.

3 TECHNOLOGIES TO SUPPORT EDUCATION

Nowadays, with the increasing use of computers, the increase of bandwidth and consequent increased use of internet professors and students have access to a great number of educational resources. However, professors need to know how to manage and use them and even more important be able to adapt their traditional resources to a new paradigm "the distance learning (e-learning)" using naturally, new technologies.

It's known that multimedia can stimulate more than one sense at a time, and in doing so, may be more attention-getting and attention-holding.

Studies support distinctive differences in ways students retain information gathered and applied using multimedia versus traditional modes of instruction. In a study conducted with eighth graders, R. Lehrer [Lehrer, 1997], found that students who learned using multimedia had made long lasting connections with the materials while students who learned traditionally had little to no retention of the material on year later. It was also noted that the level of student engagement was significantly higher.

The use of multimedia tools and the interactivity that they provide also offers students a more attractive learning. With this kind of resources they have the opportunity to create "their own learning".

This type of resources associated with the onset of teaching/learning platforms like the LMS's (Learning Management Systems), provide students learning at their own pace. They can now access contents anytime and anywhere.

3.1 *Learning Management Systems (LMS) and repositories*

Learning management systems (LMS), also known as teaching/learning platforms, are the main tools used in knowledge management in e-learning and provide access and service organization of distance learning, via the Internet, the trainees, trainers and administrators. These systems, based on Web technology have a set of functionalities, like a range of resource types and activities, to support teaching and maximize the potential of e-learning. Monteiro (Monteiro, 2011) referred students to highlight the importance of the use of e-learning platform for the following aspects:

- obtaining materials and contents of the classes, not by decreasing their presence in classes;
- the permanent availability of content and activities from anywhere with Internet access at any time;
- school use (ease of study, best ratings, …);
- contact/communication with professors;
- self-assessment tests.

In health there are some institutional LMS (usually universities) but there is an extra-university that allows any health care professional to create your own course. In fact, the MEDUCA (Medical Education) platform, has the potential to promote courses at distance with the ability to integrate resources from different thematic granularities also including learning objects.

It is possible within this LMS organize a course providing students with the educational resources through a temporal order that can be accessed by students and managed by professors.

The LMS used in UP is Moodle (Modular Object-Oriented Dynamic Learning Environment), an Open Source software based on a global development project designed to support a social constructionist framework of education.

Moreover, in order to preserve and distribute globally resources that can be integrated into existing courses in LMS's appear repositories.

The thematic learning objects repository MELOR (Medical Learning Objects Repository) has been studied and appears to be an interesting way to promote knowledge to the health area supported by the Web.

Both, LMS Meduca and the MELOR repository are potential tools to promote knowledge sharing globally by providing means of acquiring knowledge for its users.

3.2 *Learning Objects (LO)*

Currently there is no consensus definition of the term Learning Object (LO). According with the Learning Technology Standards Committee (LTSC), Learning Objects can be set to any entity, digital or not can be used, re-used or referenced in technological support for learning.

According to Wiley (Wiley, D. 2000) you can compare a Learning Object to a LEGO piece with two purposes; one is to communicate the basic idea and the second to put an interactive interface and familiar in a new instructional technology; providing differentiated learning strategies and adjusted to the needs of the students. Define as "any digital resource that can be reused as an educational support".

Cisco Systems (2003) says that "an LO is defined as having content, interactivity and metadata. It refers that each LO has a goal of learning and thus has also associated: a learning activity, exercises and evaluation, to ensure that the new skills and knowledge have been acquired".

Below, we identify the main characteristics of a Learning Object:

- Flexibility and re-use – must be simple, easy to use and store, and reusable;
- Ease of updating – can be modified over time;
- Indexing and searching – use of metadata and digital signatures to facilitate the indexing and searching of LO;
- Customization – adaptation to the user and to the course/discipline;
- Interoperability and portability – usable on any educational platform;
- Competency-based learning – great student involvement, which should be responsible for their learning, student learning center;
- Increase de value of knowledge – each time it is reused by an educational platform will see the commercial and educational value increased;
- Granularity – the "size" of the LO; the higher the level of granularity, the greater is the capacity of that object to be reused in multiple contexts. The simplest level of the object, which corresponds to the higher-level granularity – consists of the most basic features that can be stored, as audio, text, images, animations and simulations. As these resources have a low educational context are highly reusable.

4 THE RPDLO (REMOVABLE PARTIAL DENTURE LEARNING OBJECT)

There is a wide variety of LOs, which reveals to be a growing educational resource in the health area.

Mainly they are found in Universities, educational repositories, communities and even in specialized companies.

Conducted a survey on the LOs Dentistry, we found the themes of dental hygiene, mouth anatomy and health, pre-clinical fixed prosthodontics, and many others but none related with Removable Partial Denture in Dentistry.

4.1 *The problem*

After an inicial research we identified that don't exist a digital learning contente related with the teach and learn of this subject.

Taking into account that the e-learning is, actually, more popular, given that increasingly in lifelong learning and considering that students have more skills to learn with digital contents (digital documents, electronic presentations, videos, etc.) we consider that could be very useful a Learning Object on the identified area.

We believe that we can provide them a more attractive and participatory learning, and giving them the opportunity to create their own way of learning.

Taking account that a multidisciplinary team is needed we will work together as a team Dental Doctors, Professors, Engineers and multimedia specialists).

That is possible because we have a protocol of coo-peration between a research group in Learning Technologies (GILT – Graphics Interaction and Learning Technologies) of an engineering school (ISEP – Instituto Superior de Engenharia do Porto) and University of Porto (FMDUP – Faculdade de Medicina Dentária da Universidade do Porto).

Professors of the Removable Prosthodontics of discipline decided to invest in the creation of a thematic LO. All the traditional resources used in physical classes have been organized and a plan, to create new resources based on new technologies, has been planned.

The conceptual map of this LO will list procedures as:

- Introduction contents to RPD;
- Classification of the partial edentulous arches;
- RPD components;
- RPD design based on the topography according to Kennedy's Classification.

These topics are essentially "pre-clinical" and are traditionally less appreciated by students.

4.2 *The RPDLO proposal*

We propose to produce a thematic Learning Object that is being developed with the support of the clinical dental team in order to identify weather new mechanisms of teaching/learning, may be an advantage for this type of education. It has the goals of:

- Be simple and intuitive;
- Oriented for the theme of Removable Partial Denture, within the area of Dentistry;
- Available for different platforms;
- Use different media resources like: electronic presentations, videos, audio, animations, interactive 3D images with audio and text, etc.;
- Allow test knowledge acquired through an inquiry in order to provide students with the opportunity to realize their mistakes, and learning by correcting them;
- Allow the professor to create various situations of training for the student.

4.3 *The structure of RPDLO*

We are proposing a Learning Object with the subjects of the RPD discipline where several resources

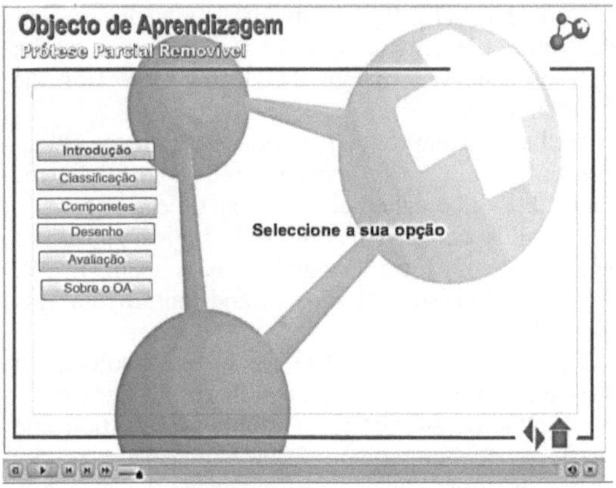

Figure 2. Example of the initial screen for RPDLO.

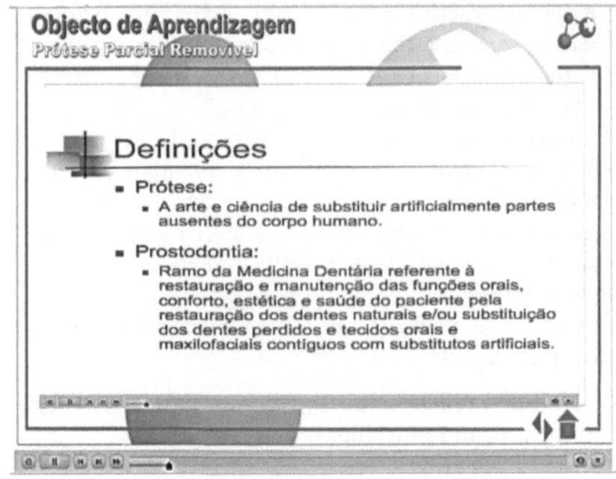

Figure 3. Electronic presentations (as PPT) will be integrated in the Learning Object about RPD.

will be organized in a pedagogical way to help students to better understand the subjects of the discipline.

RPDLO is being developed with Adobe Captivate, a software that allow us to integrate different types of resources as images, videos, audios, hyperlinks and other issues.

The RPDLO layout is presented in the Figure 2.

After initial meetings between team members identified key issues for the development of this Learning Object as:

1. Educational resources available and used by professors to teach the discipline;
2. Sequence of pedagogical themes;
3. Resources to develop;
4. Technology, media and time to develop new contents to integrate;
5. Design the layout of the Learning Object;
6. Planning activities.

Following the initial conceptual map an introduction section has been planned.

The "Introdução" (introduction) button will access all the introductory related with RPD.

The main resources of this section will be the existing electronic presentations used actually by the professors of the discipline. Also some pictures and videos will be incorporated.

The next section is classification available by the "Classificação" (classification) button and will present the different type of classifications of partially edentulous arches.

Videos and some interactive animations, according to the Kennedy classification will be integrated.

The "Componentes" (components) button presents the RPD skeletal components with their goals, functions and some 3D resources that could be manipulated and observed with greater detail using the zoom in and out tool.

The "Desenho" (design) button presents a RPD drawing based on topography according to the classification of Kennedy referring the goals of the steps witch will be supported with some videos.

Finally the "Avaliação" (evaluation) button gives the opportunity to the student do self-assessment tests to evaluate his learning.

Above, on the right corner, users will be able to navigate between pages of the RPDLO or to return home to the main menu.

On the right area of the main menu, we will available the educational resources according the selection of the user.

This is a preliminary layout that could be changed till the last version we decided to design an easy layout given them an easy interaction with contents.

All the main subjects of the discipline identified on the conceptual map will be integrated on the RPDLO.

4.4 *Type of resources to use/develop*

As mentioned, the existing digital resources being used by professors are mostly the electronic presentations that will be treated and arranged to be inserted in RPDLO as shown in Figure 3.

Another kind of resource used by the professors is video but usually they are too long. Shorter videos are more engaging than longer ones and, as known, after a few minutes, students get bored and their attention blurs up.

For instance, a 30 minutes video contains probably several tasks so it can be divided on smallest videos.

Also, we identified some new procedures to be documented in video. These videos will be done in FMDUP and edited with Adobe Premiere by the ISEP team. They will be inserted on the RPDLO as illustrated in Figure 4.

A Learning Object is composed by several resources with higher level granularity that has a low educational context but may be highly reusable.

In this curricular unit, students must know how to classify edentulous arches according to Kennedy's Classification. This subject will be available on the area "classification" represented by Flash resource.

Depending on where in the mouth teeth are missing, edentulous situations can be grouped under four

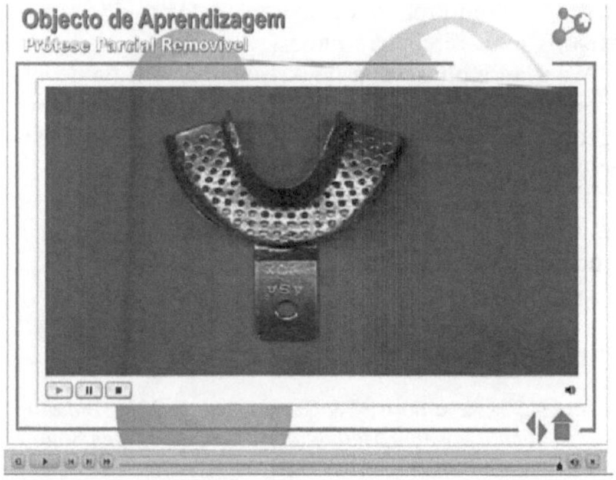

Figure 4. Video of RPDLO about taking a mold.

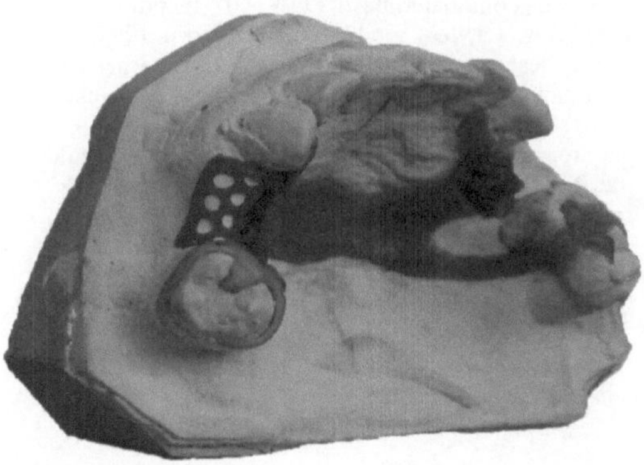

Figure 5. Virtual model of a partial edentulous arches.

different categories, as defined by Dr. Edward Kennedy in his classification of partially edentulous arches. It seems to be useful, to have an interactive resource developed in Adobe Flash, an animation software, that allows students to simulate different types of partially edentulous arches. Students will be asked to classify different edentulous arches according to Kennedy classification and professors can create several different situations of partially edentulous arches to use in classes or in other educational resources as electronic presentations or even tests.

Another technology to be used allows us to create content not immersive virtual reality, using 2D images. VR Worx is a multimedia QTVR (QuickTime Virtual Reality) authoring tool that allows users of these resources interact with content. For example, to produce an interactive resource which runs at an angle of 180° as illustrated in Figure 5.

For each type of mold we will take 7 photos that will be treated with Adobe Photoshop (photo editing software) like Figure 6.

The final immersive content will be produced using VR Worx and will allow a 180° visualization of each one with integrated zoom in and out.

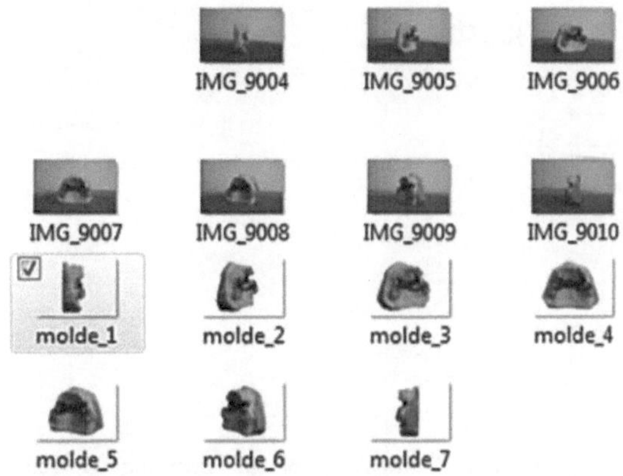

Figure 6. Necessary photos taken and edited to develop an interactive model with an angle of 180°.

5 GLOBAL DISTRIBUTION

Traditionally, before the advent of the internet, digital educational resources were usually available only to a few selected people in the form of CD or DVD.

However, everything changed quickly and is now common to find these kinds of contents in the Web.

It will resemble a large library, where users can quickly find a particular book or publication.

In the last years researchers have been working to find mechanisms to provide organization, cataloging and distribution of digital learning resources.

The use of metadata to catalog (provide information) and the emergence of digital repositories shown an important step towards knowledge sharing thematic contents.

Reusability is one of the characteristics of Learning Objects. That means that they could be used in different courses even with temporal intervals in its realization.

Online courses should be designed as a collection of digital learning resources and integrate LOs. In order to search in web and find these LOs, the descriptions of their characteristics are needed. For this purpose we must describe the LO using metadata that describes their features and is essential for addressing.

Metadata is often described as simple as data about other data, i.e., information (data) about certain content. Provide information about a each particular feature, promotes interoperability, allows identification, sharing, integration, use, reuse, recovery and administration of LOs more efficiently.

The metadata must contain a description of the LO and information about the persons who created it, so that the user can create a map of information which allows to know the source of the Learning Object.

LOs and their metadata must be stored anywhere in the web, so users can easily access it.

The LOs repositories are a kind of digital library. It enables to share, manage and use educational resources.

For our purpose we will use MELOR (Medical Learning Object Repository), Figure 7, that is thematic

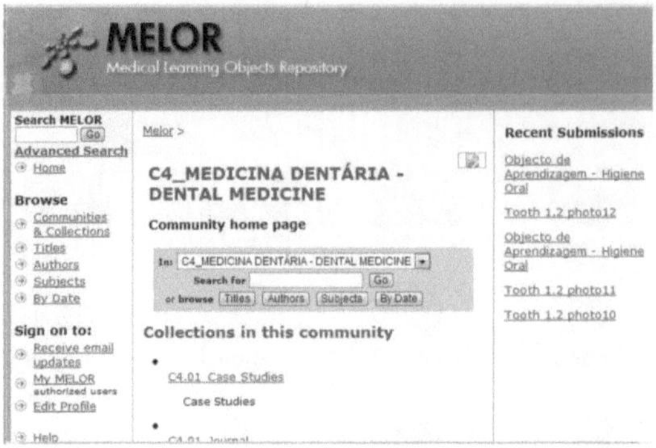

Figure 7. The MELOR (Medical Learning Objects Repository).

repository for professionals and health researchers to put digital resources that could be used on health learning, such as articles, presentations, videos, photos, theses, simulations, etc.

6 CONCLUSIONS

It's our goal to identify if the inclusion of thematic Learning Objects on the learning activities on the health area could represent a new way of teach and learn. For this purpose we are presently developing a thematic Learning Object related with Removable Partial Denture.

Actually we identified technologies that could be used to provide a better understanding of this subject as video, audio, images and 3D manipulation.

Also we required to the professors to provide us the existing educational resources.

We plan a phase that new resources will be developed and finally they will all be organized together according the conceptual map considering the pedagogical issues of the discipline.

Finally tests will be done and the LO will be delivered and catalogued (using Dublin Core) in a repository as MELOR.

REFERENCES

Castro, A.V., Carvalho, C.V. & Carrapatoso, E. 2011. *Building a Medical Learning Methodology Based on Open Source Technologies*, FIE.

Cisco Systems 2003. White paper *Reusable Learning Object Strategy: Designing and Developing Learning Objects for Multiple Learning Approaches*. Available: http://www.e-novalia.com/materiales/RLOW__07_03.pdf.

Kimberly A. Lawless, and Scott W. Brown 1997, Multimedia learning environments: Issues of learner control and navigation, Department of Educational Psychology, University of Connecticut, Storrs, CT 06269–2064.

Monteiro, A. 2011. Ph.D, Universidade do Porto, Faculdade de Psicologia e Ciências da Educação, *O currículo e a prática pedagógica com recurso ao b-learning no ensino superior*. Porto.

Wiley, D. 2000. Connecting learning objects to instructional design theory: A definition, a metaphor, and a taxonomy, in *The instructional use of learning objects*. D.A.Wiley (Ed) Available: http://reusability.org/read/chapters/wiley.doc.

Biodental Engineering II – Natal Jorge et al (Eds)
© 2014 Taylor & Francis Group, London, ISBN 978-1-138-00131-2

Multimedia tools in the teaching of removable denture prosthesis

Paula Rolino
GILT, ISEP, Oporto, Portugal

André Correia
FMDUP, Oporto, Portugal

António Vieira de Castro
GILT, ISEP, Oporto, Portugal

ABSTRACT: In the last few years the ways of teaching and learning have changed globally. One of the main reasons is the appearance of internet and digital educational resources. On the health area, and particularly on the dental, we also verify that the inclusion of thematic learning resources could be a different approach to support learning. However, there is still a lot of work to be done on this field and the main purpose of this paper is to present a study that plans to create a Learning Object (LO) focusing "Removable Prosthodontics in Dentistry".

1 INTRODUCTION

In Prosthodontics students have access to two different types of learning contents: theoretical and practical. The manufacture of a removable prosthesis has several stages. Initially the patient must spend some time in consultation with the aim of being produced a mold. This mold must be made according to the mouth of a particular patient in which the prosthesis will be placed. This is the starting point for the whole process. The mold after is sent to the laboratory where the prosthetist will manufacture the final mold. This confection becomes the focal point of the entire work, and its preparation has a high degree of precision. Later, after being confected, the mold is tried in the patient's mouth, where the dentist will assess the compatibility between the patient's mouth and the mold manufactured. If no adjustments are necessary, the molds return to the dental laboratory where the technician will resume his work. This is a time-consuming job and a delicate one too. The prosthesis is composed of top and bottom where each tooth is placed in a millimetrical way on the mold. When all the teeth of one of the parts is attached, the technician works on the other part. After all the teeth are placed, the prosthesis is covered with the finishing material and subsequently placed in an oven to be finalized. This is be a very brief description of the process which the manufacture of a removable prosthesis undergoes. Students of dental medicine must learn and understand all this process. Actually they learn and acquired this thematic knowledge in physical classes.

According with Antonio Castro (Castro, 2011) [1], given the need of continued education by the professionals in the health field and the high costs that such training entails, not only for participants but also for their institutions and not just financial but mostly humans, caused mainly by the continuous movement, absences and the exhaustion we decide to start a study with the purpose of evaluating the impact of the inclusion of new mechanisms of teaching and learning applied to the teach of Removable Prosthodontics in Dentistry" supported by multimedia technologies.

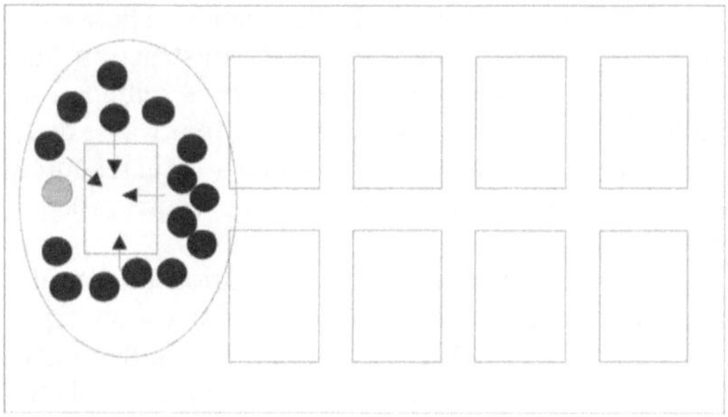

Figure 1. Students attending lab classes.

Our first step was an analysis of the actual process to teach and learn this subject on the dentistry universities. To do that we engaged ourselves with School of Dental Medicine, University of Porto.

Actually students learn this manufacturing process in real time while they attend laboratory classes (where they can observe the whole process only once, during the demonstration). The way they watch is often insufficient and leads to a not very satisfactory understanding of the process, as can showed in figure 1.

Figure 1 intents to highlight some setbacks as the angle of vision that hinders the perception of the process being transmitted, along with possible distractions because all the students are crowded up.

Above all, the main problem is that it is not possible to review or watch what has happened during the session.

In this sense, it is clear that the existence of the session in a video format could become a feature of high utility for the teaching-learning process of those students. Reconciling all components of the learning process of manufacturing a dental prosthesis in a single platform has become the starting point in the development of this thematic learning object.

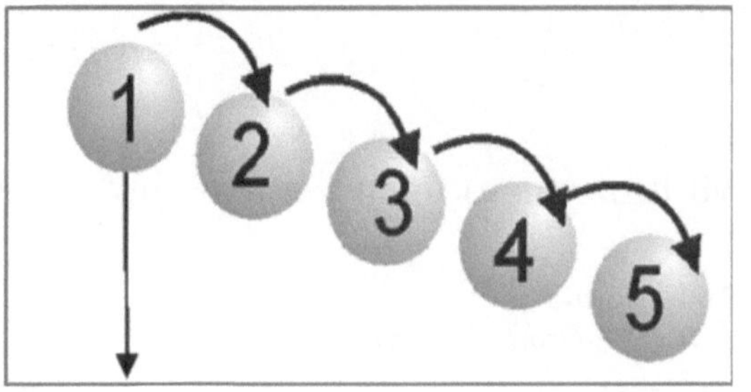

Figure 2. Stages of the learning process of the manufacture of prosthesis.

Table 1. Stages of the production film.

Time	Step
1	Clinical consultation for mold
2	Manufacturing mold laboratory sent by the dentist after time 1
3	Proof of mold made by the patient in 2
4	Completion of laboratory prosthetic work
5	Proof of the prosthesis into the patient

2 MULTIMEDIA TO SUPPORT LEARNING

Teaching and learning methods have undergone a revolution in recent years as a result of global access to the Internet and the emergence of technological resources able to provide search engines and access to information with considerable speed [2].

The use of multimedia tools to potentiate the learning environments supported by the web has increasingly been a constant on the last years. There are, however some areas in which this construction has been done in smaller steps. This work is intended to bridge the gap between the syllabus of removable dentures, and implementation of and educational resource (software) that could demonstrate the entire process related to this topic.

Our goal is to produce an application that could transmit the acquisition of this particular knowledge.

To be able to achieve our goals is fundamental to understand the entire process, people involved, sequence of procedures and pedagogical issues related with this subject.

Before start to create our learning object we defined a set of strategies and processes as:

1. Monitoring a patient throughout the procedure
2. Collect pictures and videos related procedures
3. Collect pictures and videos of parallel activities (e.g. templates)
4. Define the concept map to develop the learning object according to the teaching of the discipline Objectives
5. Analyze and select tools in productivity.
6. Assembly of the final product.
7. Evaluation and testing.

Being the conditions defined, and identified the multimedia support tools and other existing technologies, we must know use the means available to motivate students an innovative way to acquire knowledge in the classroom environment, and essentially on distance learning activities.

By establishing a bridge between the transmission of program content in the area of dental prostheses and multimedia technologies, we develop different skills in apprentice and new ways of looking at teaching the subject.

The search for new paradigms of learning to develop this educational resource in this particular area intents to be a contribution to new experiences.

The use of multimedia, as a combination of static and dynamic means provides a way of presenting information in a multisensory way, dynamic and attractive to the students in knowledge requirements in this area of dentistry.

The design of the structure has a direction vector that is the focus of this work: removable denture prosthesis. The manufacturing process in its entirety was recorded on videotape, with subsequent editing work as mentioned above. The filming went through five stages.

Each stage identifies and associates resources and other educational materials to each topic necessary for student participation in the learning process. In the following table it can be observed all the phases that, in a generic way, can be considered for the production of filming.

To follow the development of this learning object it was necessary to respond to several questions including:

- How is the subject taught?
- What kind of resources do they use?
- What are the most important moments?
- What kinds of practices are required?
- What must be done to theoretical documents?
- How to show practical activities?

After the responses are obtained and analyzed, all the necessary requirements for the development of this learning object go through the stage of the design of their interfaces. This is necessary in order to study the navigability of the interfaces that makes up the application and the necessary coordination of the different contents.

To develop this learning object we used a methodology based on various stages of the evolutionary character and called Evolutionary Prototyping Methodology. This methodology is based on the following steps: initial conception, prototyping modeling, refining the prototype and final prototype completion. This methodology is one of the best in the development of learning objects. From the beginning until the final stage, the whole process may be reassessed and improved. Despite following this type of methodology in developing this prototype, some of the assumptions in the Cascade Development Methodology (particularly with regard to testing) were taken into account. For the tests, questionnaires to students will be carried out in order to validate the tool. The main outline of the design of the interface was performed taking into account the application requirements and the objectives that are intended to be fulfilled.

The prototype will be built using the Flash Creative Suite version 6. The interfaces of each screen, after resetting end in Corel Draw and taking into account the guidelines of the screens shown in Figure 3, will be modeled with Flash. The video taken from the footage shot in the prosthetic laboratory environment was treated and edited, and had then sound and text added.

The images will be treated with Creative Suite Photoshop to touch up some imperfections that may arise. Documents shall be supplied in various formats (Word, PDF). In terms of data modeling, the database will consist of a set of xml files, using the language of Flash Action Script for interaction between pages swf and xml files.

3 STRUCTURE OF LEARNING OBJECT

The development of a Learning Object undergoes successive learning phases. The starting point is the requirements analysis. The main resources, exclusively on made to this thematic learning object are the videos made in the prosthetic laboratory of FMDUP. It is a stagger of filming that involves several times and two types of environments during clinical consultation and in the laboratory. Given these requirements, filming is held and processed at a later time, where "dead" spots of filming are removed from the videos. It should be noted that all the details involving this type of construction are documented on video.

According to the requirements of the development of a Learning Object, the design must take account the way the contents are accessed. In the case of this LO, the access to content must be a simple and effective interface and obey a simple and minimalist design. The application is divided into three parts: at the top, the logos of the institutions associated to this project and the name of the subject; on the left side, the application

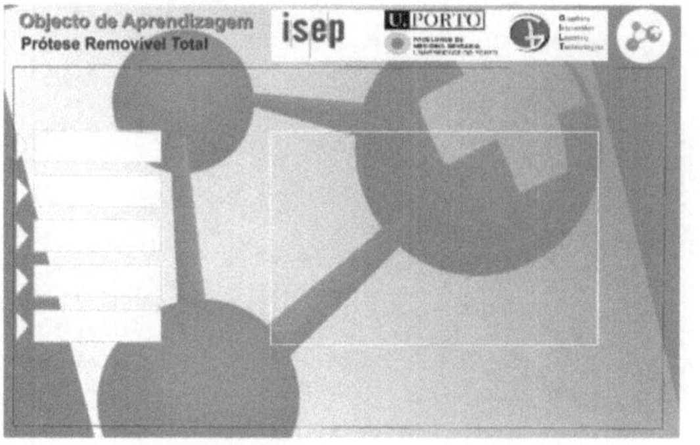

Figure 3. Main interface of the Learning Object.

menu with several buttons that, when clicked, give you direct access to the content and image; the center of the presentation, where the contents can be viewed.

The main interface displays a menu with five buttons: lectures, prosthetic, clinical, images and links. Each time they are clicked will lead to contents respectively: slides, clinical laboratory, laboratory prosthetic; equipment.

So when you click on "Lectures", you will be directed to content produced in Microsoft PowerPoint program by teachers. To view the entire process of manufacturing removable prosthesis, just click on "Prosthetic" all footage produced is available from this link. The videos have been edited after production so that the end product may show all the filming considered essential. The button "Images" leads to images that are part of the universe of the manufacture of a removable prosthesis. A minimalist design with simple lines is perchance the most suitable for this type of data taking into account the main objective of the application: learning.

3.1 *Lectures button*

This button when clicked leads the student to consult the material prepared by the Professor. This material will be provided by Professor of discipline and can be provided in three formats: pptx, docx and pdf are they prepared the application Microsoft PowerPoint or Microsoft Word and then converted into pdf.

3.2 *Prosthetic button*

This button which is divided into three buttons, leads the student to a virtual visit to the lab, the other leads to images of equipment properly labeled and a third button that leads to the videos made on the fabrication of the prosthesis in question and testifying in full its construction.

3.3 *Clinical button*

This button provides the student dental consultations and treatments and necessary medical records and performed for placement of this prosthesis. In the case of a patient whom was removed teeth and placement

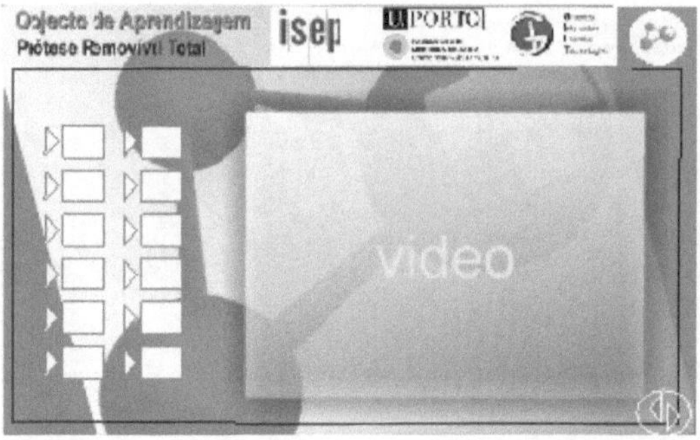

Figure 4. Interface to videos.

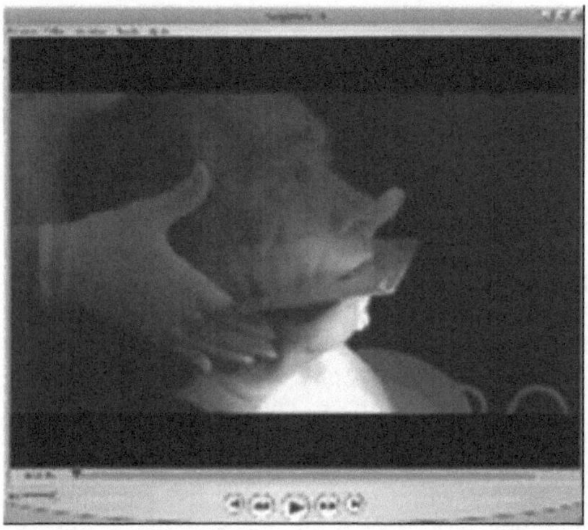

Figure 5. Video filmed in consultation clinic.

of a removable denture, the student can perceive the whole process surrounding.

The image of the interface illustrated in Figure 5 represents the result after having clicked the clinical. The scheme can be seen in the initial version of the educational resource to support the teaching of the manufacture of removable dentures. The image focus is one of the moments in which the video is shot in the manufacturing trays and which constitute the support of the prosthesis. The aim is that students can "capture" all times and steps as if they were present in the laboratory.

3.4 *Images button*

The button images allow visualization of medical images relating to all key points considered in the preparation of this prosthesis.

3.5 *Links button*

The link button leads to a set of pages related to the subject. These pages are hosted on the Internet and are repositories of information on removable dentures.

4 ADVANTAGES IN USING THIS LEARNING OBJECT

The development of an application of this kind must take into account the advantages that of the use of such an application may bring: enhancing of synthesis and understanding, of analysis and autonomy for the student, which enables greater confidence and security in the consolidation of knowledge. It is known that repeated viewing of images will allow for static and dynamic reinforcement of the various types of memory: working memory, visual memory, long term memory and short term memory.

But it is mainly in working memory and long term memory that this paper intends to contribute to the reinforcement of skills. How? The recurrent use of images and video feed allows for the cognitive circuits to work much more intensely than if the information was transmitted only once. There is an enhancement of neuronal activity that is fed to the visual and auditory memory. The details related to this type of work are increasingly improved since the application is used recursively as many times as necessary.

Whenever they wish, students may consult all the processes underlying the manufacture of this prosthesis; this way they may always answer those questions that are inevitably present in all learning processes. By using this educational resource, neuronal activity is crafted so that memories will be activated and the student may continuously have all the necessary information present in the brain. Another of its advantages is that memory works in a photographic way, i.e. the information captured in the preview of the video or image is strongly engraved in the brain, which reinforces the capabilities of the visual memory of the student and indirectly stimulates his/her cognitive abilities.

The recursive use of audiovisual media in the teaching-learning relationship combines essential cognitive abilities like concentration, schematization, memorization, comprehension, synthesis and motivation, among others. Whatever they may be, the methods and means for the teaching-learning relationship are to stimulate the response to the stimulus. And in this field, there is nothing better than using and enjoying multimedia and adding tools that allow for the improvement of this relationship. What they do is stimulate the maximum acceleration of mental processes in learning. The more we read, store and analyze information, the faster we understand. The more times we do it, the faster our brain processes the same information. We react to stimuli and respond mechanically. Viewing a video on a particular subject increases the confidence level of the student, you know that you can view as many times as desired and thus dispel the doubts. The same goes for sound, images and written documents.

By concentrating the focus on the students learning object, we enhance their ability to concentrate. The initial attitude is the same as when they go to the cinema to see a movie for fun; so they are really motivated.

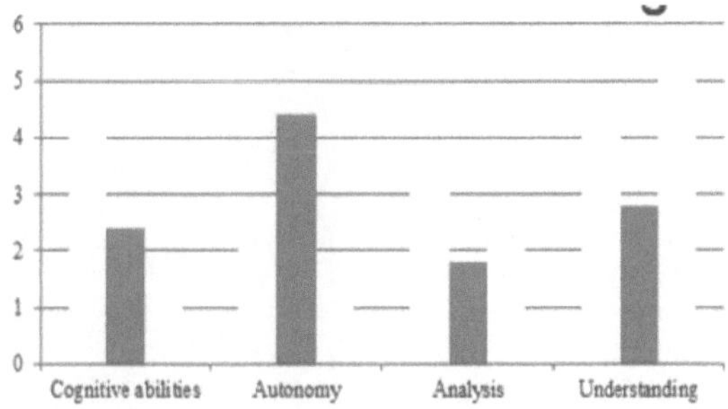

Figure 6. Improvement in cognitive domain in the use of a Learning Object.

Audio-visual media are captivating regardless of their content. If you are interested in what you will learn, you will view the videos available in the application with a circumstantially different interest, parallel to the one you have when watching a movie. The objectives are different (one is learning, the other is fun) but the kind of concentration is the same. The disturbing variables are minimized with the use of audio-visual media.

This feature educational proposes to provide dental students, all artifacts related to the construction of this type of prosthesis, being accessible from any computer. The use of such features allows for and enables its use at any time. This facility which translates into recursion, allows a better understanding.

The synthesis capabilities, comprehension, analysis, learner autonomy are enhanced, allowing you to gain greater confidence and security in medical act is known that repeated viewing of images will allow, whether they static or dynamic strengthening of various types of memory: working memory, visual memory, long term memory and short term memory.

But it is mainly in working memory and long term memory that this paper intends to revert to the reinforcement of skills. How? The recurrent use of images and video feed allows the cognitive circuits in a much more intense than if the information was transmitted only once. There is an enhancement of neuronal activity that is fed to the level of visual and auditory memory. This allows the details related to this type of work are increasingly improved since the feature is utilized recursively as many times as necessary.

This fact makes the study of the object – the construction of a dental prosthesis – is increasingly improved, since it will build a set of information available that are being reinforced. This is a key advantage in the use of this work: recursion that will enable enhanced information gained at perceptual.

By using this educational resource, neuronal activity is crafted so that the memories are activated and the student has continuously present in your brain all the necessary information.

Another of its advantages is that knowing that memory works in photographic style, i.e., the information captured in the preview of the video or image is strongly engraved in the brain, which reinforces the capabilities of the visual memory of the student and indirectly stimulate their cognitive abilities.

This educational resource aimed at meeting a technology for inclusive education where they can overcome.

The methodology that is being used for the development of this prototype is the Evolutionary Prototyping Methodology. Since this methodology based on the following steps: initial design, prototyping modeling, refining the prototype and final prototype presents a complete flexibility suited to this type of platform Thus, until the final stage of the prototype whenever he can always re-evaluated and improved. The videos will be produced and screened in this application involved filming treated and processed in Adobe Premiere. Each film is treated according one stage of manufacture of the prosthesis. If students want to see the video of the construction trays click the relevant button and you can envision the respective movie. Each film is discussed with the technical explanation on the contents of the film in question.

5 CONCLUSIONS

The teaching content related to manufacturing removable dental prosthesis, is in its essence by large in the practical classes. Because we know that there are moments that are unique and unrepeatable, this leads us to the following reflection: What to do when a student misses a class? We try to give an answer to this reflection and look at the development of this learning object as an answer to it.

We know that in many classrooms different types of audio-visual media are used for the teaching of diverse content. However, these means are not entirely interrelated and do not allow for the best use of audio-visual media in vocational education. Combining multiple formats (image, text, video and sound in a single platform) approaches the virtual environment to the real one. Apart from the fact that this provides flexibility, it presents a better use of educational resources.

REFERENCES

Castro, A. V., "Tecnologias Multimédia na Auto-Aprendizagem de Lógica e Linguagens de Programação Estudo de Caso", FEUP – Porto, 2005.

Castro, A.V., Carvalho, C.V., Carrapatoso, E. 2011. *Building a Medical Learning Methodology Based on Open Source Technologies* FIE (eds).

Author index